Joint Construction of Narratives in the Psychoanalytic Setting

Language, Discourse and Mental Health

This series is a unique resource to further knowledge and understanding of mental health from a pluralistically informed linguistic perspective.

Using qualitative and quantitative approaches to language-based analysis, the empirical and theoretical contributions in these volumes provide a compelling insight on mental health from a range of perspectives and contexts, including psychotherapeutic communication, public presentations of mental health, literary accounts of lived experiences, and language features and phenomenology associated with specific mental health problems.

To discuss your book proposal, please contact the series editors:

Laura Cariola, Lecturer in Applied Psychology, University of Edinburgh, UK (laura.cariola@ed.ac.uk)

Elvis Coimbra-Gomes, English Language Teacher, University of Lausanne, France (elvis.coimbragomes@unil.ch)

Scott Parrott, Associate Professor, The University of Alabama, USA (msparrott@ua.edu)

Or Commissioning Editor Becky Taylor (b.taylor@exeterpress.co.uk)

Mental Health Ontologies: How We Talk About Mental Health, and Why it Matters in the Digital Age

Janna Hastings, 2020

Madness and Literature: What Fiction Can Do for the Understanding of Mental Illness

ed. Lasse R. Gammelgaard, 2022

Eating Disorders in Public Discourse: Exploring Media Representations and Lived Experiences

ed. Laura A. Cariola, 2023

Child and Adolescent Migration, Mental Health, and Language: Effects of Trauma and Foreign Language Immersions

Fernanda Carra-Salsberg, 2024

JOINT CONSTRUCTION OF NARRATIVES IN THE PSYCHOANALYTIC SETTING

The Role of Shifting Perspective

Eszter Berán
and
Zsolt Unoka

UNIVERSITY
of
EXETER
PRESS

First published in 2026 by
University of Exeter Press
Reed Hall, Streatham Drive
Exeter EX4 4QR, UK

www.exeterpress.co.uk

Joint Construction of Narratives in the Psychoanalytic Setting: The Role of Shifting Perspective

Language, Discourse and Mental Health
ISSN 3049-7205 Print
ISSN 3049-7213 Online

https://doi.org/10.47788/DYQM2219

A CIP record for this book is available from the British Library

ISBN 978-1-80413-048-3 Hbk
ISBN 978-1-80413-049-0 ePub
ISBN 978-1-80413-050-6 PDF

EU Authorised Representative: Easy Access System Europe – Mustamäe tee 50, 10621 Tallinn, Estonia, gpsr.requests@easproject.com

Typeset in Caslon and Myriad by S4Carlisle Publishing Services, Chennai, India

Contents

Acknowledgements

We thank the International Psychoanalytic Association as well as the Hungarian National Research Foundation (OTKA PD 108868) for their support of this research.

We also thank Klára Soltész-Várhelyi, Pál Czobor, Sára Berán, Ajna Császár, Péter Antal-Bacsó, Tibor Pólya, Katalin Jakab, Csaba Pléh, György Gergely and Anna Póda for their help in this research and their advice on the preparation of the manuscript.

Introduction

In verbally based psychotherapies—including psychoanalysis—the client's life stories provide the basis for working through problems and discussing emotional processes during the sessions (Grecucci et al. 2017; Rottenberg & Gross 2007), building a good working alliance with the psychotherapist (Castonguay et al. 2006; Flückiger et al. 2018; Negri et al. 2019), as well as allowing for the client's exploration of their sense of self (Bucci 2002; Ulvenes et al. 2014), their experiences and the validation of these experiences on the part of the psychotherapist (Carson-Wong 2016). So, the client's life stories are the 'material' brought into the therapy, with which the psychotherapist engages, and therapeutic treatment is based on this interactive work. This—in the case of psychoanalysis—is underlined by the well-known Freudian reference to it as the 'talking cure'. Hence, we can think of the therapeutic work taking place at the session as a process of reconstructing self-narratives of the client (Adler & McAdams 2007; Schafer 1992), including the construction of new narratives from un-verbalized experiences, and the transformation (rewriting) of old narratives into new ones.

The construction of new narratives and the transformation of old ones is achieved with the help of the psychotherapist, or, in case of psychoanalytic therapy, the psychoanalyst, who is an active participant of the construction process, helping the elaboration of various aspects of the narrative by asking questions, giving feedback and interpretations. So, the client's new self-narratives are generated at the session in co-construction with the therapist, which process is termed a type of narrative interaction (Becker & Quasthoff 2005), in which, again, the therapist plays an active role.

The goal of this book is to characterize the narrative interaction that takes place at the psychoanalytic session, and relate it to the psychotherapy process taking place at the same time. We argue that narrative interaction in fact contributes to the psychotherapy process. We describe narrative interaction taking place at the session in a step-by-step manner, analysing it from a linguistic point of view, tracing changes in the analysand's narratives that in the long run—as we argue—lead to structural changes in the narrative self within psychoanalytic psychotherapy. In order to achieve these goals, we use the empirical material of transcribed psychoanalytic sessions: we have audio-recorded and transcribed psychoanalytic narratives of two Hungarian analysands undergoing psychoanalytic psychotherapy in Budapest, Hungary (see details in Chapter 4), and examined structural alterations in the narratives, namely the changes in the perspective of the narrator or, in other words, changes in their point of view. So, according to our hypothesis in this book, the work of restructuring the analysand's narrative self can be traced by describing the process of reconstructing their self-narratives, as it takes place in the psychoanalytic session. By analysing shifts in perspective in the analysand's self-narratives we can carefully trace the construction process of these narratives, so describing how changes in the narrative self have occurred in the case of the observed therapies. Since our data is based on psychoanalytic psychotherapies, we focus in this book on psychoanalysis. However, some of our conclusions may apply to other types of verbally focused psychotherapies, where narrative interaction plays a central role.

Two central concepts that we work with in our analysis of narrative interaction are the narrative self and the narrative perspective. These interrelated ideas are discussed in more detail in Chapter 3, but we shall briefly describe them here. By narrative self we mean, following Gallagher (2000: 15): 'A more or less coherent self (or self-image) that is constituted with a past and a future in the various stories that we and others tell about ourselves.' In other words, we can state that the totality of narratives of which the main protagonist is the individual themself constitutes the narrative self. The perspective from which such stories are told is termed the narrative perspective (NP), which was defined as the narrator's point of view within the story, characterizing the way the narrator sees the events and characters of the narrative (Bortolussi & Dixon 2003; Genette 1983; Uspenskiĭ 1973).

Narrative perspective is linguistically defined, and in order to examine NP within the transcribed texts of the psychoanalytic sessions we have created a discursive model of NP. This model introduces various aspects of NP, namely: 1) physical aspect, 2) subjectivity, 3) intentionality, and 4) discourse level. The physical aspect of NP gives the spatial and temporal coordinates of events of the narrative, with regard to the narrator's position. The subjectivity aspect of NP gives information referring to the person of the narrator(s) and the characters of the narrative, as well as to their position regarding the story plane (i.e. whether they are located inside or outside the story). The intentionality aspect of NP refers to the narrator's knowledge of the internal worlds of themselves and others, as well as the narrator's treatment of other characters as intentional agents. Finally, the discourse level of NP refers to the narrator's position with regard to the narration process: whether they are identifying with the narrator, a different character or talks from their current position in the therapeutic here and now (Bal & Lewin 1983; Chatman 1986; Phelan 2001).

Narrative perspective will often shift continuously in a text (Uspenskiĭ 1973; Jin & Liu 2023). This means that perspective change frequently occurs in text or in talk. So, while a given perspective may characterize a specific segment of speech or written text, the next segment could exhibit a perspective change and hence the new segment can be described as having an altered point of view. We refer to this process as the shifting of perspective. During the course of psychotherapeutic discourse, NP is shifted frequently and in addition—as we shall argue and demonstrate through our empirical studies in this book—speakers can influence each other's perspective shifts. The NP expressed in one speaker's speech unit may be repeated by the other speaker in their next turn, by shifting into the same perspective. This is what we refer to as the coordination of perspectives, or interactive regulation of NP.

By coordinating perspectives with the analysand, the analyst may influence the analysand's way of shifting perspective and hence their way of narrating, which would help in the transformation of the analysand's self-narratives. This in turn influences the psychotherapy process. For example, the psychoanalyst may express their empathy with and understanding of the analysand by shifting into the perspective used previously by them; or the analyst may shift into a perspective different from the current one used by the analysand, so drawing attention to aspects of the story that the analysand may then explore from a new perspective. By such means, the analyst may use perspective shifting behaviour to achieve certain therapeutic goals.

Shifting perspective also plays an important role in the attention regulation of the speakers. By both speakers at the same time focusing their attention on a specific speech unit—termed the intonation unit (Chafe 1994; Jin & Liu 2023)—they generate shared mental representations of the information contained within the given intonation unit. This information also includes information on perspective. Hence, speakers will both create similar mental representations at the same time in a given moment during their conversation, including information on NP. This way, perspective information is related to attention regulative processes during narrative interaction. By learning new ways of shifting perspectives, the analysand discovers new, more adaptive ways of regulating their attention during the analytic session. This helps them to create new mental representations, and to rewrite narratives (Dimaggio et al. 2003) with the help of the analyst or later, outside the session, without the analyst's help, where they can use these skills.

As we shall see in the subsequent chapters of this book, the analysis of psychotherapeutic discourse by using our method of studying NP shifting behaviour of the speakers is closely intertwined with the psychotherapy process, such as attention and affect regulation, the workings of autobiographical memory, mentalization, identification, and so on. Using our model of NP, we examine the way narratives are co-constructed during therapy, and analyse their structure and transformation, as well as their role in the psychotherapy process. We aim to:

- describe processes of narrative interaction taking place at the psychoanalytic session by analysing shifts in speakers' NP, and relate them to the psychotherapy process;
- describe the process of coordinating NP between speakers;
- analyse various aspects of the joint construction relevant to the psychotherapy process, such as the regulation of affective involvement, mentalization, empathy expressed on the part of the analyst, working in the here and now of the session, long-term changes in interpersonal relating and expressing sense of agency;
- show the analyst's active role in the reconstruction of the analysand's self-narratives.

Regarding psychoanalytic theory, the co-construction process of narratives, as well as the coordination of perspectives in psychoanalytic discourse that we demonstrate in our book can be related to the intersubjective orientation within psychoanalysis. This approach states that psychoanalysis is based on the notion that, in addition to the analysand's unconscious experiences, the psychoanalyst's subjectivity in the analytic process is crucial and essential to that very process, and countertransference and other unconscious aspects of the analyst's activity constantly influence the therapeutic work (Bohleber 2013; Renik & Spillius 2004). This view is in contrast to previous notions of the analyst's abstinence and neutrality, and the therapeutic goal of minimalizing countertransference characterizing analytic work. So, according to the intersubjective orientation, the psychoanalytic encounter includes the interaction of two subjectivities and 'the understanding gained through clinical analytic investigation is a product of that interaction' (Renik & Spillius 2004: 1054). Analytic insight is co-created by the analysand and the analyst, and this implies that the unconscious activity of both participants contributes to therapeutic change. Intersubjectivity in psychoanalytic work as presented by Lawrence Brown's theory involves the sharing of unconscious phantasies by the analytic dyad (Brown 2013), which results in a joint narrative: the intersubjectively created product. In our studies, this product is what we analyse linguistically, while recognising that what appears in language may be only the observable facet of 'intersubjectivity proper' (Bohleber 2013).

Our book is structured in the following way: Part 1, 'Theoretical background of the joint construction of narrative', consists of Chapters 1–3; Part 2, 'Methodology', consists of Chapter 4; Part 3, 'Empirical study of the joint construction of narratives in psychoanalysis', comprises Chapters 5–9; there is finally a conclusion. This third section of the book contains studies on various aspects of the psychotherapy process, such as memory process, affect regulation, identification processes, expression of empathy on the part of the analyst and alliance, interpersonal relationships, agency, and working in the here and now. Our analysis shows how the joint construction of narratives contributes to the psychotherapy process, by studying the coordinating of perspective or, in other words, the interactive regulation of the shifting of NP.

In Chapter 1, 'Narrative interaction and its development', we discuss the theoretical background of our discourse-based approach to analysing NP by summarizing some relevant literature on narrative interaction. We introduce the concept of narrative and describe the theoretical background of this concept, mainly drawing on narratology and psychology. The chapter also describes the development of the capacity of co-constructing narratives in childhood with the help of parents and care-givers, and the central role of narrative interaction in the early development of autobiographical memory and the self.

In Chapter 2, 'Psychotherapeutic discourse', we describe characteristics of psychotherapeutic discourse as a type of institutional discourse, as well as the nature of narrative interaction within such a discourse. We argue that the nature of narrative interaction within psychoanalytic discourse is determined to a great extent by its institutional frameworks, such as the psychotherapeutic contract and the interactional roles defined by it, the theoretical background and orientation of the psychoanalyst, and the interpretation of local and distant textual contexts as important factors influencing therapeutic discourse. The nature of narrative interaction, and the possible narratives themselves constructed and reconstructed in such a setting, are determined to a large degree by the factors mentioned previously. Although our studies in this book focus on psychoanalytic psychotherapy and psychoanalytic theory, we would like to generalize some of our findings concerning the way narrative interaction contributes to the psychotherapy process in the case of the observed therapies to other modalities of psychotherapy, where narrative interaction plays a crucial role.

In Chapter 3, 'A discourse-based model of narrative perspective', we introduce our discourse-based model of NP, which is used for analysing in-session verbal interaction in the subsequent chapters of the book. We describe the specific linguistic background of our model, and define 'narrative perspective' by drawing on studies from narratology and cognitive psychology. We also describe the four main aspects of our model: physical aspect, subjectivity, intentionality, and discourse level. We also explain how we operationalize our model of NP in order to analyse the transcripts of psychoanalytic discourse, utilizing the Budapest Psychotherapy Database with a focus on nine variables: verb tense, deixis, diegesis, subject number, subject person, mode of focalization, agency, patiency, and discourse level. We define these variables and illustrate their use in our analysis with in-session excerpts of analyst–analysand narrative interaction.

In Chapter 4, 'The Budapest Psychotherapy Database', we describe the methodological background of our studies: how the empirical basis of our studies was collected for the purpose of analysing psychoanalytic discourse. We have developed the database, which includes longitudinal audio data of two psychoanalyst–analysand dyads—one male and one female—collected between 2004 and 2006 in Budapest, Hungary. The participants were all native speakers of Hungarian and therapy sessions were conducted in Hungarian. This chapter briefly discusses processes of data collection, transcription and coding, as well as the ethical guidelines followed by the researchers while collecting and analysing the data. Excerpts from the Budapest Psychotherapy Database are presented throughout the book, both in the Hungarian language and in English translation.

In Chapter 5, 'Autobiographical memory and narrative perspective', we describe the interconnections between the functioning of the autobiographical self-memory system—mainly based on Conway's self-memory system theory (1992, 2001; Conway et al. 2019) and related research—and various narrative perspectives. We argue that autobiographical memories and the self-concept are closely related, and hence working on and transforming self-narratives in psychotherapy involves working on and transforming the self, which is considered a major goal of psychoanalytic psychotherapy. We also argue and show that processes of remembering and reconstructing past events at the psychoanalytic session in the form of self-narratives may be related to shifts in perspective of the story-teller, and can be described by tracing these shifts in a detailed discourse analysis.

In Chapter 6, 'Introducing a pseudo-narrator', we focus on the function of one specific perspective in in-session narrative interaction: pseudo-diegesis. This perspective characterizes the narrator's view when they introduce a new narrator by continuing the story from their point of view, without signalling the end point of the original narrative. In pseudo-diegesis the new, secondary narrator takes the place of the primary narrator. We illustrate the use of the technique of shifting into pseudo-diegesis by presenting a well-known example of psychoanalytic psychotherapy interaction involving the Hungarian analyst Sándor Ferenczi during in-session interaction as described in his collection of essays, 'Child-analysis in the analysis of adults'. We then analyse excerpts from the Budapest Psychotherapy Database to illustrate how and for what therapeutic goals this technique is used today in psychoanalytic psychotherapies, and argue that the use of pseudo-diegetic perspective contributes to the psychotherapy process by expressing empathy on the part of the analyst or identification with various characters in the analysand's story, as well as a demonstration of possible narrative positions on the part of the analyst.

In Chapter 7, 'Long-term changes in interpersonal relating', we study the data of the Budapest Psychotherapy Database using Luborsky's theory of Core Conflictual Relationship Theme (CCRT) (Luborsky & Crits-Christoph 1990) and the quantitative method of analysing interpersonal relationships in in-session narrative interaction. By analysing what the analysand expects (i.e. desires) from others, how others react to this, and how the analysand in turn responds to their reactions we can show how interpersonal relationships change over time during the one and a half years of the observation period. We also examine—using qualitative analysis—how the shifting of perspective plays a part in discussing relationship problems at the session, and how this contributes to the psychotherapy process.

In Chapter 8, 'Long-term changes in expressing agency', we use McAdam's quantitative method to analyse changes in agency and complete this by our analysis of patiency in the course of the observation period on data drawn from the Budapest Psychotherapy Database, in the case of both dyads. We also study how shifts in perspective contribute to changes in agency and patiency at the psychotherapy session, and show how this relates to the psychotherapy process.

In Chapter 9, 'Working in the here and now of the therapeutic session', we focus on the function of one specific perspective in narrative interaction as well as in the psychotherapy process, namely the here and now of the therapeutic session. This perspective is defined as discourse activities that refer to events taking place in the here and now of the session: discussion of the analysand's aroused emotions and ideas related to the narrated events, or to the analysand–analyst relationship. We argue that this perspective has an important function in the psychotherapy process, because it focuses attention on events happening in the emotional world of the client at the moment, and it encourages reflection on the self. In order to illustrate the functioning of this perspective at the session, we use excerpts from the Budapest Psychotherapy Database.

Finally, in the 'Conclusion', we revisit the original aims of this book and summarize some of the theoretical, empirical, and technical contributions that have been developed across the previous chapters. We also make some suggestions for the practical application of the findings for clinicians.

The data used in the book to analyse the function of narrative interaction within the psychotherapy process comes from psychoanalytic psychotherapy. However, we would like to suggest that our findings may be generalizable to some extent to other modalities of psychotherapy that make extended use of self-narratives. Therefore, we suggest that the studies included in this book could be useful for clinicians of various modalities of psychotherapeutic orientation, as well as for professionals such as researchers of the psychotherapy process and discourse analysis. We also recommend it to students of psychotherapy and counselling, due to the detailed analysis of several examples of psychotherapeutic interaction.

PART 1

Theoretical background of the joint construction of narratives

1 Narrative interaction and its development

This chapter discusses the theoretical background of our discourse-based approach to analysing narrative perspective (NP) in psychoanalytic discourse by summarizing the relevant literature on narrative interaction. We also discuss the way narrative skills and capacities develop in childhood. The issue of defining narrative interaction and describing its roots in childhood development is central to the main theme and argument of this book. We discuss how our capacity for constructing narratives evolves in childhood, since it serves as the basis for constructing narratives in adulthood in a variety of settings, including the psychoanalytic setting. As the development of narrative capacity is closely related to the development of autobiographical memory and the sense of self during childhood, reconstructing and co-constructing narratives at the psychoanalytic session with the collaboration of the analyst leads to the reconstructing or rewriting of memories (and related emotions) in the self-memory system (Conway 1992, 2005; Conway & Pleydell-Pearce 2000). We shall talk about the concept of the self-memory system in more detail in Chapter 5. However, we define it briefly here.

According to Conway and his colleagues, the self-memory concept states that memory is a database for the working self, which is created from autobiographical memories and active goals and self-images. We argue that, during retrieval, autobiographical memories might take the form of narratives. So, transformation of autobiographical narratives may alter the way the working-self operates. Hence, the process of narrativization may be a potential mechanism of change in psychotherapeutic treatment (Schafer 1980, 1992). In order to understand this process more deeply, it is crucial to explore how narrative and memory processes work in early development. However, we are not focusing on neural networks and brain processes in our discussion, rather on developmental evidence of the co-construction of narratives with care-givers.

The chapter first introduces the concept of narrative, as well as the concept of narrative interaction, and briefly describes the theoretical background of these concepts. The chapter further discusses the development of the human capacity of co-constructing narratives in childhood and adolescence with the help of parents and care-givers through the process of scaffolding, and the central role of narrative interaction in the early development of autobiographical memory and the self. The chapter also discusses studies of narrative interaction in various settings, including care-giver–preschool child interaction, family interaction, and adolescents' interaction with parents and peers.

Defining narrative

Oral narratives are often used in everyday conversations by speakers all around the world (Barthes & Duisit 1975; Shuman 2012) in order to discuss personal experiences, convey ideas, convince audiences, and to serve a variety of other purposes. Such narratives, or in other words 'stories', may involve the person telling it (i.e. the narrator), or may centre on other people. They often occur spontaneously or may be deliberately planned. So, we may say that personal narratives serve to organize life events in a temporal and logical order and establish coherence across past, present, and possible future experiences (Ochs & Capps 2001).

In the scientific study of narrative, in the fields of literary criticism, narratology, linguistics, psychology, and sociology, the first question that arises is how to differentiate narrative from other genres occurring in everyday communication, such as descriptions (Labov & Waletzky 1967; Schiffrin 1994) or scientific arguments (Bruner 1985). In the history of the study of narratives, various scholars' goal was to define the necessary formal criteria for what we may call narrative structure. Debates on this issue have focused on the following main questions:

1. Do we need a particular set of structural elements in order to define a well-formed narrative and, if yes, what are they?
2. Do we need a plot in order to call it a narrative?
3. Is there a required or preferred format for a narrative, such as an extended monologue-like sequence, or is it more like a dialogue or polylogue?

In the following section, we are discussing these questions, each in turn, and argue for what we would like to call a constructivist definition of narrative.

Do we need a particular set of structural elements in order to define a well-formed narrative, and, if yes, what are they? According to Labov and Waletzky (1967; Labov 2006), the answer to this question is a definitive 'yes'. According to their variationist theory, narrative is a particular way of the discursive organization for reporting past events, namely a temporally ordered set of event sequences with specific functions. (Variation analysis is a sociolinguistic approach studying variation and change within a language. The main assumption of variation analysis is that linguistic heterogeneity is related to social structures as well as to language use per se. Thus they study distribution of certain linguistic forms within the speech community.) Adult narratives of personal experience, those that are well formed at least, begin with an abstract sequence, which is the summary of the story about to be told, followed by the orientation, which describes the contextual details for the events: time, location, and characters. This sequence is followed by the complication, which consists of one or more action clauses, describing events in a temporal order, followed by the evaluation. An evaluation sequence expresses the narrator's attitude towards the events they were just told. At the end of the narrative there is a closing sequence, the coda, indicating that the narrative is over. These various narrative sequences can be observed in an illustrative example from a study based on ten self-defining memories (vivid, important, decisive memories of the life story) (Singer & Salovey 1993) using McAdams's structured life-story interview (McAdams 1997). This narrative is the 'turning point' story of one respondent:

1) When I was 18 at my high-school graduation in 2004, **Orientation**
2) I was the one who said my farewells in the name of my class, **Complication1**
3) and then following this was the announcement of the literary prize of my town, which I won. 4) The first prize was 10 thousand Forints, **Complication2**
5) I was so proud of myself, **Complication3**
6) and this is when I have started to see myself in the proper light— **Evaluation**
7) one would say I grew and aptitude to appreciate myself.
8) Therefore, the above event is a decisive one in my modest little life. (No 31) **Coda**

Similar to Labov and Waletzky, Prince (1987) argues that, in order to distinguish narratives from simple event descriptions (e.g. 'The glass fell on the floor'), it is necessary to recount at least two real or fictive events, neither of which logically presupposes or entails the other. However, contrary to structuralist descriptions of narrative such as Labov's or Prince's, according to the constructivist account, the formal requirements of narratives are a less crucial part of the definition. According to Bruner (1985, 2004), for instance, the sequential ordering of events within the narrative is only one of the devices narrators use to represent 'reality'. Moreover, Bruner suggests that what we should study is not so much the structure, but rather the function of a narrative, namely how narrative operates as an instrument of the mind in not merely the representation, but also in the construction of reality.

Fludernik (2002) further states that sequentiality, chronological order, and logical connectedness are not essential for narrative structure. What is crucial instead is the narrative experience (i.e. experientiality) and its expression in the story, which, for Fludernik, becomes the defining feature of narratives. By narrative experience, Fludernik means that the narrative expresses the narrator's, storyteller's, or another human-like character's verbalization (narrativization) of their perceptions, emotions, and evaluative thoughts related to the recounted events.

While looking at the study of narratives in psychoanalytic psychotherapy, we shall adhere to the constructivist view on narrative structure, mainly because many of the stories told in this setting will not meet Labov's criteria of 'well-formedness' (as discussed in Chapter 2). Consider, for example, the following narrative, from the psychoanalytic setting with a young female analysand:

> I had to go to the [thesis] consultation like this, basically, I did not make any progress since the previous consultation. And this was extremely embarrassing, and, like I could not tolerate it at all. And I simply don't understand why I'm unable to write it. Really. I cannot understand. Because I can't. It's not progressing now, like not at all. (Female analysand in her 20s from the Budapest Psychotherapy Database)

The woman talking here is a university student, and she is recounting her experience of thesis-writing, which causes her some difficulties. There is no orientation or coda sequence in this narrative. It draws conclusions from past experiences to the present, and the emphasis is on the client's feelings and emotions, satisfying Fludernik's criteria of containing narrative experience.

Now let us turn to the second major question regarding defining criteria for narratives: Do we need a plot in order to call it a narrative?

According to the formalist/structuralist definition (Prince 1987), the plot contains the narrative's main events and situations. It is the dynamic global organization of structural elements that determines the thematic interest of a narrative as well as its emotional effect. Prince (1987) gives a good example of the difference between story and plot. 'The king died and then the queen died' is a story (emphasis on chronology), whereas 'The king died and then the queen died from grief' is a plot (emphasis on causality). According to this view, plot is also an essential part of a well-formed narrative because of the structuralists' accentuation on story-event sequences, temporal and causal connections between them. The plot may even enchain events into typical sequences such as in folk tales or ballads (Kukkonen at al 2014).

In contrast to the structuralist view, however, the constructionist view claims that plot could be eliminated altogether from narratives. As Fludernik writes, indicating her theoretical standpoint of experientiality as the primary focus of narratives: 'In my model there can therefore be narratives without plot, but there cannot be any narratives without a human (anthropomorphic) experiencer of some sort at some narrative level' (2002: 9). So, Fludernik argues that the mere presence of a plot without the human-like experience's emotional involvement represents zero narrativity. However, according to the structuralist view, this would be a prototypical narrative. This narrative from the psychoanalytic session would serve as a good example of a narrative that does not have an obvious plot. Therefore, regarding the question of the plot, in the analysis of psychotherapeutic discourse, we again must rely on the constructivist view.

Finally, let us turn to the third question: Is there a required or preferred format for a narrative such as an extended monologue-like sequence, or is it more like a dialogue or polylogue (Sizoo 2002)?

Some structuralist scholars argue for the former; for example, Labov and Waletzky (1967), whose well-known sociolinguistic study of oral narratives focused on the danger of death experience stories before they have developed the sequential description of narrative structure we described previously. So, even in their research question, asking participants whether a life-threatening event has ever happened to them, Labov and Waletzky took it for granted that the narrating of personal experiences was an oral genre edited by the narrator into a monologue form, despite assuming, for example, that the narration must be interesting enough to the listener (i.e. narrators must try to grab the listeners' attention). However, others with a more constructivist understanding, such as Ochs and Capps (2001), as well as Quasthoff (Becker & Quasthoff 2005; Gülich & Quasthoff 1985) suggested a more interactive approach to narrating personal experience to an audience such that

> the content and direction that narrative framings take are contingent upon the narrative input of other interlocutors, who provide, elicit, criticize, refute and draw inferences from facets of the unfolding account. In these exchanges, the narrative becomes an interactional achievement, and interlocutors become co-authors. (Ochs & Capps 2001: 2–3)

It could be argued that interlocutors' so-called listener activities (Sacks 1986) creating an interactive, dialogical way of story-telling is more frequent in everyday conversation than narratives performed as a monologue. Moreover, if there is more than one interlocutor and co-teller who contribute to the construction of the narrative, we can use the word coined by Sizoo (2002), polylogue, to describe the multiple co-authorship involved in the narrative.

Habermas (2019) designates narrative interaction between equal adults as a typical way of co-narrating in everyday conversations—in other words, as a kind of default option of interactive narration. According to this view, primary narrators need to have feedback from their listeners in order to continue narrating, using non-verbal signals, or brief verbal expressions such as 'yeah!', 'uhum', 'uh-huh'. A more elaborate reaction from listeners may be what is referred to as assessment, including repetition of the narrator's words, exclamations, reformulating the narrator's stance, or even the listeners coming up with their own story, making a point similar to the primary narrator's (Habermas 2019).

So, in conclusion, we can say that personal narratives may take a monologue-like format as well as an interactive format depending on the situation of recounting the narrative, including the social context. In the context of psychoanalysis, and perhaps other modalities of psychotherapy and counselling, both therapist and client contribute to the construction of the client's self-narratives. So, we can say that narratives are jointly constructed in psychotherapy.

In the following sections, we will define the concept of 'narrative interaction' and characterize various forms of narrations, the so-called 'default' and the interactive narrative, in terms of the five dimensions described by Ochs and Capps (2001): tellership, tellability, embeddedness, linearity, and moral stance.

Narrative interaction

The interactive way of constructing personal experiences in narrative form is referred to as the joint construction of narrative (Berán & Unoka 2016), occurring in many settings in everyday life such as, for instance, family conversation, gossip, TV interview, psychotherapy, parental reminiscing with a child, school assignment for a group of children. Such activities are discussed under the label of 'narrative interaction' by Quasthoff and Becker (2005). Narrative interaction refers to recounting narratives—possibly incorporated in everyday social interactions—by jointly co-constructing them, by at least two, but often more, people.

Ochs and Capps (2001) describe a set of dimensions to characterize narratives of personal experience, as is shown in Table 1.1, ranging on the spectrum from the so-called 'default narrative' to a more interaction-based narrative.

The five dimensions of narrative defined by Ochs and Capps represent a scale between two extreme types of narratives. For tellership, this implies various degrees of involvement of conversational partners in the recounting of the narrative. So, according to Ochs and Capps, it may be the case that there is one primary narrator, who recounts events in front of a relatively passive audience;

Table 1.1 Narrative dimensions based on discussion in Ochs and Capps (2001: 20)

Dimension	Default narrative	Interactive narrative
Tellership	One active teller	Multiple active co-tellers
Tellability	High	Low
Embeddedness	Detached	Embedded
Linearity	Closed temporal and causal order	Open temporal and causal order
Moral stance	Certain, constant	Uncertain, fluid

or, alternatively, there may be more than one active co-teller who contribute information, support or challenge the primary narrator's account, or even supply narratives of experiences of their own. According to Ochs and Capps, it is possible that absent persons' thoughts and words also influence the narrator, and he/she may quote their voices. Listeners may display high levels of involvement vocally or non-vocally (through eye contact and gestures).

The next dimension, tellability, refers to the quality of the narrative as a tellable account, in other words the extent to which it reports a sequence of events and makes a point (Ochs & Capps 2001). Narratives that are highly tellable are often told on more than one occasion. Highly tellable, according to Ochs and Capps, also implies that the event is relevant and important to the interlocutors in the present or may be in the future. In contrast, low tellability is characterized by accounts of events of less import and relevance to the interlocutors, the narrator may be hesitant or awkward while telling the account, or the story has no resolution. According to Ochs and Capps, narratives with low tellability nevertheless may be told, because interlocutors often recount narratives they have never told before, or the storylines of which are not resolved, due to various communicative goals, for instance, to clarify their conclusions for themselves and others, or to regulate emotional tension.

Narratives also differ in the level of their embeddedness in surrounding discourse activities (Ochs & Capps 2001). In some cases, the narrative is detached from prior, concurrent, or subsequent discourse and is recounted in a lengthy conversational turn. Such narratives may relate content that is unrelated to the topic of previous discourse, or their rhetorical format may be different from the previously used format. According to Ochs and Capps, narratives may be embedded in prayers, explanations, disagreements, or integrated into other similar discourse activities. Embedded narratives may not have boundaries easily distinguished from surrounding discourse activities. This means that they may not have a distinct turn format, and their content may be related to the topic of discussion of surrounding discourse, for instance making a point in an argument relevant to the surrounding activity. They may also have various turn lengths; for instance, they may be recounted as a series of brief turns.

The next dimension of narratives, according to Ochs and Capps, is linearity. This term refers to the way narratives organize events into structures of time and causality. Such organization may to varying degrees be linear. Events may be represented in the narrative as either evolving with a single, closed or a diverse, open, uncertain temporal and causal path. In linearly organized narratives, events follow one another in temporal order, and one event causally leads to another, subsequent event. In non-linear narratives, temporal and causal links between events are open ended (Ochs & Capps 2001). In such narratives, the relation of one event to another regarding chronological order or causality may be obscured intentionally or unintentionally by the narrator. The narrator may give explanations for this, such as confusion, disagreement, or memory lapses.

Finally, the narrator's moral stance is inherently included in narratives of personal experience, since they do not represent an objective, comprehensive account of the events, but rather the narrator's view or perspective of them. According to Ochs and Capps, conversational narratives also serve to transfer moral worldviews: 'Narrators of personal experience evaluate protagonists as moral agents, whose actions, thoughts and feelings are interpreted in local notions of goodness. Narrators often shape the narrative to make their own comportment appear morally superior to that of another protagonist' (2001: 46). In some narratives, moral stance is relatively certain and prevails throughout, whereas in others it is indeterminate and unstable.

What Ochs and Capps call the default narrative (Table 1.1) is close to the well-formed structure as defined by Labov and Waletzky. One primary narrator (teller) tells it, and the narrative itself is rather detached from surrounding discourse activities. It has a single overarching storyline and has a closed temporal and causal order, with a certain stable evaluation. As Ochs and Capps note, such narratives are easy to identify and analyse scientifically. In contrast, at the other end of the continuum, we find narratives told by multiple co-tellers; they have multiple, divergent storylines embedded in surrounding discourse activity, they have a non-linear temporal and causal organization, and uncertain, fluid moral stance. Since they are 'full of hesitations, queries and considerations of alternative perspectives, such narratives are generally difficult to demarcate and systematically analyze' (Ochs & Capps 2001: 22).

In conclusion, we can say that the narratives co-constructed in the psychotherapy setting that we will analyse in the subsequent chapters of this book are more similar to what is referred to here as the interactive narrative. These narratives are told by more than one teller, since both the therapist and the client contribute to the narrative interaction process. The narratives have divergent storylines and are embedded in surrounding discourse activities. They may have non-linear temporal and causal organization and an uncertain or fluid moral stance.

Development of narrative capacity: an overview of the process from early childhood to adolescence

In the reminder of Chapter 1, we describe the development of the capacity of co-constructing narratives in childhood and adolescence with the help of parents, care-givers, and peers, emphasizing the central role of narrative interaction in the early development of autobiographical memory and the self. Inspired by the above definitions of narrative structure as understood by the structuralist account, the literature on children's narrative development generally assumes that children are striving to achieve a well-formed narrative (referred to as the high-point structure), and they learn this with the help of parents and care-givers through narrative interaction. This may be understood as learning an ideal type of narrative organization on the part of children, whereas in practice in later life, depending on the social context of recounting the narrative, the narrative structure may vary based on the five dimensions described by Ochs and Capps (2001).

Table 1.2 contains the main milestones of narrative development. In the beginning—at about 3.5 years of age—small children's narratives are less structured and may be rather disorganized, with less reasoning and more non-verbal expression. As children develop their narrative capacity—also acquiring more sophisticated language skills—personal narratives become longer, with more varied themes and more detailed orientation and evaluative statements.

Parents and care-givers scaffold early narrative development. As such, parents help children to construct narratives by asking questions, prompting them, repeating the child's words, and providing emotional and structural elaboration (McDonnell et al. 2016). The concept of scaffolding originates in the writings of the Russian psychologist Lev Vygotsky (1930), who claimed that parents help their children in accomplishing developmental tasks, providing assistance only as far as children needed it to achieve the zone of proximal development (i.e. the next level of development). When parents scaffold children in narrating their personal experiences, they help their children to learn to narrate, develop autobiographical memory skills, and learn about mental states (Habermas 2019).

Table 1.2 Development of narrative capacity

2nd year	referencing past events that happened to them as answers to adults' questions or prompts, with emotions and evaluations
3.5 years	narrating a simple story with a single event that happened to them in joint construction of narratives with parent/care-giver
5 years	verbal theory of mind development parallel with narrative competence
6–11 years middle childhood	during elementary school years, children develop the ability to share and discuss personal narratives of individual life events with others using high-point structure, and being familiar with well-formed narrative structure
12–15 years early to mid-adolescence	learning to narrate entire life, using autobiographical reasoning
16–18 late adolescence	developing further coherence of the life story, and autobiographical reasoning, narrative interaction with peers takes on more importance, but still narrating some life episodes with parents
19–20 young adulthood, and later life	developing further coherence of the life story, and autobiographical reasoning

By the age of 6–7, children have learnt narrative skills sufficient to tell more simple life-story episodes, and by early adolescence they have learnt to narrate sequences of such episodes to narrate their entire life. Table 1.2 summarizes the approximate rhythm of the development of narrative capacity, which we shall describe in detail in our subsequent sections.

Early childhood and preschool years: narrative development and autobiographical memory

The development of narrative capacity begins as soon as children are able to comprehend and reconstruct personally relevant past events in conversations about the past and future with the help of parents/care-givers at about 2–2.5 years of age. The process of narrative development involves 1) the development of retrieval skills necessary for reconstructing past events, as well as 2) the verbal skills necessary for constructing a well-formed coherent story. The former is closely related to the development of autobiographical memory skills, which mainly involves the kind of memory we call episodic (Tulving 2002).

According to Nelson and Fivush (2004), autobiographical memories consist of single life episodes, and the ability to reconstruct such memories emerges gradually during the preschool years, beginning regular functioning at about 4–5 years of age. Autobiographical memory 'involves basic memory abilities, understanding of temporal relations, narrative, self and others and mental states' (p. 489). Nelson and Fivush also stress the importance of language as a sociocultural tool in the development of autobiographical memory. As a linguistic genre, we may add that narrative may involve a cultural effect: learned from parents/care-givers, mediating between culture and autobiographical memory development. Nelson and Fivush claim that narrative structure and content influence and are influenced by autobiographical memory—this latter also has a reciprocal relationship with self-representation and theory of mind abilities. They write:

> Experience with different forms of narrative, in play, stories, and especially in talk about personal episodes, provides a model for organizing one's own episodic memories into the kind of narratives that emphasize personhood, motivations, goals, outcomes, emotions, and values. Practice with this organization has a two-sided outcome: The child learns to tell about personal experience in the social forms valued by the community and acquires a more coherent form that aids in the retention of a whole episode, and not just fragments of scenes. (2004: 490)

So, Nelson and Fivush argue that language skills development during the preschool period allows the development of a verbally accessible autobiographical memory (and not the other way around: the development of memory skills supporting linguistic performance). The emergence of simple narratives at about 5 years of age provides additional organization to events with a quality different from the causal and temporal organization by giving meaning, emphasizing goals and plans, motivations and emotions of characters, and their meaningful relation to the narrator (Nelson & Fivush 2004). Hence, we can conclude that narratives may also provide structure for recalling past episodes or—as some studies show—constructing future scenarios (Conway 2001; Habermas & Bluck 2000; Pasupathi et al. 2007; Sools 2020) containing and organizing recollected details into meaningful patterns.

Toddlers are able to relate a recounted event to emotions and evaluations by the age of 2 years—which may be considered the basis for subjective perspective. By the age of 3.5, they can report on a simple past event with the help of their parent/care-giver during narrative interaction when the child co-constructs the past event with the parent (Fivush & Salmon 2023; Uehara 2015). The focus of such narratives is typically 1) what happened, and 2) what is the subjective meaning of the event for the child. At this point, the child needs the parent/care-giver's active contribution in order to be able to construct a narrative of past events. Such a helpful contribution on the part of the parent in a developmental task was labelled 'scaffolding'. The following is an example of a narrative interaction from the CHILDES database (MacWhinney 2000) from the data of Peterson and McCabe (1983), with the adult (investigator) scaffolding a 4-year-old child in the task of telling a narrative (chat 3, narrative 1):

1	*CHI:	yeah <and I> [/] <and I> [/] and I bumped myself that day &-uh &-uh
2		my bathroom and my mom wasn't watching out .
3	*INV:	you bumped yourself and [//] that day ?
4	*CHI:	yeah (.) yeah .
5	*INV:	and [/] and backed up ?
6	*CHI:	no did like this .
7	*INV:	oh and you went back ?
8	*CHI:	yeah .
9	*INV:	and your mom wasn't watching out ?
10	*CHI:	unhunh .
11	*INV:	what happened ?
12	*CHI:	I go to doctor's again .
13	*CHI:	they cut it out .
14	*INV:	oh you went to the doctor's and you got them cut out ?
15	*CHI:	yeah .
16	*INV:	oh I see.
17	*INV:	these were stitches ?

Scaffolding, on the part of the adult (the investigator), consists of her asking questions of the child to move narration forward and repeating the child's statement in corrected linguistic form. Parent–child joint reminiscing about personal past events is more than a memory task for the child, however. It could provide an important occasion for them to learn the forms of personal narration, the significance of this activity for sharing personal narratives with others, and establishing and strengthening a sense of self.

Parents or care-givers differ in their style of providing scaffolding for children. When mother and child are jointly reminiscing a past event, some mothers use a highly elaborative style (Fivush 1991; Fivush et al. 2006; Fivush & Salmon 2023; Haden et al. 1997; Peterson & McCabe 1992). This consists of providing richer and more detailed narratives in interaction with the child, with greater contextual information in the orientation sequence (where and when the event happened, who was there, what they did), and more detailed evaluations about the personal relevance and meaning of the event (why the event was significant, and what is its emotional relevance for the child). Such mothers keep asking more open-ended questions about the event and give more detailed answers even if the child does not remember. They praise and confirm their children's contributions, signalling that they are valid and important. In contrast, a low elaborative style is characterized by fewer questions by mothers, repetitively asking the same questions over and over again, resulting in a less detailed narrative with fewer descriptions. Children of highly elaborative mothers can recall autobiographical narratives of past events better at a later age (Haden et al. 1997), because such elaborated narratives can be better integrated into autobiographical memory. Maternal reminiscing style (i.e. high or low elaboration) was also found to be consistent across the preschool years.

In connection with maternal reminiscing style, Fivush et al. (2006) emphasize the mutual influencing nature of narrative interaction between child and mother/care-giver:

> Maternal reminiscing style is part of an ongoing developmental process, in which mothers and children mutually influence and accommodate to each other. So, our view of development is focused on the process of interaction. The developmental mechanism of change from this perspective is language interaction (Nelson 1996); as children participate in linguistically scaffolded interactions, in which specific skills and content are co-constructed, children internalize these interactions, such that what begins as socially mediated becomes part of the individual's repertoire. (2006: 1569)

To summarize what we have discussed so far, we can say that parents–child joint reminiscing was shown to lead in children of highly elaborative mothers to the development of more elaborated personal narratives a few years later (Fivush et al. 2006; Haden et al. 1997; Reese & Newcombe 2007), and to better skills in autobiographical remembering tasks (Bauer & Burch 2004; Farrant & Reese 2000; Fivush & Vasudeva 2002). In other words, what fosters autobiographical memory development in early childhood is highly elaborative co-narrating with the parent and detailed evaluations—with parental help—at the end of narratives (Bird & Reese 2006; Reese et al. 2019).

Evaluations are related to the parent (mother)–child attachment relationship (Reese et al. 2010), such that mothers of securely attached children use more evaluations during narrative constructions with children, and children learn evaluative style from their mothers and use it in their narrative constructions in later years. Reese and colleagues use the following example to illustrate the evaluative, highly elaborative style of the securely attached dyad (evaluation is in italics, based on Reese et al. 2010: 26):

M: Do you remember what happened last, a couple of days ago, when you were playing in the sandpit?
C: No.
M: Do you remember what happened to the bird?
C: What? Yes, it [unintelligible] it died.
M: It died, didn't it? Well, how did it die?
C: Because it hurt itself.
M: How did it hurt itself?
C: It flew past it.
M: It flew past it.
C: You, and it hit it. [break in conversation] …
M: How did it hurt itself?
C: Because it, um, it, it hit meself on the nose.
M: Yeah. It flew into the window, didn't it? And it got hurt. And then what did we do?
C: What?
C: Bury it.
M: We buried it.
C: I li–, I don't like burying things.
M: No, it was a bit sad, wasn't it?
C: I don't care if it's sad, because I hate birds.
M: You were a bit upset, weren't you?
C: No, I wasn't.
M: But then you decided you weren't upset. Cos it was a bit much.
C: No, I was only sad upset because I didn't want to um, put my red flower in the little place.
M: Yeah.
C: Yes.
M: It was nice that you gave him a flower, though.

Such evaluative comments on the mother's part help the child to understand the emotionally stressful event, make sense of it, and address the difficulty of encountering death for small children. Reese and colleagues (Reese et al. 2010) also show how an insecurely attached mother–child dyad uses a low elaborative style, with little or no evaluation involved on the part of the parent. Parents with low elaborative style repetitively talk about event details, asking fewer and redundant questions compared to the more evaluative mother, and do not discuss the emotional aspects of a potentially disturbing event.

In another study (McDonnell et al. 2016), the mother's attachment style was related to maternal elaboration while reminiscing with their child and to child autobiographical memory specificity in preschool aged children. Their findings showed that emotional elements of reminiscing—such as high levels of emotional elaboration—were related to a more specific memory in children where the mother also provided high levels of structural elaboration (i.e. asking questions of the child, such as when and where the event happened, who participated in it, what has actually transpired, etc., and scaffolding the child's answers). However, if mothers did not provide high levels of structural elaboration, emotional elaboration provided children with less specific memory. Emotional elaboration has also been related to lower levels of specificity in the case of high levels of maternal attachment anxiety and avoidance (i.e. in the case of insecurely attached mothers). Autobiographical memory specificity (providing a memory of a one-time specific event for a cue word) is relevant in terms of psychologically healthy personality development. In adults, low levels of specificity have been associated with depression, borderline personality disorder, PTSD, and other trauma-related symptomatology (Barry et al. 2018; Berán et al. 2019; Van Vreeswijk & De Wilde 2004).

The parent's use of a highly elaborative style in narrative co-construction with their child also helps to develop and stabilize children's conceptions of their self in the preschool years. Children whose mothers use a highly elaborative narrative style also provide richer and more accurate narratives to others (Reese & Newcombe 2007), thus showing evidence of a better functioning autobiographical memory. Parental elaboration and emphasis on emotions, and especially on negative emotions, in narrative co-construction with their children is associated with a more organized self-concept as measured by Eder's (1989, 1990) Children's Self View Questionnaire (Bird & Reese 2006). So, children, who experience a more elaborate discussion of emotionally richer narratives are better able to draw on those autobiographical memories involved in such narratives for creating a sense of self (Reese et al. 2010). It has also been shown (Bird & Reese 2006) that it is not so much the actual events that influence autobiographical memories and the self-concept, but rather parents' emotional interpretation of those events in their reminiscing. Bird and Reese argue (2006) that reminiscing on negative events is important for helping the child to work through negative emotions. The following is an example of a mother–child reminiscing of a negative/sad event (Bird & Reese 2006: 623).

Mother: Can you think of a time when you felt sad?
Child: Um, when I fell over.

Mother: Yeah, you were a bit sad when you fell over weren't you?
Mother: And you hurt your hands, didn't you?
Child: This one went sliding like that, and this one went sliding like that.
Mother: Oh okay, and that made you feel sad?
Mother: You do feel a bit sad when you hurt yourself, don't you?
Mother: Yeah, and what happened?
Child: This one went sliding like that and flipped over …
Mother: And then, and then yeah, you felt a bit sad.
Mother: And what happened when you felt sad?
Child: Um.
Mother: What did you do?
Child: You came.
Mother: I came, yeah.
Child: And [sibling] said, are you okay?
Mother: [Sibling] looked after you?
Mother: He did too, didn't he?
Mother: He was good, wasn't he?
Mother: And what did you do?
Mother: You cried, didn't you?
Mother: That's all right. It's all right to cry when you feel sad.

In this excerpt, the mother directs the conversation from concrete details of the event towards emotion-relevant discussion, helping the child to name the emotion and connect it to the concrete events, as well as discussing behaviour related to the emotion (i.e. crying), and resolving the emotion (by seeking contact). Such elaborations of explaining and resolving negative emotions, as opposed to just attributing them, leads to meaning creation. According to the authors: 'in order for children to understand the personal meaning of a negative experience and integrate this event into a coherent autobiography, a more in-depth discussion of the causes and consequences of emotion, and method of resolution is needed' (Bird & Reese 2006: 623).

A highly elaborative parental reminiscing style is also related to children's well-being, estimated by measuring self-esteem. Emphasis on positive aspects of events is associated with higher self-esteem by age 6 (Bird et al. 2006). According to Fivush and colleagues (2006), however, there are sociocultural differences in mothers' reminiscing styles. For instance, mothers are more elaborative and discuss more emotions with daughters than with sons during the preschool years. Mothers from Western cultures have a more elaborative style of reminiscing compared to Chinese mothers (Wang 2001).

Narrative accomplishment in the preschool years is also related to theory of mind (ToM) skills, as well as to false belief understanding (FBU) (Baldwin et al. 2001; Tompkins et al. 2019). ToM refers to the human capacity to attribute mental states to the self and others, whereas FBU is based on the so-called false belief task (Wimmer & Perner 1983), involving the attribution of beliefs to others that do not match the persons own knowledge of reality, nor the actual state of affairs. According to Tompkins and her colleagues, preschool-aged children's narrative skills provide assistance for the emergence of ToM and FBU skills, because narratives describe contextual information and, most of all, reasons for goal-directed actions: why a person wants, hopes, desires, etc. (Tompkins et al. 2019). Narrative practice theory embraced by Tompkins suggests that, with the help of narratives, children can both anticipate and explain behaviour. The reason for this is that, in order to comprehend a narrative, children must attribute mental states to characters. So, during the preschool years children learn to comprehend narratives and develop narrative capacity as well as ToM skills through various discourse practices such as bed-time storytelling, reminiscing with the care-giver, watching movies, etc. However, we must emphasize here that Tompkins is discussing ToM and FBU as *verbal* skills. Several studies show existing ToM and FBU skills of pre-verbal infants as early as 13–18 months (Onishi & Baillargeon 2005; Song et al. 2008; Surian et al. 2007), and 25 months of age (Southgate et al. 2007) to understand object identity with spontaneous response tasks, such as anticipatory looking and violation of expectation.

In summary, we can say that in the preschool years children's narrative development is scaffolded by parents and care-givers in a way to help small children remember personal life episodes and to narrate them. The reminiscing style of mothers/care-givers may differ as to how elaborate it is. Mothers with a highly elaborative style discuss past events in rich detail with the child, ask many open-ended and yes/no questions of the child, and use emotional evaluation to discuss the significance of the event for the child. In contrast, mothers with a low elaborative style use less detail in recollecting the event with the child, ask fewer, repetitive questions trying to prompt the child to recall information, and do not use emotional evaluations. The mother's reminiscing style was shown to be associated with the development of autobiographical memory, self-organization and self-concept, well-being, self-esteem, and ToM skills.

Narrative development in the early school years and preadolescence (6–12 years)

By the age of 6–7 years, children develop the ability to narrate past personal events and share them with adults and peers. School becomes a major locale for narrative socialization; however, school-aged children still practise reminiscing with parents and family members. They learn how to use conventional forms of narrative—the high-point structure (Labov 1972)—and learn how to create more coherent narratives. Children also begin to acquire the use of autobiographical reasoning in their narratives, and their self-concept becomes more based on specific, rather than general, memories (Habermas 2011; Habermas & Bluck 2000).

Narrating a personal event independently or in interaction with care-givers, other adults, or peers becomes regular practice by age 6–7 years. By this time, children develop a good understanding of narrative structure: they know what an exciting story consists of and also know the conventions of what counts as a well-formed narrative (McAdams & Cox 2010) with a beginning, complication, middle, and ending/resolution.

High-point structure in a narrative refers to the fact that it contains a complication, or climax, which is followed by a resolution (Labov 1972). According to high-point analysis (Berman & Slobin 2013; Boyd et al. 2020; Peterson & McCabe 1983; Reese et al. 2011), narratives characterized by such high-point structure are more coherent. Less coherent narratives are the ones that end at the high point (missing a resolution), listing events without connection between them ('leap-frogging' narratives), narratives without orientation or high point ('chronological'), too short narratives lacking structure ('impoverished'), or incoherent narratives ('disoriented'). According to Peterson and McCabe's findings, 4-year-olds use the leap-frogging, impoverished, disoriented, or chronological narratives, whereas 5–9-year-olds use the end-at the high point or chronological structure, which is developed into full high-point structure by the age of 9. So, children learn to use high-point structure in personal narratives gradually, and their narratives become more coherent by 9 years of age.

Reese and colleagues (Reese et al. 2011) developed a coding schema for studying the development of narrative coherence, based on three dimensions of coherence: context, chronology, and theme. Context refers to the spatio-temporal orientation at the beginning of the narrative, chronology refers to the relating of events along a timeline, and theme refers to maintaining and elaborating a topic throughout the narrative. Their findings show that school-age children provide some context to their narratives, but full contextual information was provided only by mid-adolescent-aged participants. Regarding chronology, the authors found a dramatic development between the ages of 6 and 11. On the theme dimension, they found that school-age children have not yet achieved a fully elaborated narrative, which was more characteristic of late adolescents and adults. From Reese and colleagues' study, we can conclude that the development of narrative coherence takes place gradually during the early school years, and that, among the three dimensions of coherence they measured, ordering events along a timeline is the specific skill mastered at this age. For this, children must understand the causal relationship between events, and create links between them, forwards and backwards in time. In another study where participants narrated their entire life narratives, 8-year-old children were able to create a life story; however, it was not a globally coherent one—their narratives were rather a collection of interesting episodes (Habermas & de Silveira 2008). A coherent life story is shown to be created only in early adolescence (Habermas & Paha 2001). So, evidence points towards the conclusion that older children can achieve coherence in a limited sense in self-narratives, understanding temporal and causal connections between events.

Autobiographical reasoning is another aspect of personal narrative that begins to develop in pre-adolescence, and continues developing throughout the adolescent years. The concept was invented by Habermas and Bluck (2000), and refers to the links between autobiographical events and self-development in the narrative:

> Autobiographical reasoning creates links between remembered events and other distant parts of one's life and to the self and its development. It refers to the remembering subject's life as the relevant frame of reference, thereby implying the life story. Autobiographical reasoning requires an extra mental effort that goes beyond th-e effort of mere remembering. We termed this activity as 'autobiographical reasoning' to underscore three aspects: the constructive and interpretative nature of the activity, the cognitive and communicative nature of it, and its normative aspect implied by its appeal to reason and logic. (Habermas 2011: 3)

Autobiographical reasoning employs two types of connections between events and self-development: those related to 1) self-stability, and those related to 2) self-change (Habermas 2011; Lilgendahl & McAdams 2011; McLean et al. 2022; Pasupathi et al. 2007). Self-stability connections sustain continuity of the self, whereas self-change connections emphasize how past experiences have changed the self. For example, stability of the self is being emphasized in the following sentence: 'My parents have bought me a piano for my eighth birthday, and ever since I have been a lover of classical music.' In this episode, a connection is made between an event (receiving a piano as a birthday gift) and a stable characteristic of the self (becoming, and staying, a lover of classical music). Self-change is emphasized in the following statement of autobiographical reasoning: 'I have become more and more fond of classical music in the past years, instead of listening to pop music as I used to, since I have worked on my skills of piano playing.' In this episode, a connection is made between a past event (working on skills of piano playing) and characteristics of the self that emphasizes change (becoming more and more fond of classical music instead of pop music).

Habermas and de Silveira (2008) have shown in a study of narrating life stories (discussed in detail below) that causal connections between the individual's past and the current self were drawn by 20% of the 8-year-old participants, but by 75% of the 12- to 20-year-old participants. Moreover, autobiographical reasoning was evidenced from 12 years of age, and developed further on throughout adolescence and the young adult years.

During the early school years and pre-adolescence, parental reminiscing with the child still plays a major role in establishing autobiographical memory, developing self-concept, emotion regulation, and increasing well-being (Reese et al. 2010). In their study, Reese and colleagues (2010) examined mother–child reminiscing in a sample of 20–40 months of age, and in a follow-up study 10 years later, when children were 12–13 years old. they were asked to recall some of their autobiographical memories from ages of 10, 5, 3, and before 3 years. The researchers then computed correlations between the mothers' references to children's emotions at 40 months, and children's references to their own emotions at 40 months, and at 12–13 years. Results showed a moderate-strength positive relationship between the mother's references to emotions and the children's reference to their own emotions in both age groups. It was also found that the mother's references to children's negative emotions predicted richer personal perspective in life stories in early adolescence—perspective measured with the frequency of emotion words in narratives. In the authors' interpretation, these results suggest that discussing and resolving negative emotions through reminiscing in early childhood leads to the subsequent positive portrayal of the negative event. This, in turn, can lead to finding meaning in a negative experience, which may contribute to optimism, a sense of self-efficacy, and successful coping behaviour (Reese et al. 2010).

Narrating together with family members may also influence the way children and pre-adolescents learn to construct memories, identities, and the self. Bohanek and colleagues (Bohanek et al. 2006) examined family narrative interaction with respect to pre-adolescents developing a sense of self-worth and self-efficacy. They distinguished three types of interaction patterns in family reminiscing of past events with respect to whether families discussed events in integrated and validating ways: 1) individual perspective, 2) coordinated perspective, 3) imposed perspective. In the case of individual perspective, family members articulate their own views of the past event in which they have participated; however, they did not create an integrated, common 'family' perspective. In the case of a coordinated perspective, they discussed individual perspectives and then created an integrated, collective one. In the case of an imposed perspective, one family member directed the conversation in which unpleasant exchanges might also occur. Bohanek and colleagues' findings have shown that family conversations with a coordinated perspective were related to higher self-esteem in girls (aged between 9 and 12 years). Conversations with the individual perspective were related to an external locus of control in children and a higher self-efficacy in boys. Conversations with imposed perspective were associated with neither self-esteem nor locus of control.

Looking at family interaction styles more closely, the authors relate how, in the case of creating a coordinated perspective, families first engaged in detailed conversation about the event, several perspectives were taken and discussed, including children's perspective. During such conversations, one's own perspective is better understood in relation to the perspective of others. They write:

> Specifically, children's opinions are acknowledged by other family members, and children's perspectives are integrated into the evolving theory of what occurred, which is recognized by the family as the shared family story. Through the process of integrating children's perspectives, families using a coordinated perspective style provide a safe and comfortable environment for children to tell their perspectives, thus creating interconnectedness as a whole family and recognizing the individual value of the child. Because children's perspectives are validated and integrated, their self-esteem is high. (Bohanek et al. 2006: 48)

The authors explain gender differences with the stereotypical assumption that, in girls, identity, relatedness, and connectedness are valued by others, whereas in boys others value more individuality, placing more weight on achievements outside the family, such as academic and sporting achievement. Such differences may be highlighted at the beginning of adolescence, when children first begin to establish their own individual identities (Erikson 1959; Van Doeselaar et al. 2020).

In conclusion, we can say that in late childhood and preadolescence narrative structure develops further, and children learn how to create well-formed narratives of personal events, as it is defined by the structuralist approach. Their narratives become more coherent as they age, and they begin to show the precursors of autobiographical reasoning, making connections between past events and the current self. Narrative interaction with parents and family members remains important for the formation of self-narratives for this age group.

Narrative development in adolescence (13–18 years)

In adolescence, the problem of forming a stable identity (Erikson 1959; Van Doeselaar et al. 2020) becomes a central developmental task. During the adolescent years, young people develop their narrative of their entire life story for the first time in a globally coherent manner, creating a basis for narrative identity. Autobiographical reasoning develops further, making life stories and episodes even more coherent. Narrative interaction with peers takes on more importance, but narrating some life episodes with parents providing scaffolding still remains important for the adolescent's development of his/her emerging narrative identity.

According to Erikson's theory (1959) of identity development, the primary developmental task in adolescence is the formation of a stable identity that is based on the secure commitments the individual makes in three major areas of life: occupational interest, sexuality, and worldview (philosophy, religion, politics). In order to be able to reach those commitments, the adolescent has to negotiate the conflict between identity and role confusion and, so, navigate through an identity crisis, during which they reconsider and/or abandon previous, less mature childhood identity commitments, and forge new ones, based on the exploration of new possibilities.

According to narrative theorists (Branje et al. 2021; Habermas & De Silveira 2008; McAdams 1985, 2021; Van Doeselaar et al. 2020) the process of identity formation as described by Erikson parallels the development of the life-story narrative because, according to their view, in adolescence the concept of personhood becomes historically established. This means that identity becomes expressed in a narrative form (i.e. the life story), and individuals create what is referred to as a narrative identity. Habermas and De Silveira (2008) define the life story as a global coherence created among life events and circumstances, and the self, including the person's values and life decisions. They distinguish four types of global coherence in the life-story narrative: 1) temporal coherence, 2) causal coherence, 3) thematic coherence, 4) coherence with a cultural concept of biography. Temporal coherence refers to the listener's orientation of the actual sequence of events in the narrative. Causal coherence refers to the listener's orientation of causal links between biographical events and changes in personality. Thematic coherence refers to the listener's orientation of the dominant thematic strands in the narrative. Coherence with cultural expectations means that it is easier for listeners to understand a life narrative that follows their expectations of how such a biography should look.

Using this definition of global coherence, Habermas and De Silveira (2008) tested the hypothesis that the globally coherent life story evolves only in adolescence. Drawing on a sample of 8, 12, 16 and 20-year-olds, all together 102 participants, their findings show that temporal coherence increases most between 8 and 12 years of age, causal coherence increases most in those 12 and 16 years of age, whereas thematic coherence increases most between the ages of 16 and 20, thus suggesting that global coherence, and consequently life narrative, develops gradually in the adolescent years. It is an important finding that biographical arguments and connections with events explaining personality development are almost completely absent in the 8-year-old group, but they appear in older groups, suggesting that autobiographical reasoning develops only from early adolescence. Overall, evidence suggests (Habermas & De Silveira 2008; Nelson & Fivush 2020; Reese et al. 2010) that the life story and autobiographical reasoning develop gradually from the pre-adolescent years throughout adolescence and into young adulthood.

The development of narrative identity is related to other aspects of development, such as well-being and self-esteem, as well as self-development in adolescence. In their study, Reese and colleagues (Reese et al. 2010) found that the organization of the life story and the insight concerning a life-changing event in adolescents was related to higher self-esteem, independent of verbal skills, and to well-being.

Narrative interaction with parents remains an important way narrative identity develops during adolescence, and, in addition, the role of peers becomes essential in the co-construction of self-narratives, and concomitantly narrative identity at this age group. Weeks and Pasupathi (2010) conducted a study in which they examined the role of both parents and peers in narrative co-construction with adolescents regarding the manifestation of the adolescent's individuation or autonomy. For this, peers and family members can provide support while co-constructing identities in conversations. The authors conceptualize autonomy support during conversation based on Fivush's model of the power of voicing and silencing in discourse (Fivush 2004 as cited by Weeks & Pasupathi 2010).

According to this model, the voice–silence continuum refers to how much a person in a conversation is able to express their perspective. Being able to voice one's perspective in conversation means a validation of one's identity. Silencing, however, means that one's story cannot be told. The second continuum also proposed by Fivush's model is the self–other continuum, referring to whether silencing or giving voice is originated from the self (the narrator) or from the other (listener). It is possible that the narrator is able to tell his/her story; thus his/her autonomous identity is validated. However, it is also possible that the other voices the narrator's identity, imposing his/her view on the narrator. In the case of silencing, it is possible that the other silences the narrator, in which case their identity is negated. However, the narrator herself may choose to silence her identity, in which case the voicing of identity is avoided.

The authors give an example of a conversation between a mother and adolescent daughter (13 years old) about choosing classes at high school (Weeks & Pasupathi 2010). They suggest that this discussion of identity and autonomy topic takes place in a warm, positive, supporting conversation between parent and adolescent, where the daughter voices autonomy, and her chosen identity, and this act is being supported by the mother. The mother achieves this by elaborating on aspects of the daughter's identity that she seems to want to emphasize by asking questions and giving interpretations of what the daughter said means, without imposing on her.

In the study, the same topic is discussed with a peer (friend, p. 79):

> S: Anyway, when I was registering for high school, it was happy, because, because, I got to choose the classes, well, kind of, the classes I want. And, uh, it was a little bit bad, because I couldn't choose the fourteen classes I wanted. [laugh]
> Friend: [laugh] [nods]
> S: And then stay at the school till, like, 9 o'clock at night.
> Friend: More like the twenty-eight classes you wanted. [laugh]
> S: Yeah. [laugh] More like that.

In this short excerpt, the authors argue, the young girl's identity and autonomy is supported by the friend, although not in the detailed manner as in the conversation with the mother. The girl's identity is construed as an ambitious person with a wide range of interests, and she is able to communicate with her supportive friend the mixed feelings she has had about choosing classes.

The examples the authors discuss show how identity and autonomy is supported by the mother and the friend. However, this is not the case in all the examples Weeks and Pasupathi discuss in their study. They include conversations with both parents and friends in which the adolescent's identity is negated, silenced by the other, or avoided by the self, by for example forcing conversation on topics such as the moral consequences of the adolescent's behaviour, or contradicting the narrator's claim of her personal qualities. Overall, the study shows that friends and parents co-construct the same stories differently, offering complementary contexts for reinforcing various aspects of narrative identity. The authors suggest that early parent–child reminiscing practices may have continuities in adolescence, and may even influence adolescent's identity conversations with peers.

In another study, McLean and Mansfield (2011) examined adolescent's narrative interactions with their mothers, regarding three narrative processes: meaning-making, vulnerability, and resolution. According to the authors, meaning-making is related to reflecting and learning from past events in order to understand the current self. Vulnerability and resolution are related to understanding and working through negative emotions. In the study, researchers also measured mothers' scaffolding behaviour with respect to adolescents' age and gender. Their findings indicate that mothers give more supporting scaffolding to younger adolescents and boys, and less to older adolescents and girls, who may have more practice in narrating self-related past events, and constructing narrative identity. In fact, they found that, with the latter, mothers engage in more negation behaviour. Results also showed that mothers engaged in less meaning-making with older adolescents and more discussions of vulnerability and resolution. The authors conclude that mothers and their adolescent-aged children still continue to jointly construct self-narratives; however, with the age of the adolescents increasing, mothers have a less important role, and adolescents take over in constructing their own narrative identity.

In conclusion, we can say that narrative capacity keeps developing in adolescence and in the young adult years. The life story, as a coherent account of narrative identity, is established during the adolescent years, and narrative episodes develop through interactions with parents and peers. Autobiographical reasoning, as a form of meaning-making, also develops at this time. As our identity constantly evolves during the adolescent and adult years—changing with age, acquiring new elements based on new events happening, and accomplishing new developmental tasks in our lives (Erikson 1959)—narrative identity is also altered, based on the life-story episodes we construct for ourselves and/or to others (McAdams & Cox 2010).

Concluding this chapter on the developmental process of narrative interaction, we can say that it takes place from the early years of 2.5 until the adolescent years and beyond (Quasthoff & Stude 2021), as an integral part of the development of other cognitive functions such as memory, verbal skills, and theory of mind, as well as functions of emotional development such as emotion regulation, attachment, and development of the self and identity. It is clear from the earlier discussion that narrative interaction with parents and care-givers as well as with peers in the later years enhances memory specificity and autobiographical memory formation, helps to develop the self-concept and a stabilized self, and identity, and increases self-esteem and well-being. These positive developments, however, are the result of specific ways of constructing narratives in interaction: using a highly elaborate style in the early years as well as being supportive of the adolescent's autonomy later.

In this chapter we have demonstrated the importance of narrative interaction in all the mentioned developmental areas by describing a body of literature relevant to it. In subsequent chapters we shall demonstrate, through the analysis of psychoanalytic discourse, the importance of narrative interaction for the psychotherapy process in terms of the reconstruction of autobiographical memories at the session, mentalization, affect regulation, agency and representations of interpersonal relating.

2 Psychotherapeutic discourse

The interactive construction of narratives (Quasthoff & Becker 2005) may be encountered in various everyday situations, such as, for instance, friendly adult interaction, interaction among adolescents, and parent–child interactions, as we have discussed in Chapter 1. In psychotherapeutic discourse—especially in psychotherapies focusing on verbal interaction, such as psychoanalysis, short dynamically oriented psychotherapy, expressive psychotherapy, existential psychotherapy, narrative therapy, person-centred psychotherapy, to name just a few—self-narratives of the client's life story are reconstructed at the session in an interactive way, in cooperation with the psychotherapist, who also contributes to the transformation of these narratives by their responses, comments, and interpretations (De Jong et al. 2013; Deppermann et al. 2020; Pawelczyk 2012). The transformation of the analysand's self-narratives in psychoanalysis is a long-term process, which may last for years, and fragments and episodes of the analysand's life story are reconstructed at the sessions with the help of the psychoanalyst. As we aim to demonstrate in the subsequent chapters of this book, the tracking of the process of reconstruction and transformation of self-narratives in psychoanalysis allows for understanding some aspects of psychotherapeutic change, conceived as the consequence of the therapy process itself.

At the same time, psychotherapeutic discourse taking place at the session, including discussion of the client's self-narratives, is determined by its institutional frameworks, which may include many aspects of the situation and terms under which psychotherapy takes place. In other words, the psychotherapeutic situation in itself implies some characteristics that are inherent to the conversation, which could possibly be conceived within such a framework. This chapter describes characteristics of psychotherapeutic discourse as a type of institutional discourse, as well as the nature of narrative interaction within such a framework. As such, we discuss the psychotherapeutic contract and the interactional roles defined by it, as well as the theoretical background of the psychoanalyst, and interpretation of local and distant textual contexts as important factors influencing therapeutic discourse. Finally, we briefly describe some aspects of the process of transformation of the narrative self in psychotherapy, which consider an important aspect of psychoanalytic discourse. More specifically, the chapter also describes the characteristics of narrative interaction within psychoanalytic psychotherapy, including the attention of the analyst to the analysand's narratives. Here we shall argue that the analysand's self-narratives are reconstructed in psychoanalytic discourse while they are co-narrating their stories with the psychoanalyst. Tracking important aspects of this co-narration—such as the shifting of narrative perspective by the speakers—allows for the understanding of the transformation process of narratives in psychoanalytic discourse.

Psychotherapeutic contract

Discourse—as defined in the broad sense—is language use in various contexts of human interaction (Schiffrin 1998). Based on this definition, psychotherapeutic discourse was considered a kind of institutional discourse due to its determination by the institutional frameworks of its practices (Labov & Fanshell 1977). More precisely, frameworks of such discourses control and regulate the possible interactions that may take place within them: the interactional roles of the participants, the specific goals of the given psychotherapeutic practice, and the way such therapeutic goals could be achieved by the interlocutors through linguistic and non-linguistic means. One important aspect of the controlling institutional framework of such discourses is the psychotherapeutic 'contract' between the interlocutors, which also defines and regulates the interlocutors' institutional roles, and their behaviour. The nature of narrative interaction, and the possible narratives themselves constructed and reconstructed in such a setting are determined, to a large degree, by the psychotherapeutic contract.

The psychotherapeutic contract is a written or oral agreement between client and therapist—and in the case of group psychotherapy also including other group members. The purpose of the psychotherapeutic contract is to clarify and agree upon the circumstances and the legal, financial and ethical rules that apply to the behaviour of both the client and the therapist during the time-period of treatment, also determining the frameworks of psychotherapeutic conversation that differ from that of everyday conversations (Thomä & Kächele 1985). The issues that are determined by the contract are varied; they usually include the timing of the occasions, and timeframes of sessions, the frequency of meeting, the venue of treatment (if the psychotherapy takes place in person or online), its financing (which may be covered by the client's health insurance, paid privately, or be free, or state-financed), the number of participants (in case of group therapy), as well as the goals of therapy. This latter may be self-development in general, supportive therapy, or problem-solving with a specific goal (i.e. working through problems related to divorce, grief, or school behaviour in case of children, etc.), or problems related to chronic conditions such as depression, schizophrenia, or personality disorder.

It is clarified in the contract that meetings between the client and the therapist occur only with the professional aim of practising psychotherapy, as opposed to including private meetings with the aim of friendship or other kind of (e.g. romantic or sexual) relations. Steps towards creating a non-professional relationship are forbidden for both parties during the time-period of treatment, and often even following it. The rule of confidentiality and the agreement of non-disclosure on the part of the therapist are important ethical conditions, which establish the client's trust in the therapeutic alliance.

In therapeutic discourse, client and therapist occupy differing, asymmetric roles (Scarvaglieri 2020)—also determined implicitly or even explicitly by the therapeutic contract. Psychotherapy itself is a helping intervention, in which the active, helping party is the therapist, and the client is the one who is seeking help and being helped by the intervention. The exact requirements of the therapist's and the client's roles differ according to the type of psychotherapy they participate in. In long-term psychoanalytic psychotherapy, the sessions include the analysand disclosing important information about themselves and the analyst mainly listening to the client's narratives, and contributing to those narratives, without sharing their own problems, and self-narratives with the client. So, the personality of the analyst in psychoanalytic psychotherapy remains obscure to a certain degree. This is in contrast to regular conversations between friends, where after a narrative of self-disclosure it is considered to be polite for the listener to disclose a similar narrative about themselves (Habermas 2018). In dynamic group therapy, however, other members of the group (i.e. other analysands) also have a say about the analysand's narratives or ongoing group interaction, and they may also disclose narratives with a similar theme. In this sense, analysands' roles in group psychotherapy are more symmetrical with each other, whereas the analyst's role is an asymmetrical one in group therapy as well.

The asymmetries and lack of balance and mutuality in the roles of client and therapist may lead to limitations regarding the emotional closeness of the participants. As we have mentioned earlier, the development of informal friendship is largely prohibited and considered unethical between client and therapist; however, a strong alliance based on partnership and cooperation between them is necessary in order for the psychotherapy to be effective (Eichenberg et al. 2022; Zilcha-Mano & Fisher 2022). In psychoanalysis the positive and negative affective regard of the analysand towards the analyst is termed transference

(Freud 1912), and it is 'reciprocated' by the analyst, in a positive or perhaps negative way in what is termed countertransference. The emotions of transference and countertransference are interpreted within the frameworks of psychoanalysis, with the above-mentioned limitations applying to them. According to the intersubjective approach, however, countertransference is considered an important tool for the analyst, and their subjectivity together with the subjectivity of the analysand creates an ongoing negotiation of the needs of two independent subjectivities (Safran & Muran 2001).

The explication of the goals of psychotherapy is also part of the psychotherapeutic contract, and determines, to a large extent, the course of the actual psychotherapy. In psychoanalytic discourse the major goal of psychotherapy is the restructuring of the analysand's self by resolving his/her unconscious conflicts (Leonardi et al. 2022; Sandler & Sandler 1984) in order to make possible a more adoptive life on the analysand's part, by becoming more efficient, and with reduced symptoms (Cogan 2007), and to help them to

> alleviate distress, find new or improved sources of satisfaction, and know and change themselves in ways that enhance inner contentment, deepen self-confidence, open paths to new experience, and allow for self-realization. In addition, a successful analysis will enhance a patient's capacity for self-reflection and tolerance of uncertainty. (Brand Bartlett 2002: 630)

In practice, however, these goals are defined in a way that is more comprehensible for the analysand. As we described above, the goals could include self-development (Brand Bartlett 2002), problem-solving with a specific goal, or problem-solving related to chronic conditions. The asymmetrical interactive roles of the analysand and analyst can also be detected in terms of their goals within psychoanalytic discourse. The analyst often consciously works towards the major goals of therapy—which in psychoanalysis may include concrete goals such as the discovery of unconscious motifs and conflicts, the revealing of traumas in the analysand's life (childhood or later), and the restructuring of the self. Whereas the analysand with more conscious or unconscious goals may be just more spontaneously revealing what is on their mind, what they consider the major concerns in their lives at the given moment (Berán et al. 2017).

Theories at the background of psychotherapeutic treatment

Any kind of psychotherapeutic treatment is based on underlying theories and psychotherapeutic techniques included in the practical arsenal of a given kind of psychotherapeutic modality (Thomä & Kächele 1985). The effectiveness of the application of a given technique in the case of a specific client also depends on factors other than adherence, such as therapeutic alliance, patient motivation, match between patient needs and psychotherapeutic techniques, non-specific factors, and so on (Roth & Fonagy 2006). However, the set of theoretical principles and treatment techniques following from theory inarguably plays a major role in the realization and actualization of treatment and, hence, its manifestations can be detected in psychotherapeutic discourse sometimes explicitly, but more often implicitly.

Theoretical assumptions and principles are not always detectible explicitly in all kinds of psychotherapeutic discourses. For instance, in cognitive behavioural therapy (CBT) these principles are quite explicitly explained to the client at the session, and explanation of underlying theoretical principles and techniques used in therapy are part of what is referred to as the 'psychoeducation' of the patient (e.g. Cash & Hrabosky 2003). In contrast, in psychoanalytic and dynamic psychotherapies psychoanalytic theories and techniques are typically not explained, and their communication to the analysand is not considered part of treatment. So, in the case of psychoanalytic discourse, psychoanalytic theory as a background of therapeutic interventions is harder to detect and describe. In the excerpts of psychotherapeutic discourse used as examples in this book from the Budapest Psychotherapy Database, psychotherapists use an amalgamate of various analytic theories and techniques, such as classical Freudian technique (as far as concerning the setting: the analysand laying on the couch, and meeting two to three times a week, as well as using free association), Kleinian theory as well as object relations theory, and an intersubjective approach in their treatments. Although they do not describe the application of these theories at their sessions, it often can be inferred from their interventions, questions, explanations, and interpretations. In our discussion of the excerpts from the Budapest Psychotherapy Database in later chapters, we assume that analysts intervene at the psychoanalytic sessions in order to accomplish treatment goals, and such interventions are based on the theoretical convictions of the given analyst. However, in our discussions of these excerpts we are not going to include much of the specifics of psychoanalytic theory and technique, because we will focus on processes of narrative interaction and their contribution to the psychotherapy process, and we will approach psychoanalytic discourse from the angle of describing the narrative construction taking place at the session; at the same time, we shall also discuss some aspects of inter-subjectivity theory as related to descriptions of the narrative construction taking place.

With that in mind, we will discuss two major aspects of psychoanalytic technique that have implications to narrative construction taking place at the sessions in general. These are, as described by Habermas (2018), the abstinence and neutrality of the analyst, and free association.

The abstinence and neutrality of the psychoanalyst implies that they refrain from unambiguous expression of their opinions, and evaluations of the analysand's statements, views, and behaviours, thus being non-judgmental of the analysand's expression of their selves. This may have an effect on therapeutic discourse by allowing the analysand a freedom of discovering their subjectivity, as well as the questioning of their way of thinking or acting, or even narrating these thoughts and acts. So, analysands 'take a critical stance towards their stories, questioning their stories and evaluations and searching for fuller, more consistent and more plausible stories' (Habermas 2018: 280). We must note here again, however, that abstinence and neutrality emphasized by the classic Freudian view are not part of the requirement of analyst's behaviour according to the inter-subjectivist view.

Drawing from the contemporary intersubjective and relational paradigms in psychoanalysis—particularly the contributions of the Boston Change Process Study Group (BCPSG 2010), Ed Tronick's mutual regulation model (2003), and the mentalization-based approach developed by Fonagy and colleagues (2002)—a more nuanced view emerges regarding the analytic stance of abstinence and neutrality. Rather than merely refraining from judgment or influence, the analyst's 'non-judgmental' position becomes a relational offer, a holding space that fosters epistemic trust. This trust is not a passive by-product, but an active process built through ostensive cues, affect attunement, and mutual regulation (Fonagy et al. 2015; Tronick 2003). It is within this trust-saturated intersubjective field that the analysand begins to mentalize their own experiences—questioning and reshaping self-narratives, as Habermas (2019) suggests. Abstinence, then, is reframed not as withholding, but as creating room for co-authored meaning-making.

Relational psychoanalysts (Aron 2003; Benjamin 2010) have long emphasized the analytic dyad as a site of mutual influence and recognition. BCPSG's microanalytic studies (2010) affirm that therapeutic change often arises through moments of 'now-ness' and dyadic repair. In this light, neutrality does not imply absence but presence—a 'poised responsiveness' that facilitates transformation. The analyst's stance, guided by mentalizing awareness, becomes a scaffold for the analysand's epistemic openness: the analyst is neither a blank screen nor a directive figure, but a trustworthy co-participant in the reorganization of subjective meaning (Fonagy 2015). Intersubjectivity, affect regulation, and mentalization are thus tightly interwoven, and therapeutic abstinence—rather than being an ascetic ideal—is reinterpreted as an ethically charged space that invites the analysand's voice to evolve in the presence of a responsive, attuned other, by recognizing the presence of the analytic third (Benjamin 2004; Bohleber et al. 2013).

Building on the relational framework articulated by Lewis Aron and Galit Atlas (2019), the concept of generative enactment offers a vital expansion of how we understand the analyst's role beyond neutrality and abstinence. In contrast to viewing enactments solely as resistances or impasses, generative enactments are understood as co-created moments that, while often emerging from unconscious dynamics within the analytic dyad, have the potential to catalyse transformation. These enactments—particularly when recognized and worked through within the therapeutic relationship—can offer emotionally charged, 'lived' experiences that reshape the analysand's internal world. Far from being errors or lapses in neutrality, they are moments in which the analyst's subjectivity is implicitly or explicitly involved, revealing unconscious relational patterns in action. When metabolized reflectively within the analytic dialogue, such moments create space for new meanings and new ways of being. This relational understanding aligns closely with mutual regulation frameworks: the analyst's willingness to acknowledge their role in the enactment fosters trust, while the dyadic repair that follows becomes a powerful mechanism for developmental change. So, generative enactments exemplify how therapeutic abstinence can be ethically flexible, relationally engaged, and deeply co-constructed. In our analyses of psychoanalytic dialogues, we point to the inevitable version of enactment, the chosen narrative perspective that influences the patient's attention, memory retrieval processes, and affective involvement.

Free association of the analysand at the psychoanalytic session implies that they must talk at the session without restrictions, and say out loud whatever comes to their mind, without adhering to requirements of everyday conversation, such as making 'sense', or being 'relevant' (Sperber & Wilson 1986). This kind of talk—according to psychoanalytic theory—allows the analysand to convey the contents of their mind more directly, and free associations provide a web of meaning surrounding an important idea that comes up at the session, related to narratives of everyday events, childhood events, dreams, or phantasies.

The requirements of free association may have a profound effect on the recollection of events in narrative form. Considering Ochs and Capp's (2001) criteria of interactively told narratives here, we find that:

1. narrative structure may be less linear, less determined by causality, and more open, digressive and fragmented;
2. narratives may be embedded in other discourse activities such as therapeutic interventions, and discussions of emotions or other relevant events in the here and now of the session;

3. narratives may contain events not easily verbalized, or events of low tellability, such as traumas, or not clearly remembered childhood events.

Regarding (1) non-linearity, the relation of one event to another regarding chronological order or causality in the analysand's narrative may be unclear. The analysand may give subsequent corrections and attempt subsequent explanations (Habermas 2018); however, in light of free association, this is not a responsibility of the analysand, which the psychoanalyst demands or expects. Regarding 2) embeddedness, embedded narratives may not have easily determined boundaries from surrounding discourse activities. This means that, instead of a distinct turn format, the psychoanalysts may be actively involved in telling them by asking questions, suggesting possible meanings, and their content may be related to the topic of discussion of surrounding discourse, as we mentioned above. Regarding 3) tellability, it is often the case that the analysand recounts narratives in the psychoanalytic setting that have low tellability, because they have never been told before, or their storylines are not resolved (e.g. dreams). At the same time, these narratives are very meaningful to the analysand. The analysand's goals with recounting such narratives may be to clarify their conclusions for themselves, to gain a deeper self-knowledge, or to regulate their emotional tension at the session. However, they may also recount narratives at the session with high tellability.

The characteristics of psychoanalytic discourse 1, 2, and 3 render it necessary to interpret and analyse psychoanalytic narratives in their discourse contexts, and to take those contexts into consideration when examining the content or the formal qualities of such narratives.

Interpretation of local and broader textual contexts in psychotherapeutic discourse

In the interpretation of psychotherapeutic discourse, it is important to note that in a given segment of discourse the analysand and the analyst express their shared past knowledge and shared experience, including their common interaction history and their assumptions about their relationship and its development. In their seminal work, Labov and Fanshell (1977) describe various layers of meaning in therapeutic interaction that they use when interpreting a given utterance. For example, the broadest context for meaning is the 'psychotherapeutic treatment'; within this, a further layer is the 'first interview with the client'. Within this context, there is the layer of 'narrative' that the client tells about her eating disorder, and the final context is that of family discourse, which the therapist uses to interpret the meaning of the client's statements more precisely.

So, while examining and interpreting self-narratives of the client in psychotherapeutic discourse, we must consider non-explicit meanings within the broader contexts of a series of psychotherapeutic sessions and the client's psychopathology, as well as local contexts of the given segment of the given session. For example, it could be informative what phase of psychotherapy we are dealing with: the beginning, the working through (which itself might be divided into several 'sub-phases') or the final, concluding phase. Especially in the working and concluding phases, we must consider the accumulated knowledge of the interlocutors about each other, and about their interaction history, and take this into account when interpreting a given segment of discourse.

In our analysis of narrative interaction in psychoanalytic discourse, we aim to examine the shifting of narrative perspective by the speakers, in order to trace transformation of the analysand's self-narratives during psychoanalysis. In certain cases, such analysed shifts in perspective may be preceded by other, previous shifts during the narrative construction process of a given narrative theme, which may last over sections of a session, over a whole session, or even over several sessions (Habermas 2018). So, local and broad textual contexts both play a role in interpreting a given shift in perspective.

In addition to the above described characteristics of psychotherapeutic and psychoanalytic discourse, we describe two aspects of such discourses, which may influence narrative construction taking place at the session, namely: the analyst's attention towards the analysand's narratives, and the transformation of the narrative self.

Attention in psychoanalytic discourse

The analysand's self-narratives constructed during the psychoanalytic session have great significance in their development through treatment (Schafer 1980, 1992; Spence 1982). The attention itself that the psychoanalyst as listener focuses on the analysand in the psychoanalytic setting is part of the process that advances the analysand's self-discovery, emotional development, and establishes and strengthens attachment, and alliance between the client and the therapist, and also helps to establish trust between the interlocutors (Abargil & Tishby 2024; Baker 2020; Flückiger & Grosse Holtforth 2008; Housby et al.; Williams 2008). The psychoanalyst's attention expands to narratives with low and high tellability, to the act of narration as well as to narrative content. As such, we may assume that the analyst's attention helps to achieve the goals of psychotherapy, and advances the therapeutic process in psychoanalytic discourse as well.

However, in our study of narrative construction the focusing of the speakers' attention is also important in other respects in psychoanalytic discourse. By shifting narrative perspective (NP)—which is defined as the narrator's point of view within the story—the analyst draws the analysand's attention to aspects of their narrative that has not yet been discovered by them before. The analyst may bring up new perspectives related to the narrative, may comment, or ask a question shedding light on new aspects of the narrated events or the characters of the story, thereby drawing the analysand's attention to new information and giving the narrative construction process a new direction. The analyst might also emphatically challenge the analysand and validate their experiences to create therapeutic depth and deepening of the alliance. It is important to note here that this function of directing the analysand's attention to new aspects of the narrative is fulfilled by the attention regulating role of NP.

Transformation of the narrative self in psychotherapy

The reconstruction of self-narratives at the psychoanalytic session was considered a reconstruction process of the narrative self by several theorists (Avdi 2008; Gergen 1999; Habermas & Kemper 2021; Schafer 1980, 1992; Spence 1982). The narrative self is defined as the totality of narratives about the self, shaped into a coherent whole as a result of constantly changing, adoptive meaning-making processes (Gallagher 2000; McAdams 1985). Such meaning-making processes also take place during the recollecting of personal memories, in other words during the reconstruction of narratives in a variety of settings, specifically at the psychotherapeutic session. During the reconstruction process, representations related to a given autobiographical memory are reorganized, reinterpreted, and reframed in order to create 'better' or more 'livable' narratives for the client (Schafer 1980, 1992). The therapist's interventions play a central role in this process. Lane and colleagues (2015) emphasize that elements of autobiographical memory are reactivated during recollection at the psychotherapy session and, while the client is emotionally engaged with such memories by discussing them with the therapist, they incorporate new elements (new emotions and information), and reconsolidate in a different, new form. Therapeutic change occurs as reconsolidated memories are reintegrated into the self-memory system, leading to new ways of behaving and experiencing. So, in this way transformation of autobiographic memories occurs at the session, and hence transformation of the narrative self also takes place.

The transformation process of self-narratives may also be referred to as narrativization (Miskovic 2007). This concept encompasses not merely the transformation of narratives by this process of reactivation and reconsolidation of autobiographical memories, but also the narrative expression of new or old experiences that are verbalized by the client for the first time at the psychotherapy session.

As we mentioned earlier, the analyst's role in psychoanalysis is to listen and react to the self-narratives described by the analysand, and help them to reconstruct their self-narratives, and narrate previously un-told, and un-verbalized experiences. We would like to emphasize that in verbally oriented psychotherapies, the psychotherapist takes an active role in the reconstruction of the client's self-narratives at the session. The various co-constructive moves of the therapist in psychoanalytic psychotherapy as described by Habermas (2018) include clarifying what the analysand has said; naming and reformulating emotions that the analysand went through at the time of narrated events, or is going through at the here and now of the psychoanalytic session; confronting the analysand with evidence that may contradict their statements, or emotions; and interpreting the analysand's emotions based on psychoanalytic theory.

Our studies of examining narrative co-construction processes included in this book are based on describing the shifting of perspective by the speakers. This process includes the regulation of attention as well as affect in psychoanalytic discourse, and is intertwined with memory processes, which we describe in detail in Chapter 5.

3 A discourse-based model of narrative perspective

This chapter introduces our discourse-based model of narrative perspective (NP), which we use for analysing in-session verbal interaction in the subsequent chapters of the book. First, we describe the theoretical background of our model, and define narrative perspective by drawing on studies from the field of narratology and psychology. In brief, the concept of narrative perspective is used to describe the narrator's point of view: their position with respect to the story plane, the time and place of its actions, actors and characters (Genette 1983), which we shall discuss in detail below. We also outline our model of NP, based on four aspects of perspective relevant to psychotherapeutic discourse: 1) physical aspect, 2) subjectivity aspect, 3) intentionality aspect, and 4) discourse-level aspect. Moreover, we explain how we operationalize our model of NP in order to analyse transcripts of psychotherapeutic discourse using nine variables: verb tense (Ikeo 2022), deixis (Duchan et al. 2012; Green 2022), subject number, subject person (Benveniste 1971; Palmer & Frank Robert 1981; Wiebe 2012), mode of focalization (Brooks & Warren 1959; Chen et al.; Genette 1983), agency (Bal & Lewin 1983; Bremond 1973; Deppermann 2020; Van Dijk 1975), patiency (Berán & Unoka 2016), diegesis (Bunia 2010; Pier 2014; Todorov 1981), and discourse level (Berán & Unoka 2016). We define these variables and illustrate their use in psychoanalytic discourse with examples of narrative interaction from the Budapest Psychotherapy Database. Finally, in this chapter we describe the regulative role of NP in narrative discourse based on two aspects of regulation of the speakers: self-regulation and interactive regulation or, in other words, a coordination of perspectives between speakers.

The concept of NP originates from narratological theorizing (Genette 1972, 1983; Uspenskiĭ 1973) about literary works, and it refers to the point of view of the narrator, through which events, actions, and actors or characters of the story are presented to the reader/listener. The narrator's point of view expresses his/her relationship to the story plane, and actions, actors, and characters in the text. NP can also be conceptualized as a continuously *moving camera* through which we can observe the story world and its events, actions, and characters and, hence, perspective is a continuously changing, structural characteristic of narrative discourse.

The concept of NP has also been studied in the field of cognition, in experiments examining the process of reading (Erickson & Kintsch 1995; Rapaport et al. 1989; Zubin & Hewitt 1995). According to these studies, the deictic centre window is a constantly shifted and updated model or representation of the deictic information of the text in the reader's mind. The deictic centre is the spatio-temporal centrum of objects and events of the narrative, where the seen (in the case of reading) or heard (in the case of listening) information is represented. According to Deictic Centre (DC) theory, readers adjust their origo or deictic centrum to the story world, so that they can interpret deictic expressions such as 'yesterday' as referring to the story world (Sanders & Krieken 2019) instead of referring to reality. In psychotherapeutic discourse, however, the story world refers to the narrator's 'real-world' experiences, thus the deictic centrum reflects the reality aspects of the narrator world, the way they see and experience it.

Both narrative (Genette 1983; Uspenskiĭ 1973) and cognitive studies of perspective taking (Rapaport et al. 1989; Sanders & Krieken 2019) claim that NP (or DC) is constantly shifted in the text, and hence constantly shifted in the reader's or listener's model or representation of the text/conversation. The changing or shifting of perspective is defined with regard to a unit of textual analysis. In our definition of NP we use *intonation unit* as a unit of analysis. This is a segment of natural language, present in all languages, a unit that forms rhythms of about one unit per second in natural language (Inbar et al. 2023), and is best suited to articulate therapeutic discourse (Chafe 1994). Another reason we transcribe and analyse psychoanalytic discourse in terms of intonation units is because this is a speech segment that the speakers' attention focuses on during communication at a given moment (Chafe 1988, 1994). The syntactic category closest to a full intonation unit is the clause within a sentence.

Intonation unit—a formally defined speech unit—has a well-defined and distinguishable border within the speech flow. The latter consists of a well-recognizable tune character, and a final intonation contour, which could be the lowering or raising of pitch, or holding it at the same level. At the end of the intonation unit, optionally there is a small pause of a few (about 5) milliseconds in Hungarian language (Németh 1996), and in other languages as well. The length of the pause also depends on the speed of the speech-flow. Intonation units could be full or fragmented (broken). They have been shown to evoke a neural response using EEG (Inbar et al. 2023). In our study of psychoanalytic discourse, we apply the concept of perspective onto intonation units; in other words, we analyse each intonation unit with a corresponding NP that characterizes the given unit (Chafe 1988).

So, we define the shifting of perspective in terms of changing one of the variables of NP from one intonation unit to the next. In describing our model of NP we will discuss and illustrate each variable with examples from the Budapest Psychotherapy Database, and also demonstrate how the shifting of perspective occurs with respect to a given variable.

Physical aspect of NP

The physical aspect of NP positions the narrator in a spatio-temporal matrix; more specifically, it places the actual (present) position of the narrator in relation to the spatio-temporal planes expressed in the narrative (Berán 2009). The physical aspect of NP provides information on the narrator's spatio-temporal relation to the narrated events, and its characters, which may be subjective, thus differing from the objective measures of these phenomena. For example, the sense of time elapsed in narrative might be shorter or longer, depending on the way the narrator experiences it in the story. In everyday communicative discourse, there are several tools' speakers use to express physical aspects of perspective, for example verb tense—which in Hungarian is expressed in the verb suffix—deictic expressions used for place and time, verbs expressing movement and direction of movement. In our studies of narrative construction in the Budapest Psychotherapy Database included in this volume, we used two variables to study the physical aspect of NP: verb tense and deixis.

Verb tense. Since our data in the Budapest Psychotherapy Database consist of psychotherapies where both participants (analysands and analysts) speak in Hungarian as their native language, we can say that our original text (data) is in Hungarian. However, in the following chapters, whenever we analyse excerpts from the database, we will supply the English translation also. So, in our descriptions of the data and our analyses of NP use by the speakers, we will refer to the Hungarian characteristics of the text.

Regarding verb tense, in the Hungarian language there are three grammatical verb tenses: 1) past, 2) present, and 3) future (Rounds 2009). Tense information is provided by the suffix of verbs in Hungarian. In contrast, English marks tense with verb endings and auxiliary verbs across its twelve tenses (Michaelis 2020). Nevertheless, English verb tenses can also be categorized as expressing past, present, or future tenses, thus they can be mapped unto the Hungarian verb-tense categories. For this reason, we use the original Hungarian version of the text to determine verb tense for the verb-tense variable during our analysis of excerpts from psychotherapeutic discourse.

Moreover, subjective sense of time, or dramatized performance may be expressed in alteration of verb tenses (Pólya 2005; Schiffrin 1981; Tannen 2007; Wolfson 1979), which could be studied by taking into consideration longer sequences of text (i.e. by coding several consecutive intonation units).

In Excerpt 3.1 we show an example of the shifting of verb tense in the analysand's talk, from the psychotherapy of the male analysand–male analyst dyad from the Budapest Psychotherapy Database. It is from the third part of the observation period, in the working phase of therapy, when the analysand describes his visit to his mother's home, from where he just has recently moved out.

Excerpt 3.1 (F32)

1145PAT:	a múltkor is csak felugrottam egy szatyromér,	last time I have just dropped in for my bag,
1146PAT:	hogy elvigyem azt a szatyrot,	to get that bag,
1147PAT:	amiben a fürdőszoba kellékeim vannak,	in which I have my bathroom-supplies,
1148PAT:	amit még előtte vettem meg,	which I had bought earlier,
1149PAT:	tudja hogy a rudam most már van,	you know that I have already the rod now,
1150PAT:	és hogy akkor fel tudjam ott tenni,	and so that I could put it up there,
1151PAT:	meg a kis polc is abba volt,	and the little shelf was in it too,
1152PAT:	szal meg ilyenek.	so, things like that.
1153PAT:	na mindegy.	it doesn't matter.
1154PAT:	és akkor,	and then,
1155PAT:	hogy ja de hogy ő nem tud levelezni,	that oh that she cannot handle the mails,
1156PAT:	jó,	alright,
1157PAT:	megnézem neked,	I take a look at it for you,
1158PAT:	és akkor ott nekiálltam,	and then there I have started
1159PAT:	és akkor ott+...	and then I there+...
1160PAT:	+, egy órán keresztül pötyögtem be neki+...	+, for an hour, I was typing them in for her+...
1161PAT:	érti?	do you know?
1162PAT:	+, az egyre újabb címeket.	+, the ever newer addresses.

In lines 1145–48 the analysand uses past tense in the Hungarian version, which is translated as past perfect in the English version. In 1149–50 the analysand shifts into present tense, translated into simple present in English. Then in 1151–52 he shifts into past tense again, and in lines 1153–57 back to present tense, translated as simple past and simple present in English. In 1158–62 he shifts into past tense again in the Hungarian version, translated into present perfect and past continuous in English, which sequence is interrupted in 1161, when he asks the therapist if he understands what is being said in using present tense both in Hungarian, and in English.

From this sequence of shifts we can observe that tense shifts are very frequent phenomena in the above excerpts of psychoanalytic discourse (and in other types of discourses as well). As we have mentioned, verb tense in English can be mapped onto the three categories in Hungarian; however, there is one verb tense, present perfect, which may translate as present or past in Hungarian, depending on the context. So, in the case of the present perfect the category mapping is not as obvious as in the case of the other tenses.

Deixis. Deiknyani means 'to show' in Greek, referring to verbal pointing. In the use of deictic markers, or deixis, perspectival information relates to the object, person, place, and time being referred to, and deixis relates the word or phrase to the utterance context—i.e. to the speaker, addressee, time, and place of speaking (Dylgjeri & Kazazi 2013). Regarding word-class, deictic markers belong to the class of adverbs and pronouns. For example, deixis referring to place are *here* and *there*, and deixis referring to the direction of movement are *from here*, *from there*, or *to here*, *to there*. Referring to time are *at this time* or *at that time* or *then*. Deixis referring to objects are *this* or *that*, *these* or *those*. In our category system analysing perspectives of psychotherapeutic discourse, we did not differentiate deictic markers based on the above categories (i.e. referring to time, place, object, etc.) but rather, we differentiated them based on the distance of the place pointed at from the narrator's current position. Thus we differentiated 1) proximal (such as *this*, *here*, *at this time*) from 2) distal (*that*, *there*, *then*, *that time*) deictic markers, and we also used the category of 3) mixed deixis, where both proximal and distal deixes appeared in one unit of analysis, namely in one intonation unit. This differentiation of deictic markers is useful in the description of psychotherapeutic discourse. Proximal deixis describes the events and characters of the narrative as being closer to the narrator in time and place, whereas distal deixis describes events and characters of the narrative as being more distant in time and place from the narrator. Mixed deixis represents an ambivalent relationship of the narrator to the actors and events of the narrative in terms of time/space. In Excerpt 3.2 we show some examples of the use of deictic markers. This excerpt is from the beginning phase of psychotherapy, from the first part of the observation period of the male analysand–male analyst dyad. The analysand here tries to describe his complex relationship to children, which came up as a topic at the previous session. At the beginning of this session, the analysand is referring back to his thoughts about this problem following the previous session.

Excerpt 3.2 (F4)

20PAT:	meg+/	and+/
21PAT:	+, meg **amit**+/	+, and **that**+/
22PAT:	ugye **itt** szóba került ha **ez, ezek** +/	well it came up **here** if **this, these** +/
23%com:	pause 3s	
24PAT:	mér is volt-	why it has been-
25PAT:	+, **ez** mindig olyan vonzó a számomra	+, **this** has always been so
	ha gyerekekkel ugye,	attractive for me, if with the children, hasn't it
26PAT:	de csak **erre#** jutottam,	but I came to **this#** only,
27PAT:	tehát mondom **ez** hogy-	as I have been saying, **this** that-
28PAT:	+, hogy egyszerűen **az a**+..	+, that it is simply that the+…
29PAT:	+, **az a** szeretet meg a ragaszkodás	+, **that** love and attachment
	ami viszonzás képen jött,	that came in return,
30PAT:	hogy **az**+/	that **that**+/
31PAT:	+, **az** nagyon pozitívan tudott hatni rám.	+, that could affect me very positively.
32%com	pause	
33PAT:	meg **ez** a kettősség hogy+/	and **this** duality that+/
34PAT:	ami mindig is jellemzett ö,	that has always been my characteristic er,
35PAT:	hogy **ez** a-	that **this** the-
36PAT:	nagyon szeretem a gyerekeket, és, és, és, és+..	I like children very much, and, and, and, and+…
37PAT:	+, és iszonyúan taszít még	+, and I am horribly repulsed even
	a gondolata is hogy nekem+…	at the thought of me+…
38PAT:	legyen+/	having one+/

In lines 20–22 the analysand uses deictic markers: *that, this, and these* to refer to the topics that came up at the previous session. He uses both distal and proximal pronouns, in intonation units following one another. He also uses 'here' spatial deictic marker to refer to the analytic situation, or in other words to the session. In line 25 he uses 'this' proximal deictic marker to refer to his relationship with children. In lines 27–31 he describes his relationship with children and why this relationship was so attractive to him, using first proximal 'this', and then distal 'that' pronouns. In line 33 he shifts back to proximal deixis to refer to the duality that characterizes his relationship with children.

From the use of distal and proximal deictic markers in Excerpt 3.2 we can draw an inference about the narrator's ambivalent relationship with children at the time of the session. At times, he talks about this relationship, and about children as being within the same space as he is, using proximal markers, whereas at other times he differentiates himself from the children, being in a separate conceptual space than they are. Moreover, we may complete this picture by looking at the use of verb tense in the excerpt. We find that most frequently the speaker uses the past tense (in lines 20–35). The final conclusion, however, regarding his feelings of ambivalence towards children is in the present tense (lines 36–38). This makes sense, since this latter conclusion is a statement about the nature of the analysand's relationship with children that applies and holds true in general.

In summary, we can say that the physical aspect of NP was operationalized by using two variables in the analysis of therapeutic discourse: verb tense and deixis. In verb tense, we separated three dimensions of time: past, present, and future. In deictic markers we distinguished proximal, distal and mixed deixis used within one intonation unit. When coding verb tense and deictic markers in texts, however, it often occurs that there is no verb or deictic marker in a given unit of analysis. In such cases, we use the option: 'none applicable'.

Subjectivity aspect of NP

The subjectivity aspect of NP expresses the actor of the story, the subject, to whom events described in the narrative happen. In this aspect of NP, we find information on the person of the narrator and other characters as subjects of the story. In addition, the subjectivity aspect also provides information on the narrator's and other characters' relationship to the story world (i.e. diegesis) (Genette 1983; Pier 2009; Todorov 1981). So, in discussing the Subjectivity aspect of NP we distinguish three variables: 1) subject person, 2) subject number, and 3) diegesis. The former two variables involve linguistic characteristics that are, again, differently expressed in English and in Hungarian.

Grammatical subject person. The information referring to the person of the narrator or other characters of the story is included in the verb suffix in Hungarian language. For example, we can see that in the verb jön (come) we can provide a suffix *–nek* to get third-person plural:

jön → jön**nek** (they come)

In contrast, in English the person of the actor is expressed as the grammatical subject of the sentence, usually by using pronouns or other nouns. An exception from this is the third-person singular, present tense, in which case it is expressed in the verb suffix (e.g. comes).

The grammatical person of the subject, however, has the same categories in English, as well as in Hungarian: 1) first person, 2) second person, 3) third person. These perspectives are related to the narrator's position: in the case of first person, the perspective is identical with that of the narrator. In the case of the second person, the perspective is present in one conceptual space with that of the narrator's, but it is different from it. In the case of the third person, the actor or his/her perspective is not present in the same conceptual space with the narrator, representing a perspective that is different from that of the narrator's. In addition to the three perspectives mentioned, in our analysis of psychotherapeutic discourse we also distinguished 4) general subject, in cases where the subject of events were not persons or identifiable objects, but rather a subject not identified or specified by the narrator. Perspectives of subject person (referring to agents in the narrative) involve distinctive cognitive, emotional, and neurological characteristics (Brunyé et al. 2009; Brunyé et al. 2011; Ditman et al. 2010).

Grammatical subject number. Subject number refers to the plurality or singularity of narrator(s), or character(s). Taken together with the variable grammatical subject person, we arrive at six grammatical combinations: first-person singular ('I'), second-person singular ('you'), third-person singular ('he/she'), first-person plural ('we'), second-person plural ('you'), and third-person plural ('they').

The excerpt below is from the psychotherapy of the male analysand–male analyst dyad, from the second phase of the observation period. The analysand is in a bad mood, and did not enjoy coming to therapy that day. He is discussing his taking anti-depressant medication with his analyst. We can observe the speakers shifting between positions of grammatical subject person and number.

Excerpt 3.3 (F22)

32TER:	s milyen gondolatok merülnek fel ezzel kapcsolatba?	and what kind of thoughts did come up in connection with this?

33PAT:	//semmi.	//nothing.
34PAT:	hát az amit már elmondtam,	well, I have told you already,
35PAT:	hogy /persze,	that/ off course,
36PAT:	minek ennyi gyógyszert szedni,	why should one take so much medication,
37PAT:	lehet hogy nem is az segít,	it's possible that it does not even help,
38PAT:	meg mit tudom én mi,	and I do not know what,
39PAT:	és akkor úgy+...	and then like+...
40PAT:	egyszer ezt gondolom, meg máskor+/	once I think this, and at other times+/
41PAT:	és tényleg meg kell próbálni ezt úgy,	and really this must be tried,
42PAT:	ahogy a doktornő mondta,	as the doctor suggested,
43PAT:	olyan fokozatosan,	like gradually,
44PAT:	bár ő nem javasolta hogy hagyjam abba,	although she did not suggest that I should stop it,
45PAT	sőt ő nagyon kampányolt amellett hogy ezt nem szabad abbahagyni.	in fact she was very much campaigning that this should not be stopped.
46PAT:	tehát ezt én feszegettem,	so I was the one raising the issue,
47PAT:	hogy ezt kell-e,	that is this necessary,
48PAT:	ennyi kell-e,	how much is necessary,
49PAT:	így érti,	like, you know,
50PAT:	[szal ez+...]	[like this+...]
51TER:	[igen.]	[yes.]
52PAT:	tehát ne nehogy félreértés essék,	well it should not be a misunderstanding,
53PAT:	tehát nem az van, hogy a doktornő azt mondta hogy ezt ne+...	well it's not like the doctor has said that I should not do it+...

In Excerpt 3.3, we can observe a continuous shifting of subject person and number. In line 32 the analyst uses the third-person plural to refer to the analysand's thoughts. In line 33 the analysand replies in the third-person singular. then, in line 34 he shifts into the first-person singular, and in line 36 he shifts into the general subject, which he uses in relation to taking medicine. In line 37 the analysand shifts into the third-person singular to refer to medication, and in lines 38–40 to the first-person singular referring to himself (i.e. the narrator).

In lines 41 and 43 he shifts into the general subject referring to trying to take the medicine as the doctor suggested. In line 42 he shifts into the third-person singular referring to the doctor. In lines 44–45, again the analysand shifts back to the third-person singular referring to the doctor. In line 46, he shifts back to the first-person singular, referring to himself as the one raising the issue of quitting medication. In line 47 he shifts into the general subject, while recounting the necessity of taking medication, and in line 48 to the third-person singular. In line 49 he turns to the analyst in the second-person singular. In line 51 the analyst says 'Yes', answering to the analysand. In line 52 the analysand continues in the third-person singular, referring to a misunderstanding, and then in line 53 back to the third and first-person singular.

So, the above detailed analysis of Excerpt 3.3 shows that the shifting of grammatical subject person and number is frequent within the examined discourse.

Diegesis. Another variable, which captures information on the subjectivity aspect of perspective, is diegesis. This expression refers to the narrated world, or story world (Genette 1983; Pier 2009; Todorov 1981). The narrator may talk about a story world of which he is a part, for instance when the analysand talks about events that happened to him last week. Genette termed this homo-diegetic narration. In contrast, when the narrator themself is not part of the story world, we are discussing hetero-diegetic narration. This occurs, for instance, when the analysand is recounting his parent's childhood events that he has heard from his grandmother. Finally, an interesting constellation of diegesis is when several story worlds are embedded in one another, and narrators of these story worlds alternate with each other. For example, in *One Thousand and One Nights*, there are several different narrators we may encounter. The primary, or original, narrator is Scheherazade, who is telling the stories to the king, in order to entertain him and, so, save her own life. Within the primary narrative, however, there are several embedded, secondary narratives, told by various characters of the primary narrative as secondary narrators. One such a secondary narrator is the fisherman, introduced by Scheherazade in her story of *The Fisherman's Story with the Dzsin,* telling the story of King Junan and his vizir. He is introduced by Scheherazade the following way: 'The Fisherman talked like this' (Berán & Unoka 2005; Prince 2003).

The stories represented by secondary narratives—also termed pseudo-narratives—cannot be mapped onto the story world of the primary narrative. So, characters of *The Fisherman's Story* cannot be found in the story world of Scheherazade and the king. When the secondary narrative world (i.e. pseudo-diegesis) takes the place of the primary one, it replaces it, and we, as readers or listeners, lose sight of the world of the primary narrative, including the primary narrator (i.e. Scheherazade), with a new, secondary (pseudo-) narrator taking her place. So, this kind of diegesis—and the third level of the diegesis variable—is termed pseudo-diegesis.

Hence, in our diegesis variable we distinguished three levels: 1) homo-diegesis, 2) hetero-diegesis, and 3) pseudo-diegesis. In the excerpt below, we show examples of homo- and hetero-diegesis, and in Chapter 6 we give a great number of examples of the use of pseudo-diegesis in psychoanalytic discourse. Excerpt 3.4 is from a session of the male analysand–male analyst dyad, from the second phase of the observation period, during the working phase of the treatment.

Excerpt 3.4 (F22)

74PAT:	ezek itt kavarognak bennem állandóan.	these things are churning inside me constantly.
75PAT:	szóval az úgy sokat jár rajta mostanában az agyam.	to say, my brain keeps thinking about it nowadays.
76PAT:	hogy, khm hm.	that khm, khm.
77PAT:	szal ez a, ez a két dolog itt+//	to say, these these two things here+//
78TER:	és hogyha+//	and if +//
79PAT:	/kűzd bennem egymással szemben.	/they fight against each other inside me.
80TER:	abba gondolkodik hogy hogy vajon mi okozhatta ezt a betegséget,	if you think about that that what might have caused this illness,
81TER:	ezt a komoly összeomlást,	this serious breakdown,
82TER:	akkor mik jutnak eszébe?	then what comes to your mind?
83%com:	pause 2 s	
84TER:	tudom hogy ezek is +...	I know that these +...
85TER:	szóba kerültek már úgy+...	have been mentioned alreadylike+...
86TER:	többször, több alkalommal,	several times, at various occasions,
87TER:	de esetleg ha megpróbálja ezt úgy összegezni,	but perhaps if you try to like summarize it,
88TER:	akkor mik jutnak eszébe?	what comes to your mind?
89PAT:	ezt most pontosítná,	would you clarify this,
90PAT:	hogy most mire+/	that what do you+/
91PAT:	mire gondol?	what do you have in mind now?

In Excerpt 3.4, we can observe the shifting of perspective concerning diegetic shifts. In lines 74–77 the analysand narrates his own story, using a homo-diegetic perspective. This means that he narrates from inside the story world, of which he is a part of. In line 78 the analyst starts talking. He is recounting the analysand's story from an outsider position; in other words, he is not part of the analysand's story world, but rather takes a hetero-diegetic position with respect to it. He keeps this position until line 88. In lines 89–91 the analysand asks a question from the analyst, referring to his intentions, towards which he assumes an outsider position. He shifts his perspective to a hetero-diegetic position.

So, in summary, we can say that the subjectivity aspect of NP comprises three variables in our model: grammatical subject person and number, and diegesis. Grammatical subject person can be 1) first, 2) second, and 3) third person, and 4) general subject. Grammatical subject number can be 1) singular or 2) plural. In diegesis, we distinguished three levels of the variable: 1) homo-diegesis, 2) hetero-diegesis, and 3) pseudo-diegesis. The subjectivity aspect of NP shifts frequently in psychoanalytic discourse; more specifically, a given diegesis applies through several intonation units (thus shifting less frequently), whereas grammatical subject person and number shifts more frequently.

Intentionality aspect of NP

The narrator's intentions, desires, goals, will, thoughts and emotions—or, in other words, their propositional attitudes—is captured by the intentionality aspect of NP. Intentionality information in the text answers two types of questions:

1. what does the text say about the propositional attitudes of the narrator/characters?
2. to what extent does the narrator consider an event the result of intentional actions of the characters rather than chance?

Mode of focalization. To answer the first question, we use information on focalization (Bal 2004; Genette 1983). This concept refers to what the narrator/character sees and knows, and how this is displayed in the text. One possibility is that only behavioural information is seen and known by the narrator: they can only observe others from the outside, there is no information on attitudes, thoughts, and emotions. Such narration is termed the external mode of focalization (Genette 1983), or behaviourist focalization. In contrast, the narrator may know about the desires, thoughts, goals, ideas, emotions of other characters or of their own, and may display this information in the text. This is termed the internal mode of focalization (Genette 1983).

In Excerpt 3.5 we can see examples of the use of internal and external mode of focalization. The excerpt is from the female analysand–female analyst dyad, from the Budapest Psychotherapy Database, from the second part of the observation period, the working phase of therapy. The interlocutors discuss the client's problem of meeting new people—especially members of the opposite sex, and finding a good topic of conversation, such as music.

Excerpt 3.5 (L23)

846PAT:	ezért, hogy ha+..	therefore, if+...
847PAT:	ö valakivel a zenéről kezdek el beszélni,	I start talking to someone about music,
848PAT:	akkor +..	then+...
849PAT:	akkor az előbb utóbb általában előjön.	then sooner or later this usually comes up.
850PAT:	ez több emberrel is beszélgettem már erről.	this I have spoken to many people about this.
851PAT:	igen.	yes.
852TER:	és nem értik,	and they don't understand it,
853TER:	vagy unják?	or are they bored?
854TER:	vagy nem reagálnak?	or they do not react?
855TER:	mi történik?	what happens?
856PAT:	az a baj, hogy nem tudom,	the problem is that I do not know,
857PAT:	mert én annyira belebonyolódok abba amit mondok,	because I run afoul of what I am about to say,
858PAT:	hogy nem veszem észre, hogy most+/	that I don't notice, that right now+/
859PAT:	hogy a+..	that the+...
860PAT:	hogy a másik+/	that the other+/
861PAT:	tehát azt hallom,	so I hear that
862PAT:	hogy hogy reagál,	that how he reacts,
863PAT:	meg nyilván beszélgetünk.	and obviously we are talking.

In lines 846–51 the analysand is recounting her encounters with other young people at the Budapest night scene. She describes these encounters in terms of behaviour, focusing on talking, and topics of conversation, thus using the external focalizing mode. In lines 852–54 the analyst takes the floor, and shifts perspective, focusing on the mental aspects of others' reactions to the analysand; in other words, she shifts into the internal focalizing mode. In line 855 the analyst shifts back again to the behavioural aspects of others' reactions, asking 'what happens', thus using the external focalizing mode. The analysand in lines 856–60 answers the analyst's questions, by focusing on her mental state: 'I don't know because I run afoul of what I am about to say', thus using the internal focalization mode. In lines 861–63 she shifts back again to a behavioural description of the encounter with others, thus using the external focalizing mode.

This example shows that relatively frequent perspective shifts occur in mode of focalization; however, in theory, it is possible that the speaker stays in the same perspective for a longer stretch of speech. So, we can conclude that in answering the question about the narrator's and characters' propositional attitudes expressed in the text, we can use the mode of focalization variable, with two levels: 1) the internal mode of focalization, and 2) the external mode of focalization to capture this aspect of NP.

Agency and patiency. Looking at the second question, that is to what extent does the narrator consider an event a result of the intentional actions of the characters rather than chance, or a process, we can use two variables to capture this information: 1) agency and 2) patiency.

We define agency and patiency based on grammatical categories: we can consider agent any living entity or non-living object, natural, or social process, which may be taken as argument in the CAUSE function (Jackendoff 1992). An agent is the active shaper of events in the narrative, who has an effect on outcomes and results, taking responsibility for them (Habermas 2006). In contrast, a patient is the passive sufferer of events and outcomes of the narrative, being affected by the actions of agents in the story. In our analysis of agency and patiency we categorized various types of agents and patients, which proved to be relevant in psychotherapeutic discourse. Agency and patiency are independently coded from one another, applied to a given intonation unit. The types of agency and patiency we have distinguished are the following:

1. Self-agency
   - The cause of narrated events/processes/change of state is the self. In the case of self-agency the actor is identical to the narrator/character of the story.
   - Self-patiency
   - The passive sufferer of narrated events/processes/change of state is the self. In the case of self-patiency, the entity affected by narrated events is the self, who is the narrator/character of the story.

2. Self-part-agency
    - The executer of actions, the argument of the CAUSE function is an object that belongs to the narrator's physical body or psychological self—but not in its entirety; rather, it is only a part of it. For example, it could be a body part, or an emotion.
    - Self-part-patiency
    - The sufferer of an action, outcome or event of the narrative is an object, which is part the narrator/character's physical body, or psychological self—but not in its entirety; rather, it is only a part of it. For example, it could be a body part, or an emotion.
3. Other-person agency
    - The actor, initiator of narrative events, outcomes or processes is a person, who is not identical to the narrator.
    - Other-person patiency
    - The sufferer of an action, outcome or event of the narrative is a person, who is not identical to the narrator.
4. Object-agency
    - The initiator of outcomes or processes of the narrative, or the argument of the CAUSE function is a non-living object, or a natural process.
    - Object-patiency
    - The sufferer of actions, events and processes of the narrative is a non-living object, or a natural process.
5. No-agent
    - There is no agent in a given unit of analysis.
    - No-patient
    - There is no patient in a given unit of analysis.

In Excerpt 3.6 we can observe shifts among various levels of agency and patiency. The excerpt is from the psychotherapy of the female analysand–female analyst dyad from the Budapest Psychotherapy Database, from the second part of the observation period in the working phase of therapy. The analysand discusses the same problem as before: social relationships, and encountering potential love interests in Budapest night-life.

Excerpt 3.6 (L23)

688PAT:	tehát akkor meg így iszonyúan elkezdek szorongani.	so then I begin to feel terribly anxious,
689PAT:	tehát ez történik,	so this is what happens,

690PAT:	hogy olyankor nagyon-nagyon így elkezdek szorongani,	that then I start being like very-very anxious,
691PAT:	és igaziból így mm+..	and really like mm+...
692PAT:	nem nagyon tudok mit mondani.	cannot really say anything.
693PAT:	mert hogy így elkezdek szorongani,	because I begin to feel like anxious,
694PAT:	és így csak az jár a fejemben,	and the only thing I think about,
695PAT:	hogy így+/	that like+/
696PAT:	így jaj+..	like oh+...
697PAT:	így+/	like+/
698PAT:	biztos így+..	probably like+...
699PAT:	baromira unalmas ember vagyok,	I am a really boring person,
700PAT:	meg így, igaziból az is vagyok.	and like, I really am boring.
701TER:	milyen?	what are you like?
702TER:	unalmas?	boring?
703PAT:	aha.	yeah.
704PAT:	meg így nem is akar így+..	and like he does not want like+...
705PAT:	időt tölteni velem.	to spend time with me.
706PAT:	szóval+..	so+...
707PAT:	tehát akkor a végletekig tudom ezt a dolgot fokozni tényleg.	well then I can increase this thing endlessly really.

In line 688 the analysand does not mention any agents, but puts herself in the position of the patient. In line 689 she shifts these in the opposite direction: she mentions a non-living object as agent (the process of what happens), and does not mention any patients. In line 690–93 she puts herself again in the position of the patient, and mentions no agents. In line 694 she puts a non-living object as agent, and part-of the self (her head) as a patient. In lines 695–97 she does not use any patient or agent. In lines 698–700 she uses self-agency, with no patient. In lines 701–02 the analyst enters the floor, she uses other-person agency, putting the analysand in the position of the agent, and using no patient. In line 703 the analysand uses self-agency, and in lines 704–05 she shifts into other-person agency with no patient mentioned. In lines 706–07 she uses self-agency, and an in-animate object as patient.

In this analysis, we could observe how agency and patiency can be frequently shifted independent of each other in psychoanalytic discourse.

In conclusion, we can say that the intentionality aspect of NP can be expressed by three variables: mode of focalization, agency, and patiency. These three variables serve as good and sufficient indicators to study intentionality in psychotherapeutic narratives.

Discourse-level aspect of NP

The discourse-level aspect of NP—also close to what is referred to as speaker roles (Koven 2012)—focuses on the identifications enacted in narrative discourse, and its associations with different modes of remembering. This aspect of NP is operationalized by only one variable, discourse level. Discourse level comprises of three levels that the narrator can identify with, or occupy in the speech event (Hymes 1992; Wolfson 1976) of narration: 1) the here and now of the session, 2) the narrator level, 3) the character level.

Level 1), the here and now of the analytic session, is defined as interchanges between the analysand and analyst that are focusing on events, emotions, affective states, reflections etc. that occur in the actual reality and real time of the therapeutic session. Level 2), the narrator level, means that the narrator, while engaging in the speech event of narration, also manages the process of memory recall, and their own participation of the narrated events (Koven 2012) with knowledge and memories characteristic of a broader, more general 'big picture' kind of understanding and insight (Phelan 2001). The type of memory recollection associated with the narrator level is characterized by general autobiographical memories, which—in contrast to the character level—are not one time-specific events, with great sensory details; rather, they are extended lifetime periods, and repetitive events characterizing them (Conway 1992). For example, the statement 'during my high-school years I befriended Catherine' refers to an extended lifetime period, which is characterized by being friends with Catherine.

In contrast to the narrator level, 3) the character-level refers to the knowledge and episodic memories characteristic of a specific actor at a specific point in time in the narrative. The narrator during the speech event of narrative identifies with one concrete character of the narrative (which could be the former self of the narrator), recalling a one-time specific event that happened to them. Such episodic memories are rich in sensory detail, and are characterized by intense emotional reliving while being reconstructed (Conway 2001).

Excerpt 3.7 is from the female analysand–female analyst dyad, from the Budapest Psychotherapy Database, from the second part of the observation period, the working phase of psychoanalysis. The analysand discusses relationship difficulties with the analyst. She is corresponding with a young man, who seems to be interested in her. She experiences anxiety in connection to this relationship.

Excerpt 3.7 (L23)

514PAT:	egyébként ami még érdekes,	anyhow, what else is of interest,
515PAT:	hogy azóta váltottunk néhány emailt,	that since then we've exchanged a few emails,
516PAT:	de most megint nem válaszolok neki két napja.	but I have not been answering him for two days now.
517TER:	ühüm.	uhum.
518%com:	pat	laughs
519TER:	és miért?	and why?
520PAT:	mert nem+..	just because+...
521PAT:	nincs kedvem leülni neki megírni a levelet.	I don't feel like sitting down and writing to him the letter.
522PAT:	nem tudom.	I do not know.
523PAT:	azt írta, hogy ha+/	he said that if+/
524PAT:	hogy ő most mennyivel rosszul érzi magát,	that how bad he feels now,
525PAT:	meg minden,	and all,
526PAT:	ezt így részletezte,	he elaborated on this,
527PAT:	és hogy+..	and that+...
528PAT:	hát így+..	like this+...
529PAT:	hogy átértékelte az életét,	he reevaluated his life,
530PAT:	és hogy+..	and that+...
531PAT:	hogy még ezen gondolkodnia kell,	that he needs to think about this,
532PAT:	de szeretné, hogyha én segítenék neki ez ö ebben,	but he would like if I helped him er in this,
533PAT:	és hogy+..	and that+...
534PAT:	üljek le vele beszélgetni.	I should sit down to talk to him.

In Excerpt 3.7 in line 514 the analysand starts out at narrator level: she approaches her story with the young man from a general point of view, and then, in lines 515–16 she narrows it down to the one-time specific event (i.e. her not answering his emails), shifting into character level. In lines 517–19 the analyst takes the floor and asks the analysand her reasons for her behaviour ('why') shifting into narrator level again. In lines 520–35 the analysand answers, bringing up specific reasons (i.e. does not feel like writing), thus shifting into character level again, and then explaining the specifics of the young men's situation while staying at character level. In line 522 she interrupts this line of thought, by shifting into the here and now of the session, referring to her current thoughts and understanding: 'I don't know.'

So, from this analysis we can conclude that interlocutors might stay in the same perspective regarding discourse level for an extended time-period—such as it is the case here, with the analysand staying at character level for a while.

Table 3.1 summarizes the four aspects of NP.

The regulative role of shifting perspective in psychoanalytic discourse

In psychoanalytic interaction the regulative function of shifting perspective is a process with two components: 1) self-regulation, and 2) interactive regulation or coordination of perspectives (Berán & Unoka 2016). The process of self-regulation on the part of the client or therapist is the process when the speaker in their continuous speech shifts perspectives from one intonation unit to the next. Such shifts may occur in the case of any of the variables contained in our NP model; for instance, it could be a shift from the external to the internal mode of focalization, from the subject number plural to singular, and so on. In the case of interactive regulation the speakers influence each other's perspective shifts. For example, the analysand, after listening to the analyst's talk, shifts into the same perspective as the analyst used in her previous intonation unit. In other words, the analysand performs a shift of perspective in their own speech, by shifting into the same perspective the analyst used previously and vice versa in the case of the analyst.

Mutual, interactive, or coordinated regulation of NP shifting behaviour is based on the joint attentional situation of the speakers, which makes it possible to carry out joint action during the interaction (Clark 1996). Previous studies have shown that the general goal of conversational interaction is that the communicating parties should create similar mental representations (Fusaroli & Tylén 2012; Fusaroli et al. 2014a; Fusaroli et al. 2014b; Garrod & Pickering 2004; Pickering & Garrod 2006). The success of communication depends on the matching of the mental representations of the communicating parties. This higher-order goal is based on lower-level coordination, during which coordination can be achieved in various discourse activities: bodily alignment of the

Table 3.1 The discourse-based model of NP

NP components	Definition	Categories/levels
1. Verb tense / physical aspect	Grammatical verb tense of the verb included in the intonation unit.	1) Past, 2) Present, 3) Future
2. Deixis / physical aspect	Any expression related to the circumstances of the utterance expressed in the intonation unit: adverbs of time and location, and pronouns.	1) None, 2) Proximal, 3) Distal, 4) Mixed
3. Diegesis / subjectivity aspect	The narrator/character's relation to the story world, in which the narrated events take place. The narrator may be part of the story world, or may be looking at it from the outside. The narrator may identify with a character and tell the story from their point of view.	1) Homo-diegetic, 2) Hetero-diegetic, 3) Pseudo-diegetic
4. Subject number / subjectivity aspect	Subject number	1) Singular, 2) Plural
5. Subject person / subjectivity aspect	Subject person	1. First person, 2. Second person, 3. Third person, 4. General subject
6. Mode of focalization / intentionality aspect	The narrator's way of perceiving his/her own, and other character's inner world, his/her knowledge or lack of knowledge of it. Describing feelings, thoughts, desires, or just overt behaviour.	1. External mode, 2. Internal mode
7. Agency and patiency / intentionality aspect	Who is the actor in the story, who is influencing events in an active way, taking responsibility for outcomes, and who is the one who passively suffers the consequences of events and the outcomes of actions of other characters.	1. Self-agency, patiency 2. Self-part agency-patiency 3. Object-agency-patiency (i.e. other person) 4. Other-agency-patiency (i.e. non-living object) 5. No agent, patient

(*Continued*)

Table 3.1 The discourse-based model of NP (*continued*)

NP components	Definition	Categories/levels
6. **Discourse-level / psychological narrative-level aspect**	Positions the narrator in terms of whether he/she is telling the story from the narrator's point of view, or a character's point of view, or talking in the act of narration, in the here and now position of the therapeutic session. These levels are related to the cognitive process of memory recollection, based on differing memory structures. The narrator is recalling general autobiographical information or a specific episode, or recounting the thoughts and feelings related to what is happening in the present (at the therapeutic session).	1. **Here and now of the session,** 2. **Narrator level** 3. **Character level**

speakers, intonation, dialect, vocabulary, grammatical structures (Garrod & Anderson 1987; Garrod & Pickering 2009).

Based on this line of theorizing, we suggest that perspective shifts could also be matched within the speakers' representation of the interaction. The perspective actualized in the speech of speaker 1, directs the attention of speaker 2 to certain aspects of the narrative. When speaker 1 shifts perspective, speaker 2—the listener—must perceive the shift of perspective in order to comprehend the verbal information (Chafe 1994); so, speaker 2 takes on speaker 1's perspective. As a consequence, speaker 2 may realize the same perspective in their consecutive intonation unit. Hence, we may say that speaker 2 shifts into speaker 1's perspective, and thus manifests a coordination of perspectives.

The coordination of perspectives allows both analysand and analyst to influence each other's perspective shifting behaviour; however, due to their differing roles in psychoanalytic discourse, they apply the coordination of perspectives in a different manner. So, in the case of the analysand, influencing the analyst's shifting behaviour may be more spontaneous, and less geared towards achieving the goals of psychoanalysis. In contrast, the analyst might use interactive regulation in order to achieve the goals of psychotherapy; for example, recounting a given experience in more detail (shifting into character level) or realizing emotion up or down regulation. At the same time, at a later phase of treatment, the analysand may learn new techniques of shifting behaviour; in other words, they may learn to accomplish perspective shifts that were previously unfamiliar to them. Thus the 'shifting' repertoire of the analysand may become broader and more creative, and this may also have an effect on the analysand's self-regulation of shifting behaviour (Berán & Unoka 2016). The analysand can also apply these skills outside the psychotherapeutic situation, without the presence of the analyst.

Self-regulation and coordination of perspective play a role in the attention regulation as well as the affect regulation of the speaker (Berán at al 2017). As we discuss in detail in our previous study (Berán et al. 2017), several studies have shown that adopting a certain perspective is a sign of a more intense affective involvement on the part of the speaker. This characteristic of perspective allows for a regulation of affective involvement by shifting perspective into more involved levels during the session. Again, the analysand may use shifting perspective as a more spontaneous way of regulating their own affective involvement, whereas the analyst may regulate affective involvement in order to accomplish goals of treatment, by keeping affective involvement at an optimal level. Shifts aimed at regulating affective involvement on the part of the analyst may be learned by the analysand, just as in the case of attention regulation.

In summary, we can say that what we would like to show in subsequent chapters of this book is that by tracking perspective shifts by the speakers or, in other words, the sequence of changes in their perspective, we can characterize the narrative interaction process taking place at the session. We argue that this process is closely related to the psychotherapy process taking place at the same time. The co-construction of narratives by patient and therapist, and the interactive regulation of NP, allows psychotherapists to regulate attention and affect in order to achieve therapeutic goals, and allows patients to learn new types of shifting behaviours that they may be able to use to regulate their own attention and affect levels outside the psychotherapy session as well.

PART 2

Methodology

4 The Budapest Psychotherapy Database

This chapter describes the empirical and methodological background of the excerpts of psychoanalytic sessions used as data throughout this book. The authors have developed a database that includes longitudinal audio-recorded psychotherapy sessions of two analysand–analyst dyads—one male and one female dyad—collected between 2004 and 2006 in Budapest, Hungary. The participants were all native speakers of Hungarian, and psychoanalytic sessions were conducted in Hungarian.

This chapter discusses the processes of data collection, transcription, and coding of NP, as well as the ethical guidelines followed by the researchers during data collection and processing. We are also going to discuss the analysands' personal history and psychiatric and emotional problems they have suffered from during the observation period (i.e. the period of data collection and assessment), based on data collected by questionnaires filled out by the therapists.

Participants

Psychoanalysts participating in the study

Participant analysts were volunteers, and received no compensation for participating in the study. Psychoanalysts participating in the study were experienced clinical psychologists, and psychoanalysts, located in Budapest, Hungary. They were both trained in psychoanalysis, middle aged, and with decades of practice—one female analyst participating in the study with a female analysand, and a male analyst, participating in the study with a male analysand. The analysts were both working in private practice, with the male analyst additionally working in a day hospital. They were both members of the Hungarian Psychoanalytic Association and the International Psychoanalytic Association at the time of the observation period. The treatment method applied was psychoanalysis. the theoretical background of the female analyst included both traditional Freudian elements, object relations theory, and intersubjectivity theory. In addition, the background of the male analyst included the Kleinian approach.

The two participant psychoanalysts agreed to participate in the study, and signed informed consent forms. They were informed that they could withdraw their participation at any time without explanation if they felt uncomfortable, or for whatever reason they felt it necessary. The analysts filled out a clinical data form (CDF), which is a clinician report form that assesses a range of variables about the analysand relevant to demographics, diagnosis, and aetiology (Westen et al. 2003). They also filled out further scales and questionnaires that are not used in the studies included in this book.

Analysands participating in the study

Participant analysands were working with the chosen psychoanalysts, and they were at the beginning phase of their psychoanalysis at the start of the observation period. They volunteered to participate, and received no compensation for participating in the study. They also signed informed consent forms, and were informed that they could withdraw their participation in the study at any time if they felt necessary. We describe the ethical considerations in more detail below. The analysands were suffering from psychiatric illnesses that were treatable with the therapeutic methods chosen—namely, psychoanalysis. They did not suffer from psychotic symptoms, any type of organic syndrome, and mental disability. They required regular psychotherapeutic help, which they have received from their psychoanalysts. Participant analysands also filled out some questionnaires, which were not used in this study.

Analysand 1—whom we will call Sylard—is a male self-referred analysand, working with the male psychoanalyst. His treatment consisted of psychoanalysis two to three times a week, in the day hospital where his analyst works. Sylard was in his 40s during the observation period, he had a university degree, and he was of middle-class origin. He was single at the time, never married, and during the observation period of the assessment he was living alone, or for a period, with his mother. His diagnoses given by his therapist was dysthymia, panic disorder, obsessive-compulsive personality disorder, and paranoid personality disorder with narcissistic traits. His history of illness included regular childhood physical abuse. at age 12 he received psychiatric care. In his adult life he attempted suicide once, after which he required institutional care. According to his analyst, his family background was chaotic, cold and hostile, and his relationship problems with his mother contributed to his illness. He has mentioned to his analyst that his mother suffered from anxiety disorder, alcoholism, and borderline personality disorder, whereas his father suffered from anxiety disorder and mild symptoms of personality disorder.

The patient mentioned at the sessions that his romantic relationships and friendships are not emotionally satisfying for him, his previous relationships with his work colleagues are also conflictual and problematic and, during the observation period, he was unemployed. He lost his job due to interpersonal problems at the workplace. During the observation period he received medical treatment for depression and anxiety, including SSRI and benzodiazepine.

Analysand 2—whom we will call Clara in the analysis—also self-referred to treatment. She is an undergraduate university student in her 20s, living in Budapest, Hungary. Her treatment was psychoanalysis received three to four times a week. Based on the analyst's assessment in CDF, she suffered from generalized anxiety disorder, sexual dysfunction, and dependent personality disorder. Her love partnerships were unstable. She was able to develop stable friendships and was able to work and study at the same time, being rather effective in both. She perceived that her family history contributed to her emotional problems, as she grew up in an instable family, and her parents were divorced when she was 13. She disclosed that her mother suffered from anxiety disorder and eating disorder and her father suffered from alcohol dependence.

Procedures

Data collection and sampling

The data for the studies included in this book have been collected as part of the Budapest Psychotherapy Database, a systematically collected and transcribed set of psychotherapy sessions in the Hungarian language. The database consists of the audio-recording of psychoanalytic treatment in psychoanalytic psychotherapies with two analysand–analyst dyads for a period of 1.5 years into treatment from the onset of therapy. Between 2004 and 2006, five consecutive sessions at the beginning, middle, and last third of the observation period were audio-recorded, from which three transcribed sessions from each observation phase were used for the purposes of this set of studies (Table 4.1). The transcribed database consists of about 133 thousand words. Using theory-driven sampling methods, we analyse excerpts from the recorded psychoanalytic sessions to illustrate various theoretical points made in the individual chapters.

Recording of sessions

The audio-recording of sessions was carried out by participant analysts using a Sony mini-disk device. Audio-recording as opposed to video-recording was

Table 4.1 Dates of recording therapeutic sessions during the three phases of the observation period, and transcribed therapy sessions used in the studies

Analysand 1 -- Analyst 1 Transcribed sessions	Phase 1 2004 November 2004 December F4, F5, F6	Phase 2 2005 April 2005 May F21, F22	Phase 3 2006 May 2006 June F31, F32, F33
Analysand 2 -- Analyst 2 Transcribed sessions	Phase 1 2004 November 2004 December L1, L2, L3	Phase 2 2005 November 2005 December L21, L22, L23	Phase 3 2006 May L31, L32, L33

chosen in order to avoid as far as possible interference with the therapeutic work. Asking participant analysts to do the recording themselves served the same purpose of avoiding intrusion. The treatment method implied the classical arrangement of the analysand laying on the couch with the therapist sitting near their head. The consequence of this arrangement regarding the interaction was that the interactors' facial expressions were not visible to each other, body and hand gestures were minimized, thus mainly reducing the relevant communicative aspects in the interaction to verbal content, tone of voice, and pauses.

Ethical considerations

The study for creating the Budapest Psychotherapy Database, and its scientific analysis, was approved by the board of Semmelweis University Regional and Institutional Committee of Science and Research Ethics. After the procedures had been fully explained to them, the participants signed informed consent forms in which they agreed to the use of their material for scientific and educational purposes. Also, the participants were informed that they had the chance to withdraw at any point of the observation period if they felt uncomfortable. As mentioned, the recording of sessions was carried out by the participant analysts; thus researchers did not meet analysands personally. In order to preserve the anonymity of the participant analysands and analysts we deleted from the text files all personal information, such as the names of persons, places, institutions, dates of events, etc.

Data transcription

The audio-recorded analytic sessions were transcribed by the first author using the CHILDES system (MacWhinney 2000). The list of transcription codes used in this particular data-set is presented below. The talkers' speech was transcribed verbatim, segmenting the speech flow into intonation units, as defined by Chafe (1994) in English, and by Németh (1996) in Hungarian. According to this, an intonation unit was defined as a group of words bounded by silence, a short pause or final intonation contour to signal question, period, or exclamation. Single words, sentence fragments could also be considered separate utterances, or fragmented utterances. The method of segmentation was tested for inter-rater reliability, and showed high levels of agreement (Berán et al. 2011); the agreement between the two coders measured by 300 common intonation lines was 88.08% volt (chi-squared = 13, 79, $p < 0.01$). Inter-class correlation inter-rater reliability (Shrout-Fleiss reliability point) = 0, 99, $p < 0.01$.

Transcription codes

The interaction was transcribed using the CHILDES (MacWhinney 2000) coding system. Each line represents a full or broken intonation unit, realizing a given narrative perspective. At the beginning of each line there is a number signalling the place of the line within the transcript of the analytic session. The *T* or *P* following the number signals the speaker being the analyst or analysand, respectively. Transcription codes were the following:

Final intonation contour at the end of full units:

.	falling
?	rising—question
!	exclamation
,	level, continuing

Broken intonation units:

+...	broken unit, fragment
+//	interrupted by another speaker
+/.	self-interruption
+,	beginning of an intonation unit continuing a broken unit
<	false start

Final intonation contour at the end of fragmented units:

-.	falling
–,	level
-?	rising

/	emphasized word or syllable
# (1 s)	pause btw words or within words
[ ]	overlapping speech

Coding of NP

The coding of NP was based on the original transcript in Hungarian, using the coding system we created for analysing therapeutic discourse. All transcribed sessions were coded in terms of NP. We used the following variables in coding NP for individual intonation unit lines, as we have discussed in more detail in Chapter 3:

1. Verb tense: the grammatical verb tense in Hungarian includes three categories we used: 1) past, 2) present, and 3) future 4) non-applicable.
2. Deixis: Adverbs of time and location, and demonstrative pronouns. We distinguished 1) proximal, 2) distal, and 3) mixed categories, as well as 4) 'no deixis' present in a given intonation unit.
3. The narrator's relation to the story world (i.e. 'diegesis'): The narrator may be 1) part of the story world ('inside-narrator' or 'homo-diegesis'), or may be 2) looking at it from the outside ('outside-narrator' or 'hetero-diegesis'). The narrator may 3) identify with a character and tell the story from their point of view ('pseudo-diegesis') 4) non-applicable.
4. Grammatical subject: number and person. This is the same in Hungarian as in English. The subject could be 1) singular or 2) plural, 3) non-applicable, and 1) first, 2) second, 3) third person. We also distinguished two further categories of grammatical subject: 4) impersonal (general) subject, or 5) no subject present (non-applicable).
5. Mode of focalization: We differentiated 1) internal mode of focalization: intonation units expressing mental contents (emotions, desires, intentions, etc.), from 2) external mode of focalization: describing only overt behaviour and events, but not the mental world of the participants, 3) non-applicable.
6. Agency and patiency: Who is the actor in the story, who is influencing events in an active way, and who is the one who passively suffers the consequences: 1) self-agency/, patiency, 2) self-part agency/patiency, 3) other person-agency, patiency, 4) object-agency, patiency, 5) no agent, or patient included in the given unit of analysis.
7. Discourse level: Positions the narrator in terms of whether he/she is telling the story from the narrator's point of view (i.e. narrator's level), or a character's point of view (i.e. character's level), or talking in the act of narration,

in the 'here and now' position of the therapeutic session ('here and now'), or non-applicable. These levels are also related to cognitive processes of recall, based on differing types of memory structures. The narrator is recalling general autobiographical information or a specific episode, or recounting the thoughts and feeling related to what is happening in the present.

Coding was carried out by one main coder and another independent coder to test inter-rater reliability; disagreements were discussed and resolved afterwards. Coding was based on a coding manual created by the first author of this book for the coding of NP in psychotherapeutic discourse (Berán 2009). Inter-rater reliability was computed for each variable separately. Cohen's kappa for all the variables was between 0.55 and 0.8 (specifically verb tense: 0.76; deixis: 0.80; subject number: 0.69; subject person: 0.72; mode of focalization: 0.70; discourse level: 0.56; agency: 0. 67; patiency: 0.55), except for the diegesis variable, where kappa value was somewhat lower, 0.37. On average, coding showed a substantial agreement between the coders (0.63).

Translation of transcript excerpts

In the subsequent chapters of this book, we included qualitative and quantitative studies carried out based on the Budapest Psychotherapy Database, examining processes of narrative construction at the psychoanalytic session. We will analyse NP shifting behaviour in selected excerpts, based on the Hungarian versions of the transcripts; however, we are also going to present the English-language translations of the excerpts. Translation was carried out by the first author of the book, in consultation with Google translate. Translation took place by using the sequence of intonation unit, progressing from one intonation unit to the next, and keeping the original narrative perspective of the Hungarian-language text in the English version.

PART 3

Empirical study of the joint construction of narratives in psychoanalysis

5 Autobiographical memory and narrative perspective

This chapter explores the interconnections between the functioning of the autobiographical self-memory system, primarily grounded in Martin Anthony Conway's self-memory system theory (Conway & Pleydell-Pearce 2000), and the various positions implied by the narrative perspective (NP) of an intonation unit. Drawing on empirical research, we argue that autobiographical memories and the self-concept are deeply interlinked within the memory system. Consequently, the transformation of self-narratives in psychotherapy inherently involves altering the sense of self, a process that can lead to symptom reduction, which is one of the primary aims of psychoanalytic psychotherapy.

The chapter aims to propose a theoretical framework that integrates our NP shifting model with Conway's self-memory system theory. This integration aims to elucidate specific mechanisms underlying psychoanalytic techniques. Specifically, we posit that those processes of remembering and reconstructing past events during psychoanalytic sessions—expressed as self-narratives—are closely related to shifts in the storyteller's NP. By conducting a detailed analysis, we demonstrate how tracing these shifts provides insight into the therapeutic process.

Whether introduced by the analysand or guided by the analyst, NP shifts generate new retrieval cues that activate previously dormant aspects of a memory or stimulate the retrieval of related episodic memories. These processes enrich and potentially transform self-representations. Each NP taken and induced by the partner of the dialogue increasingly articulates multiple self-states in each member of the analytic dyad. NP shifts induced by the analysand or the analyst in the partner scaffold their self-memory systems' implicit memory retrieval skills and lead to flexibility in searching for multiple meanings and interpretations of their experiences. Their experience of flexible co-creation of meaning may lead to curiosity for the other's reality and for the reality of their relationship co-created by themselves.

Moreover, repeating such perspective shifts scaffolds the development of new memory retrieval skills within the self-memory system, allowing analysands and analysts to access and reorganize autobiographical knowledge more adaptively and flexibly. Changes in this implicit skill may lead to an experience of a less fragile self.

The scaffolding of flexible memory retrieval skills fosters the emergence of implicit, automatic retrieval processes that sustain modified self–, other, and we representations. These updated representations, embedded in the subconscious, inform planning, goal-setting, and imagining future scenarios. So, shifts in NP facilitate therapeutic change and have lasting implications for reorganizing the working self's implicit, automatic retrieval skill repertoire that provides the knowledge base from the analysand's autobiographical self, which is used in goal-directed action.

The NPs used by the speaker offer a point of view for the listener, who accepts or rejects it. This process represents a subconscious or unconscious defensive, transferential, and countertransferential contribution by the analysand and the analyst, respectively, to the co-created memory construction process, in which they reciprocally influence each other. We intend to reveal this previously less articulated layer of unconscious expression of the analyst and the analysand subjectivity, the linguistic choice of NP, which has an effect on the self's and the other's affect, self and autobiographic memory regulatory consequences.

In contemporary psychoanalysis—particularly relational (Barsness 2021; Levenkron 2009), intersubjective, Boston Change Process Study Group (2008)—autobiographic memory co-construction plays a pivotal role in therapeutic change. These frameworks emphasize the co-construction of meaning, mutual affect, self-regulation, and the transformation of self-narratives, aligning well with SMS theory and its focus on memory retrieval and reconstruction. To support this argument, we analyse excerpts from the Budapest Psychotherapy Database, illustrating how shifts in narrative perspective enable navigation among different levels of the self-memory system. These shifts reveal how psychoanalytic interventions may facilitate the more profound integration of episodic and semantic memories, ultimately promoting a coherent and adaptable sense of self.

Conway's theory of autobiographical self-memory system

According to Conway's self-memory system account of autobiographic memory (Conway 2005; Conway et al. 2004; Conway et al. 2019; Conway & Pleydell-Pearce 2000; Conway, Loveday, Cole 2016), the working self generates the psychological present through the goal-directed organization of different types of autobiographical information retrieved from either the episodic memory system or the long-term self, which contains the autobiographical knowledge base and the conceptual self.

Our theory of mutual or interactive regulation of NP proposes that, during the psychoanalytic dialogue, each of the analyst's and the analysand's verbal expressions in intonation units serve as a memory retrieval cue. The NP used in an intonation unit affects the content of the retrieved memory and the 'psychological presence' of each participant in the co-constructed dialogue. The perspective shift offered by the analyst may or may not evoke a new memory in the analysand, depending on the analysand's automatic cooperation or unconscious or conscious acceptance or resistance. The psychoanalyst and the analysand-induced perspective shifts evoke a modified version of the previously retrieved memory in the analyst's and the analysand's mind. One function of NP in an intonation unit is to focus the attention of the listener from a specific point of view to the intended content. Repeatedly using different NPs and perspective shifts by procedural learning may lead to changes in the automatic generation of subconscious and conscious autobiographical memory contents. As the analyst and analysand work together, they co-create different versions of stories from the autobiographical memories of the analysand. Their cooperative analytic activity is becoming the content of their own autobiographic memory knowledge base. The perspective shifts offered or rejected by the analysand and the analyst evoke or avoid content respectively and simultaneously lead to implicit relational patterns of mutual coordination of memory retrieval. One consequence of the repeated exercises of different narrative perspective shifts is the transformation of the working self and the transformation of the conscious representation of the autobiographical self.

In contemporary psychoanalytic theory, it is assumed that the analyst and the analysand mutually affect each other's activity subconsciously, unconsciously, and consciously. Our model aims to highlight a particular layer of psychoanalytic activity, similar to the model proposed by the Boston Change Process Study Group (BCPSG 2008). In our approach, we focus on NP shifts as the 'surface' level of moment-to-moment exchange. We agree that directing attention and triggering memory through narrative perspectives—where implicit relational knowing is enacted—is the foundational level of psychic life. The depth of implicit relational models is revealed in these mutual regulatory manoeuvres, and focusing on this aspect represents a significant departure from the classical psychoanalytic emphasis on making the unconscious conscious (Bruschweiler-Stern et al. 2007). Instead, our model is consistent with a relational and interpersonal focus on the 'here and now' (Levenkron 2009).

According to Tronick's Mutual Regulation Model (2003), analysand and analyst co-create dyadic states of consciousness, and these co-creative processes lead to a change in the way they make sense of the world and ways of being with others. In our model, 'The Interactive Regulation of Shifting Narrative Perspective' we aim to capture—at the linguistic level—the subtle relational processes by which NP, expressed through the verbally articulated affective involvement of both the analysand and the analyst and the mutual orientation of their attention towards various aspects of memories, gives rise to an implicit relational knowledge of manoeuvres that both self-regulate and regulate one another, thereby mutually governing attention and, concurrently, consciousness. These processes create a specific implicit relational field unique to the pair of the analysand and the analyst. During interactions between the analysand and the analyst, the narrative perspectives offered as memory retrieval cues are frequently not adopted as intended by the participants. Instead, a range of mismatches, misattunements, dissynchronies, and miscoordinations occur, which subsequently give rise to co-creative reparations. These reparative processes generate new ways of being together, ultimately fostering alternative relational configurations within the therapeutic dyad (Tronick 2003). In the following section, we define the components of the autobiographical self-memory systems, give examples of how the NP shifts affect their retrieval, and discuss the therapeutic relevance of activating memory types and shifting between them.

Interaction between the analysand's and the analyst's autobiographic memory systems

In psychoanalytic work, the memory system of the analysand interacts with the memory system of the analyst. The events of the analysand's life and the events at the session are also memories in the analyst's autobiographical memory system. In Excerpt 5.1, the analyst shares her memories about a previous session when her analysand shared a similar experience. A male analyst and a male analysand have worked together for several months. The analyst summarizes the analysand's experience of noticing a qualitative difference between the analytic sessions. In this case, within the reality they have co-created, the analysand distinguishes between two qualitatively different types of sessions. The analyst directs attention to this experience, which is present in both of their autobiographical memories.

Excerpt 5.1 (F21)

16 TER:	a múltkor említette hogy úgy érzékeli,	you mentioned the other day that you perceive,
17 TER:	hogy mások azok az órák amikor+//	that those sessions are different when+//

The analyst's capacity to recall both the analysand's life history and the shared experiences during sessions can lead to interventions that articulate his understanding and serve to frame—or reframe—the fragments of the analysand's shared memories. These interventions direct the analysand's attention towards new aspects of his experience, functioning as retrieval cues that activate previously inaccessible memories. In this way, an intervention may provide a framework for raw, unframed sensory experiences or help reframe an existing perspective, integrating previously disturbing or excluded material.

Furthermore, the analyst's summary of the session's events—for example, highlighting the shifts in the analysand's identification with different aspects of object relationship dyads, as well as transitions between various dyads—offers the analysand a new perspective from which to monitor the moment-to-moment shifts between different identifications. By integrating the analysand's fragmented series of episodic memories into a coherent whole and providing a summary interpretation, the analyst helps the analysand develop the implicit ability to adopt the narrator's perspective and to employ increasingly complex frameworks for organizing both episodic elements and individual memories.

In Excerpt 5.2, the analysand described three object-relational dyads—also known as core conflictual relationship themes—during the session, each characterized by the same affective experience of rejection. First, she spoke about her teacher and two potential boyfriends. The analyst then offered the narrator's perspective, which revealed how each relationship represents a repetitive manifestation of the rejection dyad across different interpersonal contexts.

Excerpt 5.2. (L23)

428TER:	igen.	yes.
429TER:	hát amit ma láttunk,	well what we see today,
430TER:	az az három ilyen történet.	that is that is three such stories.
431PAT:	igen.	yes.
432TER:	tanára, aki úgyis utálja.	your teacher who hates you anyway.
433PAT:	a Z., aki úgyse válaszol.	Z., who is not going to reply anyway.
434TER:	a Z., aki úgyse válaszol.	Z., who is not going to reply anyway.
435TER:	és a +..	and the+...
436PAT:	G.	G.
437TER:	G., akinél úgyse rúghat labdába.	G., with whome you don't stand a chance.

The stories the analysand recounts about her autobiographical memories—and his experience of how the analyst received them—become integrated into his own autobiographical narrative. For example, in Excerpt 5.3 he mentioned that, just the previous day, he had been contemplating what his therapist had told him in the prior session.

Excerpt 5.3 (F5)

25PAT:	Gondolkodtam ezen amit beszélgettünk.	I have been thinking about this, what we have discussed.

In summary, through their dialogue, the analyst and the analysand mutually regulate each other's recollections by employing various perspectives within their conversational intonation units, thereby collaboratively creating an autobiographical knowledge base to which they both contribute. This shared experience continues to evolve through individual recollections expressed from different perspectives. Moreover, their joint effort in narrativizing these experiences sets in motion a transformative process reflected in the revised representations of the analysand's life history, ultimately reorganizing her working self and influencing the analyst's working self.

The goal-directed nature of autobiographical memory and the characteristics of the psychoanalytic dialogue

According to Conway (2005), retrieval of autobiographical memory is goal-directed. The goal-directedness of autobiographic memory retrieval means that, when individuals recall personal past events, they do so with specific objectives in mind, such as maintaining a coherent sense of self, guiding current decision-making, or preparing for future challenges. The memories that are brought to mind are influenced by the individual's current needs and goals, ensuring that only the most relevant experiences are accessed.

What is the goal of psychoanalytic dialogue? Analysands arrive at psychoanalysis with different types of therapeutic goals, but there is one common feature of their goals, namely to have an altered future. Intersubjective and relational psychoanalysis views psychoanalytic dialogue as a mutually constructed space where both the analyst's and the analysand's subjectivities are crucial in creating meaning. The primary goal of this dialogue is to facilitate a co-creative process that transforms internal relational patterns and unconscious conflicts into more integrated and adaptive ways of being (Levenkron 2009).

Specifically, the dialogue aims to foster mutual understanding by engaging both participants in a shared exploration of feelings, memories, and relational dynamics. This collaborative process helps surface and verbalize previously unconscious material. Additionally, by collaboratively examining and reconfiguring early internalized relational templates, the dialogue promotes the co-creation of new ways of being together, enabling the analysand to develop healthier ways of relating to themselves and others (Tronick 2003).

Furthermore, as the analysand gains insight through this intersubjective exchange, they begin to integrate disparate aspects of their internal experience, ultimately fostering a more coherent sense of self. The process is not unidirectional; it also enhances the analyst's reflective capacity, as the analyst undergoes self-reflection and transformation. This enrichment of the therapeutic stance contributes to a genuinely reciprocal therapeutic relationship (Tronick 2003).

Every sentence the analysand utters to the analyst carries an implicit relational layer, promising that the dialogue is meaningful because the analyst will transform these utterances in ways that alter the analysand's future—a future distinct from both the present and the past. Since the analysand involves the analyst in this transformative process, the goal-directed retrieval of memories is influenced by various prior factors, including transference. In particular, prior beliefs about the attention of significant others, their capacity for narrativization, and cultural, local, transgenerational, or individual motivations to discuss life scenes, emotions, needs, desires, intentions, and instincts all shape what is either blocked during memory retrieval as irrelevant or obstructive to the goal, or retrieved but left unsaid or only partially expressed. Furthermore, the development of this implicit relational field of memory retrieval is also affected by the analyst's own prior characteristics—manifested through countertransference enactments and implicit relational memories.

The analyst's attention expressed by shifts in NP may be directed to details or topics irrelevant to previous others and not part of the shared autobiographical memory representations, the set of autobiographical memories recognized by others. In Excerpt 5.4, the analysand is complaining about his anxiety attacks and focuses exclusively on his bodily experiences. His analyst turns his attention to the context of anxiety attacks and, as the analysand starts discussing moving to a new apartment, he realizes that he feels rejected by his family.

Excerpt 5.4 (F5)

359TER:	de hogy a a+…	but that the the+…
360TER:	+, költözéssel időben egybeesett nagyon.	+, it fell at the same time with your moving house.

361PAT:	igen, ez utána jött.	yes, this came after that.
362TER:	hmm.	hmm.
363TER:	tehát amikor kiderült, hogy a a várakozásai nem teljesülnek,	so when it became obvious that your expectations would not be fulfilled,
364TER:	és nem tud# közölebbi kapcsolatba kerülni a családjával a gyerekekkel–	and you won't be able# to get in close touch with you family the children–
365PAT:	igen, és közben pedig amit említettem,	yes, and meanwhile in turn, as I have
366PAT:	<hogy hogy> hogy olyan/ távolabbra kerültem,	mentioned <that that> that I got like/more distant,
367PAT:	és és egyszerűen a+...	and and simply the+...
368PAT:	iszonyúan <eluralkodott rajtam egy ilyen>,	it terribly <overcame me a like>,
369PAT:	egy i:lyen:+...	a like:+...
370PAT:	+, /kitaszítottság érzet.	+,/feeling of being an outsider.

This chapter discusses the autobiographical memory system from the psychoanalytic dialogue point of view. The analysands present their memories to their analyst/prior others to change their future. The primary function of memory, specifically episodic memory, is to provide information for achieving our goals. Prior interpersonal experiences may affect this process, and one function of the repeated shifts in NP from the analyst's side is to help the analysand by procedural learning to use the working self more widely and flexibly to create representations that better serve their goals.

The episodic memory system

Definition of episodic memory

Episodic memory (EM) is a long-term, explicit/declarative experience near memory that involves conscious recollection of previous experiences and their context in terms of time, place, and associated emotions (Fivush 2011). Conway lists nine properties of EMs that distinguish them from other types of memories (Conway 2009).

Its first property is that EM is an experience-near summary record of experience, which results from sensory-perceptual-conceptual-affective processing but is not a literal copy of an experience. Some subtypes of episodic memories, like self-defining memories, 'flashbulb' memories, or trauma-related details, may contain fragments close to being literal records of experience, but some are incorrect. Recollection of these vivid details can also cause an intense feeling of reliving when brought into consciousness. It is organized and selected as a way to serve a specific goal. In psychoanalytic dialogue, the shared objective is to provide pertinent information to one another; however, this aim can be influenced by transference and countertransference dynamics.

The second property of EM is that episodic information within the memory is differentially accessible (Conway 2009; Racsmány & Conway 2006): inhibited details are difficult to access, and activated details are easily accessible. Conway suggests that the goal structure of an experience primarily determines the activation/inhibition levels of details in a specific EM. The level of accessibility of specific details in a specific EM is affected by the nature of the retrieval strategy and cues that feature it. It is also affected by the encoding, which may not be independent of the internalized working models, intersubjective goals, or the traumatic situation (Conway 2009). Different narrative perspectives, as retrieval cues used by the interlocutor, determine the level of accessibility of specific details in EM differently. There is a detailed analysis of a dream about the missing penis in Chapter 8, where the analyst's NP shifts applied in her interventions helped the analysand to access further details of her EMs. The primary function of EM is to provide relevant information for the processing of recent goals. In a psychoanalytic situation, the primary goal regarding EM is to tell the analyst about specific experiences. In the psychoanalytic dialogue, the level of accessibility of specific details is mainly affected by the goals of the analysand and the analyst. What are the participants' goals in the psychoanalytic dialogue, and what obstacles interfere with achieving these goals?

In the psychoanalytic session, the recent goal is determined by a basic rule 'which structures the analytic situation: the analysand is asked to say what he thinks and feels, selecting nothing and omitting nothing from what comes into his mind, even where this seems to him unpleasant to have to communicate, ridiculous, devoid of interest or irrelevant' (Laplanche & Pontalis 1973: 178).

Freud (1912) also provides advice for the psychoanalyst on how to listen to patients. The technical term for the advised stance is evenly suspended attention:

> Just as the patient must relate everything that his self-observation can detect, and keep back all the logical and affective objections that seek to induce him to make a selection from among them, so the doctor must put himself in a position to make use of everything he is told for the purposes of interpretation and of recognizing the concealed unconscious material without

> substituting a censorship of his own for the selection that the patient has foregone. (Laplanche & Pontalis 1973: 43)

This task is disrupted by transferential expectations formed in earlier relationships. These expectations depend on how the person's significant others in the past were able, or unable, to listen to their stories: how curious they were, how well they could regulate their own emotions, and how much detail they could tolerate (see Chapter 1 on narrative development). Regarding the goal structure of psychoanalytic discourse, there are different listening rules and theoretical effects on the abstinence rule and free-floating attention. Later, the authors argued about the impossibility of both tasks.

Donald Spence, in his paper entitled 'Perils and pitfalls of free floating attention' (1984), argued that Freud, in 'Instincts and their vicissitudes', pointed to the impossibility of listening without theory-driven preconceptions:

> The true beginning of scientific activity consists rather in describing phenomena and then in proceeding to group, classify and correlate them. Even at the stage of description, it is not possible to avoid applying certain abstract ideas to the materials in hand, ideas derived from somewhere or another but certainly not from the new observations alone ... we come to an understanding about their meaning by making repeated references to the material of observation from which they appear to have been derived, but upon which, in fact, they have been imposed. (Freud 1915: 117, cited in Spence 1984: 48)

Psychoanalytic concepts are developed not only to organize the psychoanalyst's own thinking and direct their attention, but also to provide a framework for understanding the patient's unconscious processes. Kernberg points to the concept of technical neutrality that 'implies equidistance from the patient's id, superego, acting ego, and external reality and a position of closeness to, or an alliance with, the observing part of the patient's ego' (Kernberg 2004, 2011). The analyst's attention is expressed in the narrative perspective of their interventions, which may affect the analysand's attention and function as a retrieval cue for her recollection. Repeated perspective shifts lead to changes in the working self and in autobiographical memory through procedural learning.

The third property of EM is that it is often represented in the form of visual images (Conway 2009). This means that using visual retrieval cues to explore a specific episodic memory of the analysand is a very effective tool for accessing less accessible details of the memory. However, retrieval cues of other senses could also be very effective. In the Proustian case, the taste of the madeleine cake was a very effective retrieval cue for an EM of an event at his aunt's flat that happened forty years earlier (Smith 2016). Also, it is documented that trauma-related olfactory cues precipitate traumatic EMs (Vermetten & Bremner 2003). Different sensory retrieval cues could induce affective or emotional states unrelated to the analytic situation, recontextualizing them by finding the affect-inducing EM, which may help the analysand to integrate disturbing episodic elements into conceptual frames and EMs (see later, episodic elements and conceptual frames). In Excerpt 5.5, the analysand describes an overgeneral autobiographical memory he repeatedly experiences every morning.

Excerpt 5.5 (F5)

50PAT:	nincs kedvem nekikezdeni a napnak–,	I do not feel like beginning the day–,

The therapist turns his attention to a specific episodic memory using a second-person, singular, past tense, heterodiegetic, character-level perspective:

54TER:	ma hogy kelt fel,	how did you get up today,
55TER:	milyen érzésekkel?	with what kind of feelings?

The analysand initially resists answering, stating that he does not feel anything. However, he then begins speaking in the first-person singular, present tense, and adopts a homodiegetic character perspective. This shift indicates that he has activated a specific episodic memory from that morning and has begun using a field perspective—reliving his experience through his own eyes, as if perceiving the world from the point of view of his past self in the present moment.

By persistently inquiring about the analysand's actual feelings, the analyst provides retrieval cues that elicit additional memories and further details regarding the episodic element, such as the statement, 'I do not feel like beginning the day.' For instance, the analysand typically avoids discussing himself and does not understand why it would be appropriate to do so. Later, he recalls a previous episode from his life in which he experienced similar feelings, albeit more intensely. The analyst connects this recollection with an autobiographical fact: these intense feelings were triggered when the analysand moved to a new apartment and realized that maintaining contact with his family was challenging. This new framework activated feelings of isolation and of being an outcast.

Focusing on these emotions elicits further memories related to the significance of his relationship with his niece and nephew. As they explore this topic further, the analysand comes to realize that the authentic expression of love from these children is paramount in his relationship with them—a realization that, in turn, evokes memories of not being loved by his parents. The analyst facilitates the analysand's memory retrieval process by providing varied retrieval cues and employing different narrative perspectives. As a result, the dyad transitions from the initial statement 'I do not feel anything' to the more profound expression, 'My parents did not love me, and I desperately need an authentic expression of love.'

During this process, the analyst also draws on his own autobiographical memories of conversations with the analysand. By integrating various fragmented episodic elements and frameworks, they are able to uncover a new underlying framework behind the statement 'I do not feel like beginning the day': namely, 'My goal is to receive authentic expressions of love from others, but it is hopeless because I am an outcast in my new home.'

The fourth property of visually represented EM is that it always has a visual perspective (Conway 2009). Following Freud (1915), Nigro and Neisser (1983) identified two main visual perspectives in EM: the field perspective and the observer perspective. In the observer (third-person) perspective, one sees oneself from the outside, indicating that the memory is more constructed and incorporates additional knowledge. In contrast, the field (first-person) perspective involves experiencing the scene from one's own point of view.

The fifth property of EM is that it represents a short slice of experience organized around a goal, containing information related to goal generation, plan execution, outcomes, and evaluations (Conway 2009). Through the analyst's interventions and various narrative perspective shifts, new content may be recollected, and fragments of EM can be organized, framed, or reframed, leading to new integrated representations.

The sixth property of EM is its temporal organization, which roughly corresponds to the order in which events occur. This characteristic is particularly relevant when using the EM system to plan future actions.

Although EM is subject to rapid forgetting, it can be reinstated with appropriate retrieval cues and specific retrieval techniques. In the psychoanalytic dialogue, the analyst aims to provide proper retrieval cues to help the analysand reconstruct and integrate memory fragments into their autobiographical memory.

EM makes autobiographical remembering specific. In many mental disorders, autobiographical memory tends to be overgeneral, which can cause difficulties in planning, emotion regulation, and processing. Overgeneral memory may block therapeutic change, hinder the processing of traumatic information, and impair affect regulation. Due to defence mechanisms, many patients tend to summarize autobiographical events in overgeneral terms rather than retrieving specific EMs when discussing their lives (Williams et al. 2007).

Based on the hierarchical search model of personal event retrieval (Conway & Pleydell-Pearce 2000), various mechanisms can block the retrieval process at the overgeneral level. These include capture by schematic representations of information (such as object-relational dyads), activation of ruminative thinking, or functional avoidance of unbearable emotional states (Williams et al. 2007). Developmentally, overgeneral autobiographical retrieval is influenced by a mother's reminiscing style during mother–child interactions (Valentino 2011). Longitudinal studies have shown that a mother's elaborated reminiscing style affects her children's reminiscing style years later, and training mothers in an elaborated reminiscing style has both immediate and long-term effects on the specificity of their children's autobiographical memory retrieval. Elaborated mother–child reminiscing through narrativization not only contextualizes and gives meaning to children's experiences, but also helps them understand the personal significance of negative events and integrate these into a coherent autobiography (Bird & Reese 2006, as cited in Valentino 2011). This process is also positively associated with children's self-understanding, coping skills, and a reduction in internalizing and externalizing symptoms (Valentino 2011).

Furthermore, securely attached mothers participating in adult attachment interviews—where they select adjectives to describe their past attachment relationships and use them as retrieval cues to recall specific memories—can provide specific, coherent, and integrated narratives. In contrast, parents with avoidant or unresolved, insecure attachment styles tend to have overgeneralized and incoherent memories (Sales 2009; Valentino 2011).

During the narrativization of children's emotional experiences, fragmented elements are framed within the concepts of emotions, goals, needs, desires, and actions, and are further organized into scripts, stories, and dramatic scenes where each character's behaviours, emotional expressions, goals, and desires are meaningfully integrated. Abusive parents are less likely to discuss the causes and consequences of emotions with their children (Shipman & Zeman 1999, as cited in Valentino 2011).

In the psychoanalytic dialogue, the analyst's use of NP shifts facilitates the narrativization process and the integration of fragmented elements into a relatively coherent autobiographical memory. The repeated NP shifts induced by the analyst's interventions lead to procedural learning within the working self, ultimately transforming the analysand's present experience. Many intrusive symptoms are memory fragments of traumatic or non-narrativized emotional experiences. Conway developed a theory outlining different types of representation within the EM system to conceptualize these phenomena.

Three types of representation in the episodic memory system

Conway (2009) describes three types of representation in the EM system: episodic elements, simple episodic memory, and complex episodic memory.

The first representation is the episodic element (EE), which is the most event-specific and experience-near representation of long-term memory. According to Conway (2009), EEs are similar to moments of 'now' (Stern 2018 or free radicals (Tulving 1984). In a way, they are similar to beta elements in Bion's theory.

The second representation, simple episodic memory (SEM) contains EEs organized under a conceptual frame. A single or a set of EEs may be organized under a conceptual contextualizing knowledge termed by Conway a frame (Conway 2009). EEs without a conceptual frame may intrude into consciousness, and their rawness is disturbing. For example, the following disturbing EEs may be present: tension in muscles, pressure in the head, hot feeling in the face, and the other person seems irritating, their behaviour seems to be unjust. These disturbing experiences of an analysand were fragmented sensations and memories, until they became organized under the conceptual frame of anger.

The third type of representation is based on simple EMs that can be organized into a common higher-order conceptual frame by creating a complex episodic memory (CEM, Conway 2009). For example, a self-defining traumatic memory, a memory that was life changing and consequential to the person's sense of self, such as 'my father humiliating me in front of my sister and her schoolmates because I was crying', was represented by several SEMs.

> She pulled me off the bunk bed, and I fell off. I fell with my knee into my favourite toy, which broke. My knee hurt, so I cried and shouted at my sister. My father came in and slapped me. He said a boy does not cry in front of girls. I felt it was unfair.

Exploring the SEMs in a complex EM may lead to further information that helps to understand the situation more deeply or in another way. To mentalize the story's mainly external and behaviouristic description, the analyst may use interventions that turn the analysand's attention to internal focus, to the desire, motivation, emotions, and intentions of each character in the story.

A clinically relevant question is how to access these three types of episodic representation. EEs can be typically activated automatically as intrusive experiences. EEs are also accessible when we gather further elements of EM for an activated SEM or CEM. SEM and CEM can be accessed by two different retrieval methods, either by a cue that corresponds in some way to the content of EEs or by a cue that accesses the frame (Conway 2009). We can identify a relevant SEM or CEM and let the analysand intentionally recollect memories that fit the conceptual frame, for example anger. Alternatively, an activated EE incidentally retrieves a SEM or CEM.

Based on this conceptualization, three specific clinical problems could arise. First, EEs without frames, a conceptual contextualizing knowledge for episodic elements, may lead to symptoms of somatizations or any disturbing phenomenon that intrudes into the analysand's mind. Second, a frame without accessible EEs may lead to alexithymia or overgeneral memories. Third, early capture of memory retrieval by a conceptual frame may distort the understanding of the memory. Both have relevance for psychoanalytic techniques. In the first case, the therapeutic task is to collect EEs that are intrusive or disturbing and help the analysand find the appropriate conceptual frame. In the second case, the analyst's task is to let the analysand go into one specific EM and recollect the details of the experience since recollecting specific EEs may lead to deeper processing of that experience or may lead to new frames. Rumination is a typical symptom when someone repeatedly thinks about a frame or a categoric memory: an overgeneral evaluation without the ability to go into the details of specific experiences. Third, the process of memory retrieval or imaging a future event while planning the solution of a future task could be captured too early, which may block the retrieval of other relevant details that may be needed. The analyst's task is to help the analysand to facilitate the retrieval process, which may lead to the recollection of more EEs, SEMs, and CEMs, and, based on these richer EMs, new, more appropriate frames could be formed.

Bion's (1962b, 1963) theory of alpha-, beta-elements, and alpha function describes the process of working together with the analysand on raw experiences. Bion defines beta-elements as the raw sense impressions and emotions that the analysand is aware of; however, they are not material for thought and are not ready to be integrated. Accumulated beta-elements create a beta-screen. In the case of a beta-screen, rational thoughts are cut off from emotional feelings. The raw sensory data (beta-elements) are converted by alpha-function to alpha-elements, which are part of self-consciousness and are experienced as mental, forming memory. The subject can manipulate them mentally to repress, symbolize, narrate, and use them as dream material. Furthermore, unrelated facts could be organized by the 'selected fact'. Bion defines selected fact as a phenomenon 'by which coherence and meaning are given to facts already known but whose relatedness has not hitherto been seen' (Bion 1963: 18).

EM's ninth characteristic is that it is recollectively experienced when accessed. Recollective experience is characterized by personal relevance.

EMs in therapy function by providing self-coherence or correspondence. Bluck and Habermas (2001) reason that EM's function is to serve self-coherence, that is, to have an integrated life story. Other people reason that EM corresponds to reality, and its primary function is to provide an accurate representation of reality, and serving self-coherence is secondary (Conway et al. 2004). One goal of psychotherapy is to elucidate whether the motivation for self-coherence distorts the evoked EM. Turning attention to other details of EM by perspective shifts may reveal self-contradictory data that requires reevaluating the self to regain self-coherence. Overgeneral memory (Conway et al. 2004) is another tool to maintain self-coherence, and directing attention to EMs opens the way for specific details that contradict overgeneral memories, feed a new concept of self, and require a new self-coherence.

Conway, based on previous findings, reasons that remembering the past and imagining the future take place in the same system, the remembering-imaging system (Conway 2009). One aim of the analysis is to enhance the working self's ability to flexibly retrieve the appropriate information, both from the EM system specifically and from the autobiographical memory system more generally, in order to achieve the analysand's goal.

Long-term self: the autobiographical knowledge base

Life story schemas

The life story schema is an overarching schematic mental representation of life's major components—such as life chapters and themes—organized according to culturally available narrative structures and norms regarding a proper life history. Bluck and Habermas (2000, 2001) describe four types of life story coherence: temporal coherence, cultural biography, thematic coherence, and causal coherence.

Temporal coherence involves arranging the events of our lives in chronological order. In therapeutic dialogue, both the therapist and the analysand rely on the concept of time to organize the analysand's experiences into a coherent life story.

The cultural concept of biography refers to the normative expectations for personal events that should occur during each life phase within culturally defined age ranges. Typical life events include birth, kindergarten, primary school, secondary school, high school, university, marriage, having children, work, various career stages, children leaving home, retirement, grandchildren, and death. Stressors related to the cultural concept of biography arise when an individual is delayed in reaching a certain life phase, when specific life phases (such as marriage or having children) are absent, or when there is a discrepancy between the family's and the mainstream cultural expectations.

Thematic coherence means that a specific theme organizes the life story. For example, life might be metaphorically framed as a war, a journey, or a learning process (Lakoff & Turner 1989).

Causal coherence refers to the logical flow in narratives, where events are connected through cause-and-effect relationships. In life stories, individuals often rely on culturally accepted explanations to understand how people's goals, desires, emotions, and intentions lead to specific actions and long-term outcomes. When reflecting on personal experiences, individuals employ these culturally endorsed causal theories to make sense of their lives. The causal frameworks embedded in life story schemas provide tools for understanding oneself and predicting both personal and others' behaviours over time. Moreover, the perceived predictability of others' behaviour, as inferred from their life story schemas, plays a crucial role in sustaining long-term cooperation within groups.

Lifetime period

Lifetime periods are cognitive structures that organize information about the goals, relationships, locations, activities, and evaluations that are common to a given phase of life. On the one hand, a lifetime period can serve as a retrieval cue, enabling us to access general events; from these general events, specific episodic memories can be retrieved (Conway 2005). On the other hand, as a cognitive structure within autobiographical memory, a lifetime period contributes to the temporal organization of specific episodic memories. This aspect is particularly relevant in psychoanalyses, where lifetime periods serve as a tool to anchor episodic memories within their proper context in the overall memory system.

For example, in work with post-traumatic flashbacks—specific episodic memories that have not been fully integrated into the life story schema—the therapeutic task is to help the analysand locate the flashback within its appropriate lifetime period. It is important to note that self-representations related to goals, relationships, competencies, skills, and knowledge differ across various lifetime periods. In analysis, it is crucial to compare the characteristics of the lifetime period activated by a flashback with those of the analysand's current lifetime period. For instance, one might compare a flashback from the period of a vulnerable, weak child whose goal was to cooperate with and obey an abusive father, with the present lifetime period of a strong, autonomous, and educated adult whose goal is to protect themselves.

General events

General events are conceptual representations of repeated or categorical occurrences (for example, playing music with friends), extended events (such as attending summer school), and mini-histories (like learning to ski; Conway 2005). These general events contain more event-specific information—about goals, interpersonal relationships, locations, activities, and evaluations—than lifetime periods do. In psychoanalysis, general events can serve as effective retrieval cues. Recalling a general event within the context of a lifetime period can provide insight into the goals, evaluations, and beliefs of that particular version of the working self, while also facilitating access to the episodic memories associated with that period.

Long-term self: the conceptual self

The conceptual self comprises explicit, declarative, and semantic memories. Representations of the conceptual self define both oneself and others through trait-like characteristics and offer predictive models for typical interactions with people and the surrounding world. These representations are abstract, non-temporally specified knowledge structures—including personal scripts, object-relational dyads, conceptual aspects of internal working models, attitudes, values, beliefs, and schemas (Conway 2005). Although semantic memories are accessible independently of specific autobiographical events, they remain connected to autobiographical knowledge and the episodic memory system. In fact, semantic memories can serve as retrieval cues that activate specific episodic memories that exemplify, contextualize, and ground their underlying themes or concepts.

In analysis, exploring these specific episodic memories within their unique contexts and lifetime periods can be particularly illuminating. By linking these memories to their autobiographically specific origins, the analysand may realize that this semantic knowledge does not represent an immutable truth about themselves. Rather, it was learned in a specific context during a particular phase of life, when they were different. By collecting and examining episodic memories that do not align with this abstract knowledge, analysts can help analysands develop new conceptual frameworks, beliefs, or schemas that more accurately describe their experiences.

Furthermore, culturally available schemas and categories provide cognitive tools for the autobiographical memory system. These tools are embedded in family stories, fairy tales, literature, drama, film, and other media. Individuals internalize culturally available concepts through parent–child narrativization of personal events, as well as through family and peer interactions and institutional experiences such as school, work, and religious evaluations of personal experiences. In psychoanalyses, one of the key goals is to reconstruct the representations of the conceptual self so that they align more closely with the goals and realities of the patient's present lifetime period (Benjamin 2013).

6 Introducing a pseudo-narrator

This chapter focuses on one specific type of narrative perspective playing a decisive role in psychoanalytic narrative interaction, namely pseudo-diegesis (Genette 1980; Prince 1987). As we described in our definition of the discourse-based model of narrative perspective (see Chapter 3 for details), pseudo-diegesis is a perspective having to do with the subjectivity aspect of our model of NP, more specifically with the world or 'diegesis' of the narrative. It is based on the original primary narrator (Narrator P) introducing a new, secondary narrator (Narrator S) within the original narrative world. After the introduction of a new narrator, however, the story continues from the point of view of Narrator S, creating a new story world (i.e. a new diegesis), so that the listener loses his/her sight of the original Narrator P, and representations in the world of the secondary pseudo-narrative cannot be mapped onto the world of the primary narrative.

In Chapter 3 we distinguished and defined primary and secondary narrations in detail. We gave an example of Scheherazade in *One Thousand and One Nights*, who introduced secondary narratives embedded in one another, when introducing several levels of secondary narrators within the primary narrative. In such cases Scheherazade gave an introductory sentence to the secondary narratives (e.g. 'and thus the Fisherman talked') and from that point on she continued with the new narrative. In the psychotherapeutic setting, such elaborated embedded structures of secondary narrations are rare. Pseudo-narrators take the floor for a much shorter extent, perhaps for a few sentences, and such shifts are usually accomplished by using the first-person singular, and direct speech, as if quoting the talk of a person other than the analysand or the analyst (i.e. the primary narrator), and talking in their voice (i.e. in the voice of the secondary narrator).

How do analysands and analysts use this perspective in psychoanalysis? And what is the function of shifting in and out of pseudo-diegesis from the point of view of the psychotherapy process? We will discuss these questions through examples of the use of pseudo-narrators taken from the Budapest Psychotherapy Database.

Before presenting examples of pseudo-diegesis from our database, we first note an early instance in the work of Sándor Ferenczi, who was using a shift to a pseudo-diegetic perspective as early as the turn of the twentieth century.

Sándor Ferenczi and the child analysis of adults

Sándor Ferenczi (1873–1933) was the main figure and founder, in 1913, of the Budapest School of Psychoanalysis, which operated between the early twentieth century and the Second World War. He also was one of the founders of the International Psychoanalytic Association. He had a great number of followers (e.g. Alice and Michael Balint, Géza Roheim, Melanie Klein, Sándor Radó, Margaret Mahler, René A. Spitz, Imre Hermann) and has influenced the way psychoanalysis has been practised ever since. Ferenczi was the first to emphasize the development of the relationship between analysand and analyst, and its mutual, interactive nature, as well as shedding new light on the problem of countertransference (Haynal 2011). Members of the Budapest School were also the first to focus on analytic work with children (practising child-play observation), and on early, pre-Oedipal influences, as well as on the role of the mother in infant and child development. During the Second World War, many of the members of the Budapest School emigrated to the US, Great Britain, or France due to the rise of anti-Semitism and fascism in Hungary. After the Second World War, the Budapest School was dissolved due to pressures from the communist regime (Haynal 2011). Today, the psychoanalytic traditions of the Budapest School are carried out in Hungary by the Hungarian Psychoanalytic Society and the Ferenczi Sándor Society.

In his essay entitled 'Child-analysis in the analysis of adults'—which Ferenzci first read before the Vienna Psycho-Analytical Society at a meeting to celebrate Professor Freud's seventy-fifth birthday on 6 May 1931—Ferenczi talks about a novel technique he introduced into his practice with 'deeply regressed' analysands. He writes about the inadequacy he discovered in the traditional analytic technique:

> Now in certain cases it transpired that the analyst's cool, waiting silence and his lack of any reaction had the effect of disturbing the freedom of association. The patient has barely reached the point of really forgetting himself and yielding up everything that is going on in his mind, when he suddenly rouses himself with a start from his absorbed state, and complains that he really cannot take the movement of his emotions seriously when he sees that I am sitting tranquilly behind him, smoking my cigarette and at most responding coolly

> and indifferently with the stereotyped question: 'Now what comes into your mind about this? (1931: 470)

Ferenczi goes on to say that he has tried to think of a better method for allowing the analysand more room for his repetition tendency to manifest spontaneously:

> But it was a very long time before the first suggestions came to me of how to do this and, once more, they came from the patients themselves. For example, a patient in the prime of life resolved, after overcoming strong resistances, and especially his profound mistrust, to revive in his mind incidents from his earliest childhood. Thanks to the light already thrown by analysis on his early life, I was aware that in the scene revived by him, he was identifying me with his grandfather. Suddenly, in the midst of what he was saying, he threw his arm round my neck and whispered in my ear: 'I say, Grandpapa, I am afraid I am going to have a baby!' Thereupon I had what seems to me a happy inspiration: I said nothing to him for the moment about transference, etc., but retorted, in a similar whisper: 'Well, but why do you think so ? (1931: 471)

In the dialogue reproduced by Ferenczi, his technique appears as a direct response to the analysand's shift into a character-level identification with his childhood self; Ferenczi mirrors this by speaking, also at the character level, in the role of the analysand's grandfather. In other words, the analyst responds to the analysand's perspective by taking the perspective of the grandfather and by shifting into pseudo-diegesis, and continuing talking to the analysand from that position.

Ferenczi further explains how he uses this technique:

> As you see, I was entering into a game, which we might call a game of questions and answers. This was perfectly analogous to the processes described to us by those who analyze children, and for some time this little device was quite successful. But you must not suppose that I am able in this kind of game to ask every sort of question. If the question is not simple enough, not really adapted to a child's comprehension, the dialogue is soon broken off, some patients even reproaching me straight out with having been clumsy and having, so to speak, spoilt the game. Often this has happened because I introduced into my questions and answers things of which the child, at that time, could not possibly have known. I met with even more decided rebuffs when I attempted to give learned, scientific interpretations. (1931: 471)

The technique of shifting into various pseudo-perspectives Ferenczi referred to as 'play-analysis'. According to his view, with this technique he was able to reach deep levels of involvement on the part of the patient. His analysand 'in the attempt to uncover the origin of his illness, suddenly lapses into a childish or child-like attitude' (1931: 471). He argued that psychoanalysis must aim at the reproduction of traumas associated with primary repression and symptom formation. In order to accomplish this, he used his technique of play analysis, which helped the analysands to shift into a deep regressive state. In his essay, Ferenczi questions the legitimacy of his new technique, arguing that simply shifting into the child-like state is not sufficient. The analyst later must accomplish the intellectual work with the material that has surfaced. He also argues that the technique of play analysis is not completely different from the way analysis is regularly practised:

> I think it is expedient to uncover the hidden tendencies to enactment as fully as possible, before setting about intellectual work on them and the training in self-control, which goes with this. You must catch your hare before you can cook him. So do not think that the analyses, which I sometimes bring down to the level of a game are fundamentally so very different from analysis as hitherto practiced. (1931: 473)

Ferenczi describes in the study how play analysis should be practised:

1. During the therapeutic hour after recounting events during the previous day or a regular dream analysis the analysand falls into a regressive state—that is when enactment may be used.
2. The enacted material must be worked on, and analysed intellectually, during the session.
3. During the enactment both analysand and analyst must stay in their roles.
4. The analyst must react to the patient differently than he/she had been treated in his/her family—'knowing himself safe from the repetition of such situations, he has the courage to let himself sink down into a reproduction of the painful past' (1931: 474).
5. Sometimes the analysand produces stories, little poems, drawings during play analysis, which the analyst should later analyse.
6. The phantasy play is similar to free association, and it should be encouraged by simple, open-ended questions on the part of the analyst. Hypnosis should not be used, but a kind of auto-hypnotic state may be achieved by the analysand.

So, Ferenczi outlined the basic requirements for his play therapy, which consists of an intense emotional, regressed trans-like state and an intellectual analysis of the material that surfaces during the enactment. The intense emotional state of the analysand may occur spontaneously, marking an important moment in the therapeutic process, by not merely remembering a childhood trauma, for instance, but in some way enacting it, reliving emotional reactions in a child-like state.

In this chapter we shall show, and argue, that pseudo-diegetic perspectives similar to that used in Ferenczi's play analysis spontaneously occur in psychoanalytic practice today, and analysts and analysands shift into such perspectives at times during narrative interaction taking place at the psychotherapy session. Both analysands and analysts use pseudo-diegetic perspectives in a variety of ways, and either of them may initiate the use of this perspective with differing functions in terms of the psychotherapy process. Further, we shall argue that the use of pseudo-diegesis marks an important moment of the therapeutic process, just like in Ferenczi's work, despite the fact that this technique is not consciously used by analysts in a premeditated way today (at least not by the analysts participating in the collection of the Budapest Database).

Among the forms of diegesis analysed in our studies, pseudo-diegesis is by far the least frequently used perspective (3–4% of the total use of diegesis variable). The spontaneous usage of this perspective by both analysand and analyst suggests that shifting into pseudo-diegesis expresses on the part of the speaker an identification with the person whose perspective they voice. At the same time, the functions of using pseudo-diegesis may be different in the case of the analysand and the analyst. When pseudo-diegesis is carried out by the analysand, identifications also provide a clue for the analyst that the voiced other plays an important role in the given narrative. When a pseudo-diegetic perspective is accomplished by the analyst, it usually has a function of furthering the psychotherapy process in an indirect way (e.g. expressing empathy, demonstrating a certain type of behaviour or thought process, wishing to achieve a corrective emotional experience with it).

From Ferenczi onward, the emergence of trauma and its associated dissociative states, along with the involuntary reactions and enactments they trigger in the analyst, as well as the manifestation of the analyst's own dissociative states in the analytic process and their impact on the analysand, have become central to relational work (Bromberg 1996). The decentred self, the multiplicity of self, individual self-states, or object-relational dyads and their interplay between the analyst and the analysand have, on the one hand, become a central focus of analytic attention and, on the other, a potential tool for intervention. This occurs when the analyst refrains from delivering interventions from the perspective of the analytic primary narrator and instead speaks on behalf of one of the figures in the analysand's narrative—talking in their voice (i.e. in the voice of the secondary narrator).

Recognizing the use of pseudo-diegesis on either the analysand's or the analyst's side can serve as a technical tool for identifying the activation of an individual self-state. When one participant begins speaking in the voice of the secondary narrator, it may indicate a shift towards a less integrated part of the self.

Lacan, in Seminar I of *Freud's Papers on Technique 1953–1954* (1988), poses the key question 'Who speaks in analyses?' He emphasizes the distinction between the subject of the enunciation (the unconscious 'speaker') and the subject of the statement (the conscious 'I' who speaks). This raises the question of who is the subject of the enunciation? It depends on the analyst's theoretical background and how they conceptualize the subject of enunciation. Whether the analysand or the analyst is speaking from the ego, superego, or id perspective; from a part-object in the here and now (Steiner 1984); from a particular self- or object-representation (Jacobson 1964); or from one side of an object-relational dyad (Kernberg 2016). Additionally, Ogden (1989) highlights the potential for shifting between the paranoid and schizoid positions, while others suggest that a person may speak from multiple subjective points of view or experience multiple subjectivities (Arnold 2005; Stolorow et al. 2002). As Bromberg proposes, these shifts can reflect varying degrees of dissociated self-states, ultimately leading to a multi-perspectival sense of personhood (Arnold 2005; Bromberg 1996).

Differences and similarities between play analysis and current use of pseudo-diegesis

The current use of pseudo-diegesis in psychoanalytic therapies today has some similar and some different features to the way it was used by the Budapest School therapists in the time of Ferenczi. In Table 6.1 we summarize the characteristics of currently used pseudo-diegesis compared to play analysis:

Examples of using pseudo-narration on the part of the client from the Budapest Psychotherapy Database

Our first example of the use of pseudo-diegesis is from the beginning phase of analysis with the female analysand–female analyst dyad. In Excerpt 6.1 the analysand describes a situation when she has applied to college for the second time (since she did not get in the first time), and she realized that high-school grades would not be required or counted into her total entrance scores. Upon learning this, she felt a strong sense of relief, since her scores from high-school

Table 6.1 Differences and similarities between Ferenczi's play analysis and the current use of pseudo-diegesis

	Play analysis	Current use of pseudo-diegesis
Differences	premeditated technique that the therapist aims to use at the session	spontaneously occurring technique
	initiated by analysand, responded to by analyst	may be initiated by analysand or analyst, the other interlocutor may respond or may not
	a relatively long role play during therapy, lasting for several utterances by both interlocutors	lasting for a relatively short extent, for one or two utterances
	deep trans-like state, intense emotional involvement	could be a trans-like, hypnotic state, or a state of mind, or a dissociative state, or somewhat intense emotional involvement
Similarities	the speaker shifts into pseudo-diegetic perspective	
	the speaker may use the first, second or third-person subject in pseudo-diegesis	

grades were not very good, and calculating them into her total scores would have lowered her chances of getting into her preferred university.

Excerpt 6.1 (L3)

574PAT:	hogy amikor én megláttam december hatodikán felvételi tájékoztatót,	that when I saw the entrance prospectus on December 6th
575PAT:	és bele volt írva,	and it said
576PAT:	hogy a hogy a Z-re nincsen hozott pont,	that that at Z. university there are no scores brought from high-school
577PAT:	a a az így+...	th that like...
578PAT:	akkor én így elsírtam magamat.	I cried then,
579PAT:	tehát az így nekem olyan volt,	well, for me it was like,
580PAT:	mint egy ilyen második esély az életben.	getting a second chance in life.
581PAT:	minthogyha így levettek volna minden keresztet a vállamról.	as if all crosses had been taken off of my shoulders.

582PAT:	tehát hogy így nem nem kell továb hurcolnom magammal a+…	well, that like I did not did not have to continue carrying it with me the+…
583PAT:	azt hogy én így még ilyen béna vagyok,	that I am like still such a a cripple,
584PAT:	aki nem tud tanulni,	who is unable to study,
585PAT:	és nem tud teljesíteni,	who is unable to achieve,
586PAT:	és egyébként is,	and anyways,
587PAT:	csak így halálra szorongja magát,	she is only worrying herself to death,
588PAT:	tehát hogyha bármilyen témáról van szó.	well, about any topic under discussion.

At the beginning of the excerpt (lines 574–80) Clara describes her sense of relief, when she learned that she might indeed have a chance of getting into university (if high-school scores were not required). As she states, it was for her a second chance in life. The fact that she felt so strongly about this might be explained by her family background: a middle-class intellectual family, where university education was considered necessary—as becomes obvious from the rest of this session (not quoted here). In lines 574–80 she uses the first-person singular, homo-diegetic perspective, past tense. The analyst does not interrupt the analysand's monologue. The analysand, however, explains why she had felt so strongly about her university education: it was a proof that she was not a 'cripple'. In lines 584–88 she describes what this word means to her, and she—while talking about herself—shifts into the third-person singular, present tense, pseudo-diegesis. She speaks about herself as if talking in the voice of someone else, who expresses a very harsh criticism of her. We do not know from the text who these authority figures might be, whose hypothetical words are quoted by the analysand. It is also possible that this shift of perspective signals an activation of a dissociated part of herself. So, the pseudo-diegetic perspective here signals an important distinction between her past self (the 'cripple'), and her present self after being accepted to the university.

In a previous study (Berán & Unoka 2005) with an analysand suffering from dissociative personality disorder, we have shown how memories related to various personality states are expressed using different character-level positions and can be reunited using the narrator-level perspective. In Clara's case, she is already using the narrator-level perspective here. So, in order to question her negative beliefs about herself, she needs to reevaluate some autobiographical episodic memories to challenge her beliefs—and, therefore, she needs to work on those memories at the character level. So, her global negative self-evaluation could be questioned by activating character-level episodic memories, which contradict or modify the negative view of herself. For example, the repeated failures in high school may lead to a negative view of her learning abilities, which could be modified by doing well on her university entrance exam and getting into her chosen college. It is interesting to note here a social and cultural aspect of the analysand's view of herself, which is based on, or influenced by, the system of calculating university entrance scores. The recognition of a pseudo-diegetic manifestation serves as a technical warning sign for the analyst, indicating that the analysand is speaking on behalf of someone else. This carries the risk that the unintegrated part may become conflated with the analyst as the 'other'. When such a strongly self-critical self-part is activated in the analytic dialogue without the analyst drawing attention to it or responding to it, there is a risk that the analyst, as someone positioned ahead of the analysand in academic achievement, may implicitly signal agreement with this self-part through their silence.

Excerpt 6.2 is also from another session of the female analyst dyad from the beginning phase of analysis. By taking on her perspective in the form of pseudo-narration, we can see that the analysand is identifying with her envied sibling. In the excerpt below, the analysand is recounting her feelings of envy towards her younger sister, K.

Excerpt 6.2 (L2)

743PAT:	és amikor így irígykedek,	and when I am envious like this,
744PAT:	akkor így+…	then like,
745PAT:	nagyon csúnyán viselkedem.	I act very badly.
746PAT:	nem.	no.
747PAT:	én+…	I+…
748%com:	pause 21 sec	
749PAT:	nem is tudom.	I don't know.
750PAT:	keresek egy jó példát.	I'm looking for a suitable example.
751TER:	jó.	OK.
752%com:	pause	
753PAT:	tehát nem tudom például,	so I don't know, for example,
754PAT:	nagyon sokáig így semmit nem +…	for a long time I did not,
755PAT:	+, nem osztotam meg a K.	I did not share anything with K.

756PAT:	gyerekkoromban.	when I was a child.
757PAT:	tehát hogy+...	well, like
758PAT:	hogy nem engedtem hogy használja a színes ceruzáimat,	like I did not let her use my colored pencils,
759PAT:	meg +...	and+...
760PAT:	meg nem olvashatta a könyveimet,	and she was not allowed to read my books,
761PAT:	meg nem vehette fel a ruháimat,	and she could not put on my clothes,
762PAT:	meg így ilyenek.	and the like.
763PAT:	és aztán meg így arra emlékszem,	and then like I remember,
764PAT:	hogy így egyszer megyünk az utcán, down the street,	that once we are like walking
765PAT:	és így a K. úgy mondja hogy így	and like K says, like that
766PAT:	hogy de hogy+...	that but that+...
767PAT:	csak így mondja +...	she simply says+...
768PAT:	hogy akkor használd nyugodtan az én ceruzáimat.	that it's cool if you use my pencils,
769PAT:	meg hogy így vedd fel nyugodtan and az én ruhámat.	that it's cool if you put on my clothes.
770PAT:	és hogy így akkor nagyon így belém nyilallt,	and it suddenly occurred to me,
771PAT:	hogy én akkor így lehet hogy őt nem szeretem?	that then is it possible like that I do not love her?

In this narrative the analysand is recounting an episode from her childhood, when she has questioned her feelings towards her sister. This seems to have been an 'aha' moment for her, perhaps even a turning point in her relationship with her sister, which she remembers very vividly. As she recollects her episodic memories of the event and reconstructs the scene, she is able to directly quote her conversation with her sister, especially her sister's words, as we can see in lines 768–69. Here the analysand uses a pseudo-diegetic perspective not only as a rhetorical device (Tannen 2007) in order to recreate past events for the listener (i.e. the analyst) more vividly and accurately, but also identifying with the point of view of her sister, and taking on and expressing K's point of view—shifting into her perspective for a short while. In addition, in order to reconstruct the episode even more vividly, the analysand uses the present tense instead of the past tense in describing a past event in lines 764–69. This use of verb tense signals more intense emotional involvement on the part of the narrator and is also supposed to serve as creating more involvement on the part of the listener (Pólya et al. 2007; Schiffrin 1981; Tannen 2007; Wolfson 1979). The analysand also uses character-level perspective while recollecting a one-time specific event, an episodic memory she experienced with her sister. This also points towards a more intense affective involvement on the part of the narrator, as we discussed in our previous study (Berán, Czobor & Unoka 2017).

Regarding the psychotherapy process underlying Excerpt 6.2, we argue that by identifying with her sister's perspective, their emotional relationship became available for the analysand, and she began to use mentalization—shown by the internal focalization mode used in lines 770–71—understanding her sister's kind feelings towards her. This made it possible to compare her own feelings towards her sister with her sister's feelings towards herself, leading to a questioning of her own emotions. The therapist's openness to listening to the analysand's emotions towards her sister reflects the reciprocal process of active engagement with the states of mind of 'the other'. This engagement enables the patient's present-moment perception of self to integrate and coexist with previously dissociated, incompatible self-narratives (Bromberg 1996).

Excerpt 6.3 is from the same session; continuing the topic of sibling rivalry, the analysand recounts memories of aggression and jealousy between her and her sister, and summarizes their parents' attitude:

Excerpt 6.3 (L2)

873PAT:	hogy nálunk az volt a szlogen,	in our house the slogan was
874PAT:	otthon,	at home,
875PAT:	hogy azt vallotta a mama,	believed by Mama
876PAT:	meg a papa is,	and by Papa as well,
877PAT:	hogy+…	that+…
878PAT:	+ahány pofon elcsattan gyerekkorban,	+the more slaps are banged in childhood,
879PAT:	annyi utálatos veszekedést és gonoszságot spóroltok meg felnőtt korban.	you guys, save yourselves many repulsive quarrels and evil-doings in adulthood.

In lines 878–79 we can see that the parents' handed-down wisdom is quoted by the client word by word, using present tense and direct speech as if they were telling it to her at the present moment, in the here and now. This is, again, used as a rhetorical device, making the parent's voice more vivid and authentic, as well as displaying identification with the parents' point of view by quoting their words and taking their perspective.

So, examining Excerpts 6.2 and 6.3, we can differentiate two main functions of shifting into pseudo-diegesis by the client at the session: 1) a rhetorical function, and 2) an identification function. The rhetorical function of pseudo-diegesis is related to recreating the scenes or past events more authentically and vividly. The use of pseudo-diegesis is often accompanied by the use of the present tense and character level, and thus the heightened emotional involvement of the interlocutors: the narrator (analysand) and the listener (analyst). Whereas the function of identifying with the persons quoted in direct speech signals the importance of the memories reconstructed and their heightened relevance to the topic of discussion, namely dealing with sibling rivalry, as well as the aroused negative emotions of envy, jealousy, and aggression. This may also point to the activation of an unintegrated self-state.

Both the rhetorical and the identification functions are contributing to the therapeutic process in an inter-related way:

1. Shifting into pseudo-diegesis recreates the past event more vividly and authentically. The use of pseudo-diegesis is associated with perspectives signalling higher levels of affective involvement by the narrator and the listener (e.g. the present tense, character level, first person). As we discussed in our earlier study (Berán et al. 2017) affect regulation and alternation of high and low levels of affective involvement of the analysand's and the analyst's self during the psychotherapy session is one of the key elements of effective psychotherapy. It has been shown by previous studies that emotionally rich and more abstract or intellectual sequences alternate during the psychotherapy session (Bucci 1995, 2001, 2018; Buchheim & Mergenthaler 2000; Mergenthaler 1996; Thomä & Kächele 2006; Yalom 1995). The analyst and the analysand aim to regulate the affective involvement of themselves and the other, trying to keep it at an optimal level at a given moment of the session (Berán et al. 2017). High levels of affective involvement allow for the intense reliving of past experiences involved in the reconstruction of memories, whereas lower levels of involvement and more abstract discussions allow for the elaboration of thoughts and associations related to the memories reconstructed at the session and allow for a calmer discussion of relevant issues. The task of affect regulation may be accomplished by the shifting of NP on the part of the therapist and the analysand—as we discussed in detail in our previous study (Berán et al. 2017). Shifting into pseudo-diegesis may

be used as a rhetorical device to help relive memories with more intense affect precisely because the narrator identifies with a character of the narrated story, namely the person whose words are directly quoted by them.

2. Identification with the quoted characters and taking the perspective of those characters allows for an emotional and cognitive reaction in the narrator as well as in the listener. As we have seen in Excerpts 6.2 and 6.3, the persons the analysand identified with using the perspective of pseudo-diegesis were highly relevant regarding the theme under discussion in this part of the session (i.e. sibling rivalry): her sister and her parents. The two cases of pseudo-diegesis involve these persons, with decisive ideas about their attitude towards sibling rivalry, which the analysand seems to consider very important and arguably different from (in Excerpt 6.2) or identical to (in Excerpt 6.3) her own attitude about the subject. The representations of these ideas in the narrative episodes the analysand recollects in association with the rivalry between her and her sister are in the form of concise quotations. However different her own attitude might be from the views of her immediate family, she identifies with their view in pseudo-diegesis, thus showing continuity or a lack of boundaries with them.

The analyst's reaction to the analysand's pseudo-diegetic perspective is rather minimal in the case of Excerpt 6.2, reducing her responses to listening cues (*hm, yes*), whereas following Excerpt 6.3 she asks the analysand several clarifying questions about the parents' '*ideology*':

Excerpt 6.4 (L2)

885TER:	ez a testvér kapcsolatokra vonatkozik?	Is this applied to sibling relations?
886TER:	ez a+...	this+...
887TER:	+, ideológia?	+, ideology?
888PAT:	ezt nem tudom.	I do not know.
889PAT:	ez ránk vonatkozott.	it was applied to us.
890TER:	te tehát hogy testvérek ha+...	so so that the siblings, if
891TER:	gyerekkorban püfölhetik egymást,	they can beat each other up in childhood,
892PAT:	aha.	uhm.
893TER:	akkor felnőtt korban már nem+/	then they won't do it in adulthood+/
894PAT:	jóba lesznek.	they will have a good relationship.

895TER:	jóba lesznek.	they will have a good relationship.
896TER:	aha.	uhm.

The analyst's questions show that she considered this information important for therapeutic progress, which, again, supports our previous point: the use of pseudo-diegesis may reveal important information about the analysand's identifications, and its use contributes to the psychotherapy process. This later point is, perhaps, even more unequivocal in the analyst's use of a pseudo-diegetic narrator, towards which we will turn now. By repeating the parental message expressed by the patient in the dissociated self-state after posing a question to the analysand in the position of the primary narrator, the analyst creates an opportunity for the analysand to reflect on the statements of the dissociated self-state from the position of the primary narrator.

Examples of using pseudo-narration on the part of the analyst from the Budapest Psychotherapy Database

Continuing the analysand's utterance

There are various discursive situations in which the analyst may use pseudo-diegesis: they may end the analysand's utterances, identifying with the analysand; repeat the analysand's utterance; use the same pseudo-narrator the analysand used previously, taking on their perspective.

In Excerpt 6.5 (Berán & Unoka 2015)—with the male client and male therapist dyad—the analysand and analyst discuss the analysand's relationship with workplace colleagues at the session from the beginning phase of therapy. The analysand is unemployed at the time. Following the analyst's initial orienting questions, the analysand talks in great detail about his various conflicts at his previous jobs. He emphasizes that he had a very complicated relationship with female bosses in comparison with male ones.

Excerpt 6.5 (F4)

565PAT:	az életbe is úgy van,	in life it's also like that,
566PAT:	hogy nincs az, hogy mindenkit szeretünk,	it's not like that we like everyone
567PAT:	vagy mindenkivel jól ki tudunk jönni,	or that we get along with everybody.
568PAT:	nem?	no?

569PAT:	vagy mindenkivel szimpatikusak vagyunk kölcsönösen egymásnak.	or that we are mutually, sympathetic with everyone.
570PAT:	de hogy férfi főnököknek ez az arány ez úgy kábé megfelelt a+...	but with male bosses this proportion was about+...
571TER:	az átlagnak.	average.
572PAT:	az átlagnak.	average.
573PAT:	tehát hogy a társadalomban átlagosan előfordulóan ló aránynak.	that is, the average proportion it occurs in society.
574PAT:	de női főnökökkel nem.	but not with female bosses.

In Excerpt 6.5 at the beginning the narrator (analysand) talks in general terms, using the narrator level. During his analytic conversations, it was characteristic for this analysand to use the narrator level in the beginning phase of therapy (Berán & Unoka 2017). In line 571 the therapist interrupts the client's sentence by finishing it with a suitable word: 'average', which the analysand repeats in his next utterance. This type of discourse activity is not uniquely characteristic of therapeutic discourse, it occurs in everyday conversation as well (Coates 1998; Tannen 2007) and suggestive of the listener's attention and anticipation of what the speaker will say in the next few milliseconds; so, it is evidence of the attunement of the interlocutors, as well as empathic relating on the part of the listener. Such indirect expression of his close attention on the part of the analyst may encourage the analysand to continue talking, and may contribute to a warm atmosphere where the analysand feels important and accepted as a person, being validated by the analyst.

Excerpt 6.6 (Berán & Unoka 2015) is another example of the same discourse strategy: we can observe how the analyst continues the analysand's sentence when he is confronted by difficult negative emotions related to the sensitive issue of having his own children:

Excerpt 6.6 (F4)

110TER:	<mely>melyik /része,	so, <which> /part
111TER:	ennek az egész komplex szituációnak az ami leginkább taszítja?	of the whole, complex situation repulses you most?
112TER:	(te)hát teszem azt az hogy akkor magának egy /utódja keletkezik,	well, let us say that you have an /offspring,

113TER:	aki hasonlít magára,	who looks like you.
114TER:	/vagy.	/or.
115%com:	ter cough	
116TER:	az, hogy+//	that+//
117PAT:	maga a tény úgy általában,	the fact itself in general,
118PAT:	és hogy ennek mi az oka az+/	and what causes this is that+/
119PAT:	(de)hát a multkor már itt érintettem, hogy+...	but last time I have already mentioned that+...
120PAT:	hogy amit úgy rá tudtam eddig élni magamban–,	that what I could experience experience in myself–,
121PAT:	az az /ez hogy +..	that that /this that–...
122PAT:	hogy+/	that+/
123PAT:	igen ez nagyon erős hogy+//	this is very strong that+//
124PAT:	hogy egy utód aki hasonlít rám,	an offspring, who is similar to me,
125PAT:	hogy az ne +..	**that should not+...**
126TER:	+, hogy (az) ne keletkezzen?	**+, should not be created?**
127PAT:	igen.	yes.

In Excerpt 6.6, answering the analyst's question (lines 110–16) the analysand is talking about himself and his emotions in general terms, using the narrator level (lines 117, 120–23). He has difficulty expressing his views (lines 118–23), several times interrupting himself while attempting to formulate precisely how he feels about having children, with a broken intonation unit (line 125), when finally the analyst jumps onto the floor (line 126) and finishes the analysand's sentence, providing the missing words: 'should not be created'. The analyst's help, the completion of the sentence, expresses a very serious statement, created in cooperation with the analysand, at the narrator level. The analysand agrees with the analyst's choice of words (and probably meaning), which he expresses in line 127, again at the narrator level. This latter perspective is suitable for expressing long-standing, general views or states of affairs and also for integrating various aspects of experience. At this level, the analysand is able to formulate into symbols (i.e. words) one major concern of his, which would be worked on during much of the remaining part of the session. The analyst's move in line 126, again, shows evidence of a fine attunement between the interlocutors, and ensures the analysand about the analyst's attention, and his emotional support in dealing with difficult emotions.

In order to reveal the importance of the statement of lines 125–26 from a clinical point of view, we will follow the continuation of this discussion in

Excerpt 6.7—although there is no pseudo-diegesis used in this section. In the continuation, the analyst helps the analysand to a deeper understanding of his emotions towards having or not having children:

Excerpt 6.7 (F4)

128PAT:	tehát nem érzem magam # # # # +..	so I don't feel like# # # # +..
129TER:	&=pant (hogy) itten ilyen [<] <amerikaiassan> fogalmazzunk+...	to put it in the American way+...
130PAT:	+, olyannak+//[>]	+, such+//[>]
131TER:	annyira nem szereti /magát,	you do not like /yourself as much
132TER:	hogy # # ebből nem kell még egy /másik példány? # #	as to need /another copy of this?
133PAT:	nem hogy úgy annyira /nem szeretem magam-'	It's not that I do not like myself as much–,
134PAT:	hanem hogy /annyira nem szeretem magam.	but rather that I dislike myself so much.
135TER:	aha.	uhm.
136PAT:	tehát,	well,
137%com:	pause 4s	
138PAT:	gondolom érti hogy mire ér [/] gondolok,	I guess you know what I'm mea[/] thinking,

In Excerpt 6.7, the analysand is aiming for a more exact reformulation of what was said previously about his feelings towards having children of his own. However, he is being stalled again (line 128) and, after a few seconds of silence, the analyst interrupts his utterance, there are a few seconds of overlapping speech, after which the analyst formulates in lines 131–32 what he considers to be the analysand's ideas. At this point, the therapist uses hetero-diegesis (not pseudo-diegesis), talking to the analysand in the second person, staying at the narrator level. By using this perspective, the analyst points to the analysand as an agent of his own, without 'fusing' with his perspective, as he did when using pseudo-diegesis. In lines 133–34 the analysand reformulates what the analyst said in a way that he feels more precisely fits his emotions, also at the narrator level. This clarification adds another layer to the analysand's self-understanding, because now he states clearly that the reason he does not want to have children is his self-loathing. Since this session takes place at the beginning phase of psychotherapy, this insight on the part of the analysand is very useful for deciding on further directions of treatment, and opens up further questions regarding the self-hate of the analysand (e.g. its sources and manifestations in other areas of functioning). We would like to argue that the use of pseudo-diegesis in Excerpt 6.7 has contributed to this realization of the analysand and hence advanced the therapeutic process.

Continuing the analysand's utterance is one frequent way the analyst can express their close attention, helpfulness, and indirectly his understanding of what the analysand is trying to communicate. This can further the therapeutic goals, especially with difficult topics, or when the analysand has difficulty formulating what they want to say. Continuing and completing the analysand's utterance also expresses an identification with the analysand, with the analyst taking on their perspective. This indirectly expresses a feeling of empathy with the analysand, which may even strengthen the therapeutic alliance, and hence contribute to the therapeutic goals.

Repeating the analysand's utterance

Another way for the analyst to use pseudo-diegesis is speaking for and in the voice of the analysand: repeating his/her sentence verbatim, indicating empathic relating and careful listening. Excerpt 6.8 (Berán & Unoka 2015) is from the psychoanalysis of the male analysand and male analyst dyad, from the working phase of therapy, at the end of the observation period. The analysand has a conflictual relationship with his mother but, after moving away from her apartment, he recounts some friendly interactions between him and his mother, showing a positive aspect of the relationship. The story, which he narrates to the analyst, is that he has bought some new chairs into his new apartment that he had shown to his mother. She liked the chairs, and so he had promised to buy a few for her.

Excerpt 6.8 (F32)

1043PAT:	azt mondja hadd próbáljam már ki,	she says, let me try it then,
1044PAT:	és tényleg kipróbálta,	and she indeed tried it
1045PAT:	azt mondja hű ez tényleg kényelmes.	she says well, this is indeed comfortable.
1046PAT:	ő is vesz majd ilyet a konyhába.	she will also by this for her kitchen.
1047PAT:	mondom ne vegyél,	I say don't buy it.

1048PAT:	majd én elmegyek veszek.	I will go and buy it.
1049PAT:	azt tényleg elmentem vettem.	and I really went and bought it.
1050PAT:	odavittem.	I brought them there.
1051PAT:	tegnap odamentem.	I went there yesterday.
1052PAT:	ja és kiderült közbe hogy anyáknapja van,	oh, and it turned out that it was Mother's Day,
1053PAT:	mondom akkor ezt megkapod anyáknapjára.	Then you can get this for Mother's Day says I.
1054PAT:	érti?	You know?
1055PAT:	és akkor meg se tudott+//	and then she could not even+//
1056TER:	és mit szólt hozzá?	and what was her reaction?
1057PAT:	hát hogy köszöni szépen,	well that she thanks it very much,
1058PAT:	meg hogy+/	and that+/
1059PAT:	érti?	do you understand?
1060TER:	meg hogy?	and that?
1061TER:	meg hogy?	and that?
1062PAT:	hogy köszöni szépen,	and that she thanks it very much,
1063PAT:	és hogy örül,	and that she is happy,
1064PAT:	és hogy de jól néz az ott ki.	and that it looks so good over there.
1065TER:	ühm.	uhm.

In Excerpt 6.8 the analysand recounts the episode with his mother with an intense vividness. The perspective he uses at the beginning of the episode is that of the character level (lines 143–48), using both the present tense—when quoting his mother or his own words—and the past tense. In lines 1043 and 1045 the analysand uses pseudo-diegesis, talking in his mother's name. These perspectives suggest an intense affective involvement on his part. While the analysand continues recounting the events, the analyst in line 1056 asks about the mother's reaction to the gift, interrupting the analysand's story-telling, using an outside point of view (hetero-diegesis), the third-person singular and past tense—and, by doing so, he down-regulates the analysand's heightened level of affective involvement. The analyst's question in line 1056 on the one hand signals his close attention towards the client's story, and on the other hand draws the analysand's attention to the importance of the mother's reaction, which, at this time have had an emotionally positive tone.

In lines 1057–58 the analysand continues his story, but he is stalled again, and in line 1059 he stops recounting the mother's reaction and reaches out to the analyst, asking for a confirmation from him: 'do you understand?' By doing this, he steps out of the story world to the here and now of the analytic session. The analyst at this point repeats the analysand's previous statement in line 1058, repeating it twice in lines 1060–61 in question form. By repeating the analysand's words, he takes on the analysand's point of view, using the same perspective the analysand has used previously. This use of perspective expresses an identification with the analysand, and a form of empathy on the part of the analyst, which he may use in order to encourage the analysand to continue the story, and to answer the analysand's question: 'do you understand?' in an indirect way.

In lines 1062–64 the client answers the therapist's question, recounting his mother's positive reaction to his gift in the form of indirect quotations of what the mother has said—which signals a more distant position from his mother than the complete identification of pseudo-diegesis he used at the beginning of recounting this story (lines 1043–45).

This story represents an important achievement regarding the client's psychotherapy process, because at this time he talks about an understanding mother, who is grateful for his son's gifts, while previously he mainly recounted his adversarial relationship with her. After the recounting of this 'chair story' the analyst and analysand discuss in great detail the possible conclusions that could be drawn from this episode, the analyst emphasizing the positive side of the interaction with the mother, whereas the analysand gives a more sceptical explanation: her mother only behaved kindly towards him because other people were present as well. The analyst, however, also emphasizes the analysand's ability to recount past events with his mother in a more positive light, which suggest a less negative view of the analysand's relationship with her.

Using the same pseudo-narrator the analysand has used previously

Another opportunity for the analyst to use pseudo-diegesis in his interaction with the analysand is repeating their use of the pseudo-narrator, in other words using the same pseudo-narrator they have used previously.

Excerpt 6.9 (Berán & Unoka 2015) is an illustration of this opportunity. It was taken from the beginning phase of psychoanalysis, with the male analysand–male analyst dyad. The excerpt is from the same session we have quoted above (F4), when the analysand discusses difficulties related to his job and work colleagues, especially female bosses. Later in the session, however, he talks about his experiences with a male boss, with whom he recounts numerous conflicts and negative experiences at work. In this job, where he held an important position, he felt his male boss disliked him, treated him unjustly, and embarrassed him in front of his colleagues at workplace meetings.

Excerpt 6.9 (F4)

660PAT:	az ilyen összhivatali értekezleten a beszéljük meg a K.S. ügyét típusú témák.	in like the fused office meetings topics like let us discuss the issue of S.K.
661TER:	aha.	uhm.
662TER:	mond- mondjon egy példát,	give me an example,
663TER:	hogy például mi volt mi volt egy ilyen ügy.	what it was like, such an issue.
664TER:	milyen volt a K.S. ügye?	what was it like the issue of S.K.?
665PAT:	hát ilyenkor aztán+...	well, in such a situation+...
666PAT:	+, állandóan olyanok voltak,	+, it was always like,
667PAT:	és mondom hogy ilyen összhivatali értekezleten+...	and I am telling you at the fused-office meetings +...
668TER:	aha,-	uhm,-
669PAT:	+, amik engem úgy arra emlékeztettek,	+, which reminded me,
670PAT:	amit persze csak ilyen olvasmány élményekből,	of course only from what we know from reading experiences,
671PAT:	vagy filmélményekből tudunk,	or from movie experiences,
672PAT:	így az ötvenes évekről,	about the fifties,
673PAT:	amikor igy a vállalati értekezleteken+/	when at company meetings+/
674PAT:	nem?	no?
675PAT:	most akkor jól megbíráljuk a+//	now we are going to criticize properly the+//
676TER:	szégyenpadra ültetjük+...	we let him sit at the dunce's seat+...
677PAT:	igen.	yes.
678PAT:	teljesen ilyen volt.	it was completely like that.

In Excerpt 6.9 the analysand talks about situations when he had been humiliated at his workplace. It is not about one specific event (i.e. the character level), but about repeated episodes of such events (the narrator level). In line 662 the analyst asks for a concrete example of humiliation in order to clarify what the analysand meant by such a situation. In other words, the analyst is attempting to make the analysand shift his perspective into the character level. However, the analysand remains at the narrator level, and in lines 665–75 he explains his situation with the help of a parallel from what was a well-known practice in the 1950s.

In 1950s Eastern Europe, criticism by Communist Party members was used as a method to point people who supposedly diverged from mainstream party ideology and behaviour in the right direction. This practice also took place at workplaces and in schools. There was a general tendency to distrust people who talked or behaved differently from party directives and guidelines—suspecting them of being traitors, spies, or simply preferring capitalist values to those of communism. Divergence from party guidelines in speech, ideas, or behaviour was taken seriously and was punished by criticism, humiliation or—in the worst cases—imprisonment.

In line 675 the analysand uses pseudo-diegesis, talking in the voice of hypothetical members of the Communist Party, quoting their hypothetical words directly. The analysand's allusion to the 1950s was understood and picked up by the analyst, which is evidenced by his statement in line 676. In this utterance, just like the analysand, he also refers to a statement by a hypothetical Communist Party member, similar in content to the analysand's quotation. So, the analyst's statement is a continuation of the analysand's, using the same pseudo-diegetic narrator as voiced by the analysand. In this way, the analyst expresses his understanding of what the analysand is trying to convey by using the pseudo-diegetic perspective. In addition, he also expresses his empathy with the analysand's situation being humiliated in such a way—unjustly, as the allusion to movies and books implies, which usually condemn or make fun of such practices in the 1950s—by taking on the analysand's perspective.

In lines 677–78 the analysand agrees with the analyst, and refers back to the atmosphere and his own situation at the workplace meetings by saying that 'it was completely like that'. By this statement, he also implies that the analyst understood and interpreted his situation correctly.

Speaking in the voice of the analysand

Another way of the analyst using pseudo-diegesis is when they speak in the voice of the analysand, not repeating or continuing their utterance, but creating a completely new statement in their perspective, using the first-person singular ('I' as a subject). Excerpt 6.10 (Berán & Unoka 2015) is from the psychotherapy of the male analysand–male analyst dyad, from the middle of the observation period, and from the working phase of psychotherapy. At the beginning of the session, the analysand is complaining about the use of the audio-recorder used for the purpose of this research. He dislikes it, and he thinks that it is bothersome even for the analyst, disturbing the therapeutic work. He describes in detail distortions of the therapeutic conversation that he attributes to the therapeutic hour being 'listened in on' by strangers (i.e. the researchers), who do not understand what is going on, and therefore may misinterpret his words, or what he wants to say. Later, he associates to his childhood, being misinterpreted by family members as a form of invalidation. He argues that, if one is used to their words being intentionally misconstrued by family member, they will be very careful in formulating their ideas while talking. In Excerpt 6.10 he continues to elaborate on that point.

Excerpt 6.10 (session F.21)

478PAT:	tehát hogy az úgy,	well, that like,
479PAT:	az úgy+…	that like+…
480PAT:	az úgy azér hoz egy ilyet,	that like brings such a thing
481PAT:	hogy az ember olyan–,	that you are like–,
482PAT:	jobban fél tőle azér.	you are even more worried.
483PAT:	tehát rögtön arra gondolok,	so I immediately think,
484PAT:	hogy hú de a másik abba mit fog tudni belemagyarázni.	wow what will be another able to misconstrue into that.
485TER:	szóval egy ilyen alapállás,	well, there is such a basic stance,
486TER:	hogy bele akarnak magyarázni valamit abba amit mondok.	that they want to misconstrue what I say.
487PAT:	igen, ilyenem van.	yes, I have such a stance.
488TER:	hmm.	hmm.

In Excerpt 6.10, in lines 478–82, the analysand refers to his previous statements describing his being 'jumped on' in case he says something that can be misconstrued or misunderstood. In lines 483–84 he uses the present tense and the level of here and now of the session to express his constant fear of being misconstrued by others. In lines 485–86 the analyst reformulates the analysand's words, shifting into the first-person singular, pseudo-diegesis, speaking for and in the voice of the analysand: 'they want to misconstrue what I say'. By taking the analysand's perspective in the present tense, the analyst here enters the world of the pseudo-narrative identifying, almost fusing with the analysand's position.

This expresses his very strong empathy towards the analysand and an understanding of his situation and acceptance of his feelings. At the same time, this is also a demonstration to the analysand of the acceptance of his basic beliefs, showing that he can embrace his potential shortcomings. By expressing this latter message to the analysand, the analyst provides an example of a perspective, which the analysand can take on, in case he chooses to. In line 487, the analysand responds to the analyst in a lower, almost whispering voice, and admits that he has such a stance, taking on the analyst's perspective. The analyst confirms the analysand's position in line 488 in the form of a minimal response, a listening clue.

Conclusion

Through the examples of the use of pseudo-diegesis in this chapter, we have demonstrated how varied the use of this perspective is in form and function in current psychotherapeutic practice, and how the use of this perspective contributes to the psychotherapy process. The analysands and analysts of the Budapest Psychotherapy Database use these formulations spontaneously, and unplanned—in contrast to how Ferenczi used his play-therapy technique. In summary, we can say that we have found several different forms of using pseudo-diegesis by the analysand and analyst: quoting/voicing a character from the analysand's self-narrative by the analysand, continuing the analysand's utterance by the analyst, repeating the analysand's words by the analyst, talking in the analysand's voice by the analyst, using the same pseudo-narrator the analysand used previously. We have also distinguished the two main functions of the use of pseudo-diegesis in the Budapest data: 1) the rhetorical function, and 2) the identification function. The rhetorical function serves to express and relive emotions, and involvement, as well as express authenticity. The identification function on the part of the analysand serves to express empathy or fusion with a character of his/her stories, and on the part of the analyst to express empathy for the analysand and/or demonstrate possible ways of behaviour or modes of thinking.

The use of pseudo-diegesis may reflect the activation of a self-state, which represents a more or less dissociated part of the self. Drawing on Sándor Ferenczi's concept of child analysis in the analysis of adults, we have identified the presence of pseudo-diegesis in both the analysand's and the analyst's speech. This phenomenon may indicate that internal object relations and multiple self-states are unconsciously dramatized and brought to life within the analytic process. The enacted aspects of these self-states contribute to the relational, intersubjective field, shaping how the analyst and analysand engage in a system of mutual regulation (Aron & Atlas 2019).

7 Long-term changes in interpersonal relating

The study of structural change in long-term psychoanalytic psychotherapy includes the examination of change in the quality of interpersonal relationships by examining markers of how the self functions in interpersonal relationships: how much joy the analysand finds in relationships, how they operate in important relationships, whether they find others generally well intentioned and helpful or malicious and problematic, and so on, before and after the psychotherapeutic treatment (McFarquhar et al. 2018; Solbakken & Abbass 2015; Weiner & Exner 1991). Other studies examine the working alliance between analysand and analyst (e.g. Fried et al. 1990; Gelso & Hayes 1998; Luborsky 1994; Norcross & Lambert 2018), which may also undergo changes during treatment. While psychotherapeutic outcome research aims at measuring these dimensions, psychotherapy process research focuses on the question of how and why the change in the quality of relating to others occurs during psychotherapy (Spence, O'Shea & Donovan 2016; Thomä & Kächele 2007). Research on both of these questions has become increasingly significant in the past few decades as it has been shown that one strong predictor of adult well-being is social support in everyday situations and in crisis (Burt 1987; Eisenberger & Cole 2012; Walker & McGlone 2013); thus the improvement of relationship quality is an important goal for various types of psychotherapies, including psychoanalysis, and it is also a signal of successful treatment (Lambert & Barley 2001).

This chapter explores how interpersonal relationships can be described in in-session narratives and whether changes in such narrative structures are detectible in the data of the Budapest Psychotherapy Database by the end of the 1.5-year observation period. Further, the chapter also discusses the discursive strategies analysts use to promote change in interpersonal relating in terms of shifting perspectives during the joint construction of narratives of relationship episodes. Below, we first describe Luborsky's theory of Core Conflictual Relationship Theme (CCRT) (1977, 1990) and the quantitative method of analysing interpersonal relationships in in-session narrative interaction. Following this, we describe the methodology of applying Luborsky's method to the Budapest Psychotherapy data to analyse long-term changes in the analysand's way of relating to others and the self. We illustrate the psychotherapy process behind long-term changes by analysing narrative perspective (NP) shifting in excerpts from the female analysand–female analyst dyad.

As for our research strategy, we first highlight sessions where a change in relating to others or the self is evidenced by using the CCRT method. This step is followed by a more contextualized discourse analysis of the sessions, where the change in patterns of NP occurs in the speech of both the analysand and analyst. We also give examples of how the analyst may influence the unfolding of the analysand's narrative through her interventions, using the coordination of perspectives or, in other words, the interactive regulation of NP.

Luborsky's Core Conflictual Relationship Theme method

According to Luborsky and colleagues (Barber et al. 1990), repetitive experiences of interpersonal relationships over a long period of time become crystallized into stories they have labelled 'relationship episodes'. Relationship episodes are short narratives about our social interactions often told during everyday conversations and in psychotherapeutic settings, such as psychoanalysis. Luborsky's method organizes these narratives according to a specific schema. According to this view, the analysand's narratives of interpersonal relationships are organized by prototypical subject–object–act relations, focusing on three important aspects of such narratives:

1. desire or wish: What does the analysand expect from others?
2. object's reactions: How do others react to the desires and expectations of the analysand (subject)?
3. subject's (self's) responses: How does the analysand respond to others' reactions?

Based on the answers to these three questions, a frequent (statistically the most frequent) answer emerges as a typical desire, object reaction, and response of the self that characterizes the analysand's interpersonal experiences in the long run. Luborsky calls this a core conflictual relationship theme because, between the subject's expectations and others' reaction, there is usually a problematic or conflicting element. Originally, Luborsky used this method for studying transference (Barber et al. 1990); however, this method can also be applied to study the analysand's view of their interpersonal relationships, the relations of the partners in marriage counselling, the development and improvement of interpersonal relating in long-term psychotherapy, and so on (e.g. Abargil & Tishby 2021; Abargil et al. 2023; Grenyer & Marceau 2022; Rocco et al. 2022).

Using Luborsky's content-analytic method, we classify the analysand's relationship episodes in psychoanalytic session transcripts according to three criteria. It is important to note that the picture we gain from this analysis is based on the analysand's subjective view of how they have experienced a given event or other people. An important characteristic of relationship episodes is their idiosyncratic processing on the part of the experiencer, which allows us to draw conclusions about the psychic world of the analysand (Thomä & Kähele 2006).

Luborsky and colleagues (Barber et al. 1990) created a standard category system in which they listed standard categories of desires (thirty-five standard categories), reactions from others (thirty standard categories), and responses of the self (thirty-one standard categories). They examined the frequencies of these standard categories (Luborsky et al. 1990) using a clinical sample (N = 33). Their findings showed that the most frequent wishes in their sample were: 'to be close and accepting', 'to be loved and understood', and 'to assert self and be independent'. The most frequent reactions from others were: 'rejecting and opposing' and 'controlling'. The most frequent responses of the self were: 'disappointed and depressed', 'unreceptive', and 'helpless'. In this study, Luborsky and colleagues also examined the contexts of the two most frequent wishes in terms of their related 'reactions from others' and 'responses of the self'. They found that the wish 'to be loved and understood' most frequently appeared in the context of 'rejecting and opposing' as a response from others (24.4% of the cases) and 'helpless' or 'disappointed and depressed' as a response of the self (in 44.2% of the cases). The wish 'to assert the self and be independent' was related to 'rejecting and opposing' as the response of others (25.4% of the cases) and was related to 'helpless' and 'disappointed and depressed' as the response of the self (42.4% of the cases).

Study objectives

We have applied Luborsky's CCRT method to the data of the Budapest Psychotherapy Database. We present here the results from one of the two cases in our database, namely the sessions of female therapists and female client dyads. Our main research question during this analysis was whether relationship narratives had changed in their structure during the three phases of the observation period—as analysed by the CCRT method. So, we have hypothesized that change has occurred in the structure of relationship episodes, namely in terms of

1) what the client expected from others, 2) how others reacted to these expectations, and 3) how the self responded to others' reactions during the three phases of the observation period. According to our hypothesis, changes in the structure of relationship episodes should align with the aims of psychoanalytic treatment. In the interpersonal domain, this chiefly means bringing the analysand's unconscious conflicts about how she relates to others into awareness, thereby improving the quality and dynamics of her relationships.

Another question we have asked in this research was if there had indeed been a change in the structure of relationship episodes, in which aspects it occurred, and how it was related to other aspects of narrative construction taking place in the psychotherapeutic setting, such as the shifting of NP by the speakers. So, we have examined, using qualitative discourse analytic methods, how changes in relationship-episode structure were interconnected with the NP shifting behaviour of the speakers. We have analysed this by studying patterns of NP use and NP shifting behaviour.

Finally, we also wanted to show how the NP shifting behaviour of the analyst might have affected NP shifting on the analysand's part, thus influencing the narrative construction process. Again, we hypothesized that this process was in harmony with the objectives of psychoanalytic psychotherapy.

The methodology applied in the analysis

In order to study changes in the analysand's perception of her interpersonal relationship patterns—namely, in what she desires from others, how she experiences others react to her desire, and what her own response is to others' reactions—we have applied Luborsky's method to our data.

Data selection

We coded nine sessions using the CCRT method from the psychoanalysis of the female analysand, choosing randomly three sessions from the beginning, middle, and final phases of the observation period; thus the chosen sessions fall approximately six months apart.

Coding

The demarcation and identification of relationship episodes was carried out by one main coder, as described by Luborsky & Barrett (2007), whereas two additional coders—trained psychotherapists and psychoanalysts—coded the CCRT in relationship episodes. Coders first coded each session independently, and then discussed disagreements in their coding, and came to a common decision in each case.

In order to code CCRT we completed the following steps:

a. Determining the *type* of relationship episode based on the main relationship character in the episode. These could fall into the following categories: 1) self, 2) therapist, 3) mother, 4) father, 5) siblings, 6) children, 7) sexual partner or romantic relationship, 8) male authority figures, 9) female authority figures, 10) male friends, 11) female friends, 12) other. According to our coding method, it was possible that one relationship episode contained more than one central character. In such cases, CCRT was coded for all characters separately for the given episode. Inter-rater reliability calculated for relationship types was based on the proportion of correspondence between the two coders (correct identification) and errors. We have distinguished two types of errors: a) minor (the episode type was correctly identified, but one of the coders indicated more main characters than the other), and b) major errors (the episode type differed).
   - total correspondence: 72%
   - minor errors: 20%
   - major errors 8%.

   Since, after coding independently, the coders discussed disagreements and came to a common decision regarding episode type, these error rates have not affected our actual results.
b. Rating the completeness of each relationship episode on a scale of 1–4 (measuring whether the three structural elements of the relationship episodes were present and described in enough detail: see Table 7.1) was carried out by the same two coders in the same manner as the relationship type. First, coders identified the completeness of each relationship episode independently. Then they discussed disagreements and came to a common conclusion. Inter-rater reliability (measured before discussing differences) for completeness using Krippendorff alpha (Hayes & Krippendorff 2007) was good, $\alpha = 0.81$ (CI: 0.440–1.00). This result was tested by computing Kendall's tau for reliability: $\tau = 0.82$, which also falls into the good category.

   Judges rated all episodes based on completeness, as shown in Table 7.1. Since the majority of episodes fell into the 'vaguely outlined episode' category (83.5%), and much fewer episodes were more developed by the client, and in order to be able to carry out statistical computations, we included

Table 7.1 Completeness of CCRT episodes in phases of the observation period

	First phase	Second phase	Third phase	Total
No episode components	1.3%	8.9%	2.8%	**4.1%**
Vaguely outlined episode components	87.8%	81.5%	79.8%	**83.5%**
Acceptable with all three components	10.9%	8.1%	16.5%	**11.6%**
Three components are more explicit and detailed	0%	1.6%	0.9%	**0.8%**

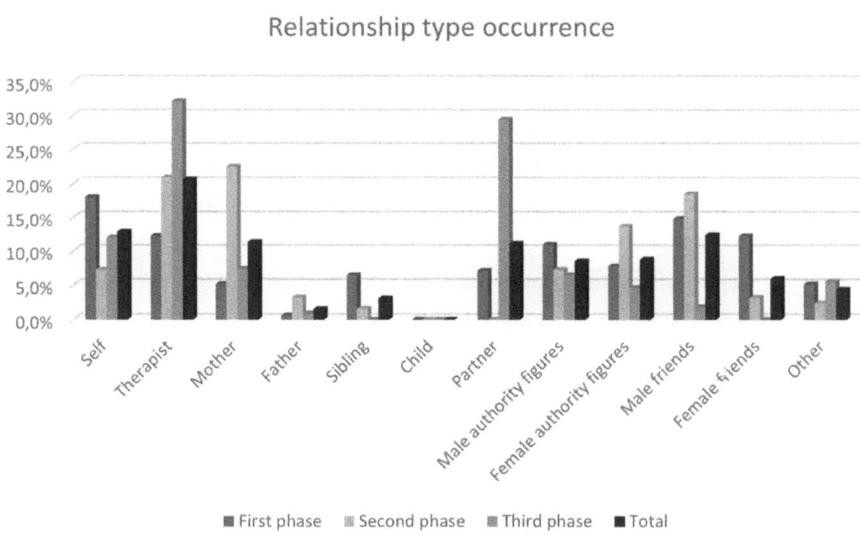

Figure 7.1 Occurrence of relationship types in relationship episodes

all episodes except for the ones missing episode components; these were excluded from the study.

Considering completeness as an ordinal variable, the difference between psychotherapy phases can be computed using the Kruskal–allis test. Based on this, there is a significant difference between the phases $\chi2(2, 389) = 6.89$ $p = .03$. Based on a follow-up Mann–Whitney test, we found that there was no significant difference between the first and second phase ($U = 8918.5$ $Z = -1.805$ $p = .07$ $r = .01$); however, there was a difference between the second and third phases ($U = 5920$ $Z = -2.38$ $p = .018$ $r = 0.16$), and there was no significant difference between the first and the third phase ($U = 8056.5$

$Z = -1.16$ $p = .248$ $r = .07$). These results show that, in terms of completeness, there was a small decrease occurring in the second phase, which returned to its original level in the third phase of the observation period. This small amount of variability in completeness is not relevant from the point of view of our study.

c. Coding relationship episodes based on the three components described by Luborsky

- Desires, needs, intentions, and expectations: what does the narrator expect from others? This was coded based on the standard categories and clusters described by Luborsky, using the second addition to his list (Barber et al. 1990). The authors described thirty-five wishes; the coders could select the one they felt best matched the desire of the client. For example, such desires are to be understood, to be accepted, to be respected, to accept others, etc. In order to reduce this large number of categories, and their redundancy, Luborsky, and his cow-orkers mapped these categories onto eight standardized clusters. For example, to assert self and be independent; to oppose, hurt, and control others; to be controlled, hurt, and not be responsible, and so on (see Table 7.3).

  The coders first rated desire independently based on Luborsky's standard categories, which were then mapped on to Luborsky's standard clusters. Next, the coders discussed disagreements and came to a common conclusion. Inter-rater reliability for desire was tested using Krippendorff's alpha (Hayes & Krippendorff 2007), resulting in $\alpha = 0.73$ (CI: 0.5513–0.9103), which is an acceptable level. This result of inter-rater reliability was tested by Cohen's Kappa, which showed an acceptable, but moderate level of agreement ($\kappa = 0.73$).

- How does the client experience others' reacting to her desires and wishes? This was coded based on the standard category system, including thirty concrete reactions and eight standard clusters (Barber et al. 1990). Examples of others' reactions are: 'others are understanding', 'others are not understanding', and 'others are accepting'. Examples of standardized clusters are: 'others are strong', or 'controlling', or 'upset'.

  The strategy for coding others' reactions was identical to that of desire. The same two coders first coded independently, then discussed differences and came to a common conclusion in the case of each relationship episode. Inter-rater reliability using Krippendorff's alpha (Hayes & Krippendorff 2007) before discussing disagreements showed an acceptable but moderate level of agreement between the coders

(α = 0.67, CI: 0.4670, 0.8360). Inter-rater reliability was tested by using Cohen's Kappa, which showed an acceptable but moderate reliability (κ= 0.67).

- What was the analysand's response to others' reactions? In other words, what were the 'responses of the self' to others? Self-responses were also coded into thirty-one standard categories and then into eight standard clusters, as suggested by Luborsky. Examples of standard categories are: 'understand', 'don't understand', 'feel accepted', and 'feel respected'. Examples of the standard clusters of responses of the self are: 'helpful', 'unreceptive', 'respected and accepted'.

  The responses of the self were also first coded independently by the two coders, which was followed by a discussion and coming to an agreement on how to categorize self-responses. Inter-rater reliability was computed by using Krippendorff's alpha (Hayes & Krippendorff 2007), α = 0.71 (CI: 0.4961, 0.8740), which is an acceptable level of agreement.

  Inter-rater reliability has also been tested by using Cohen's Kappa, which shows an acceptable but moderate reliability (κ= 0.70).

d. Statistical analysis took place using the Statistical Package for Social Science (SPSS) version 25.

e. coding narrative perspective
We also coded and analysed NP at sessions, in which change in personal relationship patterns was identified by CCRT methods. Coding NP was carried out by a third independent coder, as described in Chapter 4.

Results and discussion of CCRT analysis

Our results show, in general, that with the CCRT method we can identify changes in the analysand's relationship episodes. Comparing the three phases of her psychoanalysis during the observation period (one at the beginning and two in the working phase), we show changes in relationship episodes with important others. Table 7.2 shows the number of relationship episodes in the three observation phases, and Figure 7.1 shows the proportion of relationship types in relationship episodes occurring in the three phases of psychotherapy, divided by approximately 6 months.

There is a significant change in the proportion of the relationship types mentioned during the three phases of the observation period ($\chi2$ (10.265) = 68.27, p < .001, φ = .51). The change in occurrence of the various relationship types are summarized in Figure 7.1. Changes in occurrence were significant in the categories of therapist, mother, sibling, partner, male friends, and female

Table 7.2 Number of relationship episodes

Session	Number of episodes	%	Phase	Number of episodes	Total%
1	60	14.81			
2	62	15.31	First phase	167	41.23
3	45	11.11			
4	46	11.36			
5	35	8.64	Second phase	125	30.86
6	44	10.86			
7	33	8.15			
8	45	11.11	Third phase	113	27.90
9	35	8.64			
Total	**405**				

friends. Based on this, we can say that in terms of the occurrence of relationship type, the three phases of the observation period show great heterogeneity. The occurrence of relationship types in analytic discourse is closely tied to the themes and problems discussed at any given session. For instance, the mother is mentioned in 5.1% of relationship episodes in the first phase, whereas she is mentioned in 22.4% of relationship episodes in the second phase, and this increase is significant ($\chi2(1, 281) = 18.53$ $p < .001$ $\varphi = .26$). So, accordingly during the second phase, we find several discussions related to the analysand's problems with her mother. Similarly, discussion of the analysand's relationship with her partner has increased by the third phase, being present in 7.1% of the relationship episodes in the first phase, 0% in the second phase, and 29.4% in the third phase, which is a significant change among the three phases ($\chi2(2, 390) = 55.34$ $p < .001$ $\varphi = .38$). So, in the case of the significantly differing relationship types (as we can see in Figure 7.1) there are large differences in occurrence between the three phases of the observation period, suggesting that relationship themes that had been discussed during a given phase have varied greatly.

The analysand's wishes, desires, and goals: what the analysand expects from others

The first characteristic of the relationship episode structure, according to Luborsky's model, is what the analysand's wishes for or expects from others.

Table 7.3 Distribution of clusters of wishes

	First phase	Second phase	Third phase	Total
To assert the self and be independent	9.2%	4.6%	1.1%	5.6%
To oppose, hurt, and control others	11.3%	0%	0%	4.7%
To be controlled, hurt, and not be responsible	2.8%	8.3%	18.3%	8.8%
To be distant and avoid conflicts	16.3%	13.0%	5.4%	**12.3%**
To be close and accepting	11.3%	14.8%	10.8%	**12.3%**
To be loved and understood	18.4%	41.7%	40.9%	**31.9%**
To feel good and comfortable	9.9%	2.8%	5.4%	6.4%
To achieve and help others	20.6%	14.8%	18.3%	**18.1%**

In Table 7.3 we summarize the proportion of the eight standardized clusters of wishes (Barber et al. 1990) during the three phases of psychotherapy.

The wish with the highest proportion for this analysand was 'to be loved and understood' (31.9%), which had been shown to be one of the most frequent wishes in a previous study of a clinical sample (Luborsky et al. 1990). According to Luborsky's coding schema, the wish of the cluster 'to be loved and understood' is composed of the standard categories of to be 'loved', 'respected', 'understood', 'accepted', and 'liked' (Barber et al. 1990). 'To be loved' refers to being romantically involved; 'to be respected' refers to being valued, being treated fairly, and to be important to others. 'Being understood' refers to being comprehended, being empathized with, and being seen accurately, whereas 'to be accepted' means being approved of, not being judged, and being affirmed. 'Being liked' refers to others being interested in the self (Barber et al. 1990). As we can see from Table 7.3, the analysand expressed the wish 'to be loved and understood' mainly in the second and third phases of the observation period. These were the phases in which relationship episodes included the mother (second phase: 22.4%), the partner (third phase: 29.4%), and the analyst (third phase: 32.1%) in an outstanding proportion. We will return to the question of target persons for the wish 'to be loved and understood' below.

The analysand's second highest wish was 'to achieve and help others' (18.1%). According to Luborsky's coding schema (Barber et al. 1990), the cluster of 'to achieve and help others' is composed of the standard categories of 'to achieve', 'to better the self', 'to help others', 'to be good'. More specifically, 'to achieve' in Luborsky's coding schema refers to being competent, doing well, and winning; 'to better the self' refers to improving and getting well; 'to help others' refers to nurturing others and giving to others; and 'to be good' refers to doing the right thing, being perfect, and correct (Barber et al. 1990). The wish 'to achieve and help others' reached its highest proportion during the first phase of the observation period (20.6%), in the beginning phase of psychotherapy. Out of all wishes directed towards the self, this wish made up 43.5%. So, we can speculate that beginning psychotherapy might have inspired the client to want to better herself, to improve herself, to do the right thing, and to perfect herself.

The analysers' wish, with the third greatest proportion, was 'to be distant and avoid conflicts' and 'to be close and accepting' (12.3%). The cluster of 'to be distant and avoid conflicts' is composed of the standard categories of 'to avoid conflicts', 'not to be hurt', and 'to be distant from others'. More specifically, 'to avoid conflicts' refers to compromising, not making others angry, getting along, and being flexible; 'not to be hurt' refers to avoiding pain and aggravation, avoiding rejection, protecting/defending the self; and 'to be distant from others' refers to not expressing oneself and one's feelings, and being left alone (Barber et al. 1990). The wish 'to be distant and avoid conflicts' peaked in the first phase (16.3%). This suggests that at the start of psychotherapy the client adopted a distancing, conflict-avoidant stance in relationships, which then declined over the observation period (5.4%), in the working phase of psychotherapy.

The cluster of 'to be close and accepting' is composed of the standard categories of 'to accept others', 'respect others', 'to be open', 'to have trust', 'be opened up to', and 'to be close to others'(Barber et al. 1990). More specifically, 'to accept others' refers to being receptive to others; 'to respect others' refers to valuing others; 'to be open' refers to expressing oneself and communicating; 'to have trust' refers to others being honest and genuine; 'to be opened up to' refers to being responded to, being talked to; and 'to be close to others' refers to being included, not being alone, being friends (Barber et al. 1990). The wish 'to be close and accepting' showed a tendency to be stable over the three phases of the observation period; thus, it did not exhibit a tendency for change. This suggests that this wish on the client's part was expressed systematically throughout the observation period in about equal proportion.

Having the wishes 'to be distant and avoid conflicts' as well as 'to be close and accepting' in equal proportions suggests that the analysand wishes to be distant from others so much as she wishes to be close to others. These contradictory wishes resurface and reverberate in the analysand's relationships with her closest loved ones in connection with her most important wish 'to be loved and understood', as we shall show in our discourse analysis of the relevant psychotherapeutic sessions, in which this latter wish occurred at a particularly high level.

Changes of wishes and expectation from others during the observation period

Change was significant between the three phases of psychotherapy regarding the proportion of wishes ($\chi 2(14, 342) = 71.16$ $p < .001$ $\varphi = .46$). The following analysis contains an examination of these changes regarding the proportion of wishes, which means that we will compute a series of $\chi 2$ tests, examining all response categories separately. The multiple testing increases the chances of type one error; however, using the Holm procedure, we decreased the acceptable level of significance to 0.01. So, the results will only be significant if they are below this level. If a response category is significant, there is no need for further correction; so, we can use the original, $\alpha = .05$, significance level.

The wish 'to assert the self and be independent' shows no significant change in the three examined phases of psychotherapy ($\chi 2(2, 342) = 7.34$ $p = .03$ $\varphi = .15$). The wish 'to oppose, hurt, and control others' shows a significant change in its occurrence during the three phases ($\chi 2 = 23.93$, $p < .001$, $\varphi = .27$). This means a significant drop in occurrence during the second phase. The wish 'to be controlled, hurt, and not be responsible' also shows a significant change among the three phases ($\chi 2 = 16{,}74$, $p < .001$, $\varphi = .22$). This change originates in the increase between the second and third phases, as well as between the first and third phases ($\chi 2(1\ 201) = 4.39$ $p = .04$ $\varphi = .15$, and $\chi 2(1, 234) = 16.36$ $p < .001$ $\varphi = .26$ respectively). The wish 'to be distant from others and avoid conflicts' does not show significant change during the three observed phases ($\chi 2(2, 342) = 6.289$ $p = .043$ $\varphi = .136$), neither does the wish 'to be close and accepting' ($\chi 2(2, 342) = 0.959$ $p = .619$ $\varphi = .053$). The wish 'to be loved and understood' shows a significant change ($\chi 2 = 19.948$, $p < .001$, $\varphi = .242$), which is due to the increase between the first phase and the second phase ($\chi 2(1, 249) = 16.19$ $p < .001$ $\varphi = .26$) as well as between the first phase and the third phase ($\chi 2(1, 234) = 14.18$ $p < .001$ $\varphi = .25$). The wish 'to feel good and comfortable' does not show significant change during the three phases ($\chi 2(2, 342) = 5.43$ $p = .066$ $\varphi = .13$), neither does the wish 'to achieve and help others' ($\chi 2(2, 342) = 1.37$ $p = .505$ $\varphi = .06$).

In summary, we can say that there were three wishes that showed significant change during the observation period: 'to oppose, hurt and control others' (decrease); 'to be controlled, hurt and not be responsible' (increase); and 'to be loved and understood' (increase). So, among the four most important wishes (i.e. the most frequent ones), only the wish 'to be loved and understood' shows significant change during the observation period. Changes are due to an increase in the occurrence of the wish during the second phase of psychoanalysis from approximately 18% to 40%, thus doubling the occurrence of this wish. The highest proportion of this wish occurs at sessions 6 and 8, which are sessions we shall examine closely using the qualitative methods below. Before we turn to that, however, we shall examine 1) who the target persons are towards whom the wish 'to be loved and understood', and other important wishes—the ones that show change—are directed during the three phases of the observation period, and 2) the distribution of various wishes according to relationship type, concerning important relationships such as the analyst and the self.

Wishes directed towards various target persons

We can see from Table 7.4 that the wish 'to be loved and understood' is mainly directed towards the analyst and the partner in the first phase, towards the analyst and the mother in the second phase, and towards the analyst and the

Table 7.4 Recipients of the wish 'To be loved and understood'

	First phase	Second phase	Third phase	Total
Self	3.8%	6.7%	5.3%	5.5%
Analyst	**53.8%**	**28.9%**	**42.1%**	**39.4%**
Mother	3.8%	**22.2%**	2.6%	**11.0%**
Father	0%	4.4%	2.6%	2.8%
Children	0%	0.0%	0.0%	0.0%
Sibling	0%	0.0%	0.0%	0.0%
Partner	**30.8%**	0%	**31.6%**	**18.3%**
Male authority figures	0%	0%	10.5%	3.7%
Female authority figures	3.8%	15.6%	2.6%	8.3%
Male friends	0%	17.8%	2.6%	8.3%
Female friends	3.8%	2.2%	0%	1.8%
Other	0%	2,2%	0%	0.9%

partner again in the third phase. So, we can say that, first of all, the most important recipient of this wish is the analyst (approximately 40% of the proportion of the relationship episodes containing it). Secondly, the wish is directed towards the partner (approximately 18%) and, finally, towards the mother (11%). These three target persons with the wish 'to be loved and understood' receive approximately 70% of this wish within the total number of relationship episodes, and all other target persons receive only approximately 30%.

An interesting wish showing change during the observation period is 'to oppose, hurt, and control others', which occurs only in the first analysand phase and is mainly directed towards male authority figures, siblings, and female authority figures, as we can see in Table 7.5.

The wish 'to oppose, hurt, and control others' includes resisting domination, competing against others, getting revenge, rejecting others, expressing anger towards others, dominating others and having power over them according to Luborsky's coding schema (Barber et al. 1990). The analysand might express these wishes towards authority figures in general as a way of defying, and competing with, them; similarly, she expresses these wishes towards her younger sister due to their competition and sibling rivalry. These results may be related to the analysand's specific problems and concerns with expressing aggression and asserting the self. The fact that it occurs only in the first phase suggests

Table 7.5 Recipients of the wish 'To oppose, hurt, and control others'

	First phase
Self	0%
Analyst	0%
Mother	6.3%
Father	0.0%
Sibling	**25.0%**
Children	0.0%
Partner	0.0%
Male authority figures	**31.3%**
Female authority figures	**18.8%**
Male friends	0.0%
Female friends	6.3%
Others	12.5%

that the analysand's aggression-related problems might have been alleviated by the second and third phases, so much so that she does not exhibit the wish 'to oppose, hurt and control others' in relationship episodes.

Another wish that manifests change during the observation period is 'to be controlled, hurt, and not be responsible', which occurs only in the third phase of psychoanalysis, directed towards the mother, and towards other, less frequently mentioned, people, who did not play a significant role in the analysand's relationship episodes.

The cluster 'to be controlled, hurt and not be responsible' is composed of the standard categories of 'to be hurt', 'to be controlled by others', 'to not be responsible or obligated', and 'to be like others' (Barber et al. 1990). More specifically, 'to be hurt' refers to being punished, being treated badly, or being injured; 'to be controlled by others' refers to being submissive, dependent, or passive, and to being given direction; 'to not be responsible or obligated' refers to being free, not being constrained; finally, 'to be like others' refers to identifying with others, being similar to others, modelling after others (Barber et al. 1990). The fact that this wish occurs in the third phase of the observation period suggests that relationships and events discussed during this phase may have an adverse effect on the analysand's way of relating to others, most of all towards her mother (approximately 29%). At the same time, it is also possible that by the third phase

Table 7.6 Recipients of the wish 'To be controlled, hurt, and not be responsible'

	Third phase
Self	17.6%
Analyst	5.9%
Mother	**29.4%**
Father	0.0%
Sibling	0.0%
Children	0.0%
Partner	0.0%
Male authority figures	5.9%
Female authority figures	11.8%
Male friends	5.9%
Female friends	0.0%
Other	**23.5%**

the analysand is able to mention, and to be aware of, her problems, and become capable of discussing them at the session.

We must also mention that the wish 'to oppose, hurt, and control others' and the wish 'to be controlled, hurt and not be responsible' show opposite tendencies in terms of their changes in occurrence. Whereas the former shows a decrease in frequency, the latter shows an increase during the course of the observation period. So, this suggests that the analysand instead of hurting and controlling others (at the beginning phase of psychotherapy), had been hurt and controlled by others (at the working phase of psychotherapy), which can be interpreted as a decrease in aggressive and controlling behaviour on her part, as described by the relationship episodes narrated during treatment. So, the direction of change in connection to these two wishes shows a consistency in the client's behaviour towards others as described in her narratives.

Important relationships and related wishes

In order to understand the interconnection between wishes and target persons better, we examined the distribution of various wishes according to relationship type. The examined relationships included the ones mentioned in greatest proportions in relationship episodes, namely the therapist, the self, the mother, and the partner.

As we can see in Table 7.7, approximately 20% of wishes in all relationship episodes are directed towards the analyst. Most of these (approximately 70%) include the wish 'to be loved and understood', and a great deal less (approximately 15%) include the wish 'to achieve and help others'. This can be understood as the analysand, above all, expecting love and understanding from the analyst, which may be considered a frequent wish of analysands (Thomä & Kächele 2007). This finding is in congruence with the analyst's role in psychoanalysis, as well as with the good working alliance and positive relationship between analysand and analyst, which supports the goals of psychotherapy in the long run.

Another important relationship type is the analysand's relationship with herself, more specifically the relationship with the self. In order to examine this, we computed the proportion of wishes directed towards the self. In other words, we examined what the analysand expected from herself during the three phases of the observation period.

As we can see in Table 7.8 wishes directed towards the self in relationship episodes amount to approximately 13% of the total number of wishes. A larger portion of this sum, 44%, includes the wish 'to achieve and help others'. So,

Table 7.7 Wishes directed towards the analyst

		First phase	Second phase	Third phase	Total
Analyst	N	19	26	35	**80**
	Percent	12.2%	20.8%	32.1%	**20.5%**

	First phase	Second phase	Third phase	Total
To assert the self and be independent	0%	0%	0%	**0%**
To oppose, hurt and control others	0%	0%	0%	**0%**
To be controlled, hurt, and not be responsible	0%	6.3%	3.8%	**3.3%**
To be distant and avoid conflicts	10.5%	6.3%	0%	**4.9%**
To be close and accepting	0%	0%	0%	**0%**
To be loved and understood	**73.7%**	**81.3%**	**61.5%**	**70.5%**
To feel good and comfortable	10.5%	6.3%	3.8%	**6.6%**
To achieve and help others	5.3%	0%	30.8%	**14.8%**

Table 7.8 Wishes directed towards the self

		First phase	Second phase	Third phase	Total
Self	N	28	9	13	**50**
	Percent	17.9%	7.2%	11.9%	**12.8%**

	First phase	Second phase	Third phase	Total
To assert the self and be independent	16.0%	12.5%	0%	**10.9%**
To oppose, hurt and control others	0%	0%	0%	**0%**
To be controlled, hurt, and not be responsible	0%	0%	23.1%	**6.5%**
To be distant and avoid conflicts	8.0%	0%	0%	**4.3%**
To be close and accepting	4.0%	0%	0%	**2.2%**
To be loved and understood	4.0%	37.5%	15.4%	**13.0%**
To feel good and comfortable	28.0%	0%	15.4%	**19.6%**
To achieve and help others	**40.0%**	**50.0%**	**46.2%**	**43.5%**

we can conclude that the analysand most of all wants to be agentic. Hence, she wants to be competent, to do well, to win, to improve, to get well, to nurture others, and to give to others, as well as to do the right thing, to be perfect, and to be correct (Barber et al. 1990). Substantially less of the analysand's self-directed wishes, about 20%, include the wish 'to feel good and comfortable'. From this, we can conclude that the analysand wants to 'have stability', to 'feel comfortable', to 'feel happy', to 'feel good about herself'—based on Luborsky's coding schema (Barber et al. 1990). More precisely, to 'have stability' refers to being secure and having structure; to 'feel comfortable' refers to relaxing and not feeling bad; to 'feel happy' refers to having fun, enjoying, and feeling good; to 'feel good about herself' refers to being self-confident, accepting oneself, and having a sense of well-being. Thirdly, the analysand expects herself to turn towards the self lovingly and understandingly (13%), which means that she wants 'to be comprehended', 'to be empathized with', and 'to be seen accurately' (Barber et al. 1990).

Another important relationship type for the analysand is that of the mother. Wishes directed towards the mother are 11.3% (N = 44) of the total number of wishes.

Table 7.9 Wishes directed towards the mother

		First phase	**Second phase**	**Third phase**	Total
Mother	N	8	28	8	44
	Percent	5.1%	22.4%	7.3%	**11.3%**
		First phase	**Second phase**	**Third phase**	Total
Assert self, and be independent		14.3%	12.0%	0%	**10.5%**
Oppose, hurt or control others		14.3%	0%	0%	**2.6%**
To be controlled, hurt, and not be responsible		0%	16.0%	83.3%	**23.7%**
To be distant and avoid conflicts		0%	0%	0%	**0%**
To be close and accepting		42.9%	16.0%	0%	**18.4%**
To be loved and understood		14.3%	**40.0%**	16.7%	**31.6%**
To feel good and comfortable		0%	4.0%	0%	**2.6%**
To achieve and help others		14.3%	12.0%	0%	**10.5%**

The distribution of wishes towards the mother is only substantial in the second phase of the observation period, and therefore cannot be interpreted in the other two phases.

Looking at the second phase, about 40% of the wishes directed towards the mother is the wish 'to be loved and to be understood', 16% is the wish 'to be controlled, hurt, and not be responsible', and 16% is the wish 'to be close and accepting'. So, here again, we see the recurrence of the analysand's most frequent wish: 'to be loved and understood'. The wish 'to be close and accepting' is directed towards the mother, signalling that she wants to have a good intimate relationship with her. It is interesting, however, that the wish 'to be controlled, hurt, and not be responsible' is also directed in relatively large proportion towards the mother. More specifically, as mentioned earlier, according to Luborsky's coding schema, this wish means 'to be submissive', 'to be dependent', 'to be passive', 'to be given direction', 'to be punished', 'to be treated badly', 'to be injured', 'to be free', and 'not to be constrained' (Barber et al. 1990). So, the latter wish somewhat contradicts the other two wishes directed towards the mother, which characterize a healthy, good relationship with a parent. Expecting 'to be controlled, hurt, and not be responsible' from one's parent may be the sign of an overly punishing super-ego, and a somewhat masochistic attitude. So, based on the analysand's wishes, we may conclude that her relationship with her mother is an ambivalent one. Such a way of relating in her primary relationship may lay the foundation to the analysand's latter relationship behaviour with important loved ones. So, we may expect these to be problematic as well.

Finally, an important relationship type is that of the partner. 11% (N = 43) of total wishes are directed towards the partner. However, the partner is not mentioned at all during the second phase of the observation period.

The occurrence of wishes towards the partner is substantial only in the third phase; therefore, it cannot be interpreted during the first and second phases.

The wish with the highest proportion directed towards the partner is 'to be loved and understood', 41.4% in the third phase. The second highest proportion of wishes directed towards the partner is 'to be close and accepting', 31% in the third phase. Thirdly, the wish 'to be distant and avoid conflicts' makes up 17.2% of the wishes directed towards the partner in the third phase. This wish means, more specifically, not to express feelings, to be left alone, to compromise, not to anger others, to get along, and to be flexible (Barber et al. 1990). So, the analysand seems to direct somewhat ambivalent wishes towards her partner, although the wish 'to be distant and avoid conflicts' is present in a much smaller proportion than the wish 'to be loved and understood' and 'to be close and accepting'.

Table 7.10 Distribution of wishes directed towards the partner

		First phase	**Second phase**	**Third phase**	Total
Partner	N	11	0	32	43
	Percent	7.1%	0.0%	29.4%	**11.0%**
				First phase	**Third phase**
Assert self, and be independent				0%	3,4%
Oppose, hurt or control others				0%	0%
To be controlled, hurt, and not be responsible				0%	0%
To be distant and avoid conflicts				27.3%	17.2%
To be close and accepting				0%	31.0%
To be loved and understood				72.7%	**41.4%**
To feel good and comfortable				0%	6.9%
To achieve and help others				0%	0%

In conclusion, we can say that the analysand's most important wish during the observation period, based on the statistical analysis presented above, is the wish 'to be loved and understood', which is directed most frequently towards the analyst, the mother, and the romantic partner (love relationship). During psychoanalysis, there is a significant increase in this wish due to the difference between the first and second phases, as well as the first and third phases of the observation period. The increase of this wish is congruent with the aims of psychoanalytic psychotherapy; at the same time, however, wishes with similar aims, for instance 'to be close and accepting', do not show an overall increase during the same period. The reason for this may be that the analysand wishes to be loved, but does not know how to achieve this aim—for instance by being emotionally close and open towards others. These problems manifest in discussions at the sessions we will examine using qualitative methods.

Figure 7.2 shows that the two salient sessions that cause an increase in the wish 'to be loved and understood' are sessions 6 and 8. In the sections below we will discuss the events of session 6, and examine the narrative construction process taking place, using (as in previous chapters) the shifting of NP as a methodological tool.

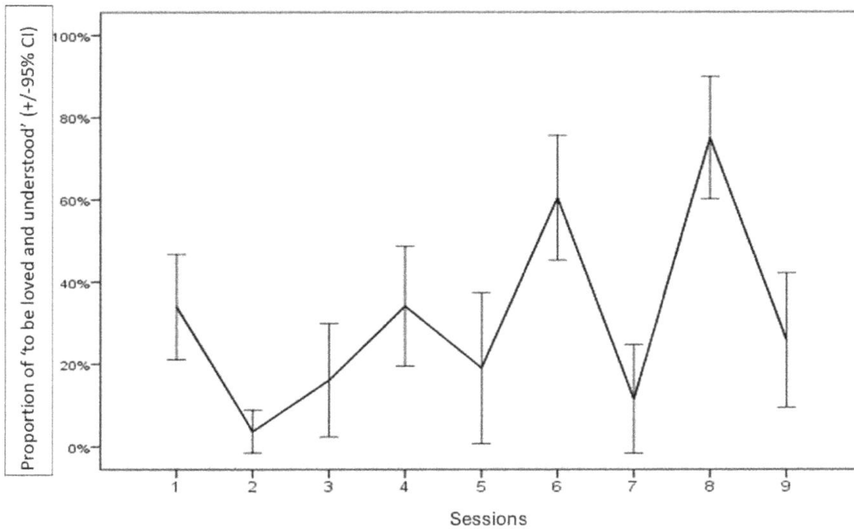

Figure 7.2 Changes in the wish 'to be loved and understood' during the observation period

Session 6 (L23) in terms of the wish 'to be loved and understood'

During this session from the second phase of the observation period, discussions of Clara's relationships took centre stage. The interlocutors discussed relationships with authority figures and potential romantic partners (coded as male friends). Based on our statistical analysis, we know that what is relevant to the wish 'to be loved and understood' is most of all the relationship with Clara's actual romantic partner—with whom she had an on/off relationship—as well as the analyst and her mother. however, one of the sessions when this wish reaches statistically salient proportions is session 6, where the analytic dyad discusses the analysand's relationships with potential romantic partners. We will focus on this topic here, including four excerpts from the session, because this session is very revealing about the analysand's ambivalent way of relating to romantic partners. We try to examine the emotional context of the wish 'to be loved and understood', and its dynamic in the analysand's inner life.

In session six, Clara narrates her experiences with Z and G, both representing potential love interests where mutual desire remains unrecognized or deferred. The central relational conflict is not merely about romantic partners but about Clara's difficulty in registering affective acknowledgment in relationships—a pattern that is re-enacted in the analytic field.

In session six, the analysand recalls two relationship episodes—first with a young man, Z, then with G. Z is an acquaintance whom Clara met recently. Studying abroad, he found her through a Hungarian social media site and initiated an email correspondence. In the session (Excerpt 7.1), she describes how he first contacted her.

Excerpt 7.1 (session 6, L23)

324PAT:	mert hogy nekem nincsen+/	because I do not have+/
325PAT:	vagy most már megvan,	or now I have already,
326PAT:	de hogy nekem nem volt meg,	but that I did not have his,
327PAT:	és neki sem volt meg az én email címem.	and he did not have my email address.
328TER:	ühüm.	uhum.
329TER:	és így egymásra akadtak ezen a hálózaton keresztül.	and you found each other through this network.
330PAT:	hát ő rám.	well, he found me.
331TER:	aha.	uhum.
332TER:	és ezért írt.	and that is why he wrote.
333TER:	és erre föl,	and then you,
334TER:	maga ennek ellenére maga úgy reagál,	despite this, you react like,
335TER:	hogy ő úgysem válaszolna magának.	he would not respond to you anyway.
336PAT:	igen.	yes.
337TER:	miközben ő kezdte a levelezést.	meanwhile, he has initiated the correspondence.
338PAT:	igen.	yes.
339%com:	analysand laughs	
340TER:	tanulságos.	it's edifying.
341PAT:	miért?	why?
342PAT:	miért az?	why is that?
343%com:	analysand laughs	
344PAT:	mondom, ennél sokkal jobb sztorim van.	I am telling you, I have a much better story.

From lines 324–30, the story of a male friend or potential love interest is introduced by the analysand. Clara uses homo-diegesis. She tells her story from an insider point of view, whereas the analyst uses hetero-diegesis, looking at the events and characters of the story from the outside—this being a typical point of view of listeners who are not participating in the narrator's story. From 332–36, the analyst summarizes the situation while the analysand agrees with her conclusion. While discussing this, both interlocutors use external focalization. In other words, they give a behavioural description of events and characters without mentioning the internal states of the story's characters (e.g. emotions). This perspective suggests a lower level of self-involvement on the part of the narrator, thus keeping an emotionally 'safe' distance between the analysand's formal narrated and current narrating selves. In line 340, the analyst tries to direct the analysand's attention to the contradictory nature of her behaviour, again using hetero-diegesis, the third-person singular subject: 'it's edifying'; however, in lines 341–43, the analysand does not elaborate on the problem. Instead, she challenges the analyst, using the same perspective as she did—so, evidencing the coordination of perspectives: 'why? why is that?' The analyst offers the opportunity for the analysand to draw conclusions about her own behaviour, which would mean an integration of her difficulties with relationships and a reasoning of why such situations may have occurred in her life—drawing a conclusion or 'moral' from all of this. Instead, however, the analysand begins another story with another potential love interest of hers, with the analyst listening and not pressuring her to elaborate on her preceding point.

The analyst's intervention in Excerpt 7.1 (lines 332–37) emphasizes Clara's contradictory stance: she dismisses the possibility of Z's genuine interest in her, even though he was the one who initiated contact. The analyst's reflective intervention (line 340: 'It's edifying') serves as a mirroring response (Winnicott 1971), which highlights the paradox in Clara's experience—she is desired, yet internally she cannot recognize this.

Clara's reaction to this interpretation is defensive—she laughs (line 339), questions the analyst's comment (lines 341–42: 'Why? Why is that?'), and deflects by moving to a different story. This response can be understood as a subtle enactment of the very pattern being interpreted: instead of exploring the emotional implications of her unconscious assumption (that she is ultimately undesired and unrecognized), she shifts to a new topic. This avoidance strategy preserves psychic equilibrium by defending against the vulnerability of recognition.

Excerpt 7.2 (session 6, L23)

380PAT:	és mondja mondja a M,	and M says says
381PAT:	hogy+..	that+...
382PAT:	hát hogy én miért nem meséltem el nekik,	well, that why I did not tell them,

383PAT:	hogy én milyen jó kis sztorikat tartok vissza,	that I hold back such nice little stories,
384PAT:	hogy hát hogy a+..	that well that the+...
385PAT:	hogy mondta a D,	that D told him,
386PAT:	hogy hát hogy mondta neki a G,	that well that G told him,
387PAT:	hogy ő halálosan szerelmes volt belém.	that he fell fatally in love with me.
388%com:	pause	
389TER:	na tessék!	well, now!
390PAT:	hát hogy ha így+..	well if like this+...
391PAT:	öö+..	erer+...
392PAT:	szóval ez egy kicsit így+..	so this a little bit like+...
393PAT:	rosszul esett.	felt bad.
394%com:	pause	
395PAT:	úgy hogy ö m+..	well then er m+...
396TER:	igen.	yes.
397TER:	és ez nagyjából azonos időbe esett azzal hogy maga is halálosan szerelmes volt.	and this happened around the same time when you were fatally in love also.
398PAT:	persze.	sure.
399PAT:	persze.	sure.
400TER:	és akkor hogy alakul úgy,	and then how does this happen that way,
401PAT:	nahát ez az.	well, this is it.
402TER:	mindig.	always.
403TER:	mindig?	always?
404PAT:	[mindig.]	[always.]
405TER:	[mindig,]	[always,]
406TER:	hogy ez nem derül ki egymás számára.	that this does not emerge for each other.

In Excerpt 7.2, Clara tells a story about a love interest, G, who has also been 'fatally' in love with her. So, they fell in love with each other at about the same time; however, they did not know about each other's feelings. She has only learned later, from a friend of a friend, that her love had been reciprocated. In line 380 she starts recounting her conversation with M, beginning in hetero-diegesis, present tense, but shifting into homo-diegesis, past tense, in line 381, and keeping up this perspective until line 383, when she shifts into hetero-diegesis again until line 387. These shifts in perspective show some reluctance on the part of the analysand to describe events from an insider's point of view. She indirectly quotes M's words—thus showing the two lovers' real situation from an outsider's point of view. In addition, throughout recounting the story, the analysand uses external focalization, except for line 387: 'that he fell fatally in love with me'. This shift into internal focalization emphasizes even more the importance of G's feelings for the analysand. The small pause after the analysand's utterance also emphasizes the importance of line 387, which seems to be surprising information for the analyst. She interrupts in line 389: 'well, now!' indicating her interest in the new facts, and emphasizing her emotional reaction to it. The analysand continues her story in lines 390–93, using homo-diegesis, and internal focalization relating her own emotions to the turn of events, so expressing heightened self-involvement in her story. Then again, the interlocutors are silent for a few seconds, stressing the relevance of the analysand's statement. In line 395, the analysand tries to explain her story further, but this attempt fails, and the analyst intervenes in lines 396–97. She shifts into hetero-diegesis, past tense, narrator level. The use of these perspectives establishes the analyst's distance from the story. at the same time she also uses internal focalization, naming the analysand's emotions (being in love with G).

In lines 398–99 the analysand agrees with the analyst's point, accepting her interpretation of the events, so, again coordinating her perspective with the analyst. In line 400 the analyst continues, and asks the analysand directly how this kind of things can happen to her, implying her surprise at the events, shifting into external focalization, present tense, and staying at narrator level—thus showing a lesser involvement of the self. The analysand, agreeing with the analyst's meaning, says: 'well, this is it', suggesting that she is aware of the importance of this event and she is not able, at this point, to explain, or elaborate on it. In lines 402–03 the analyst repeats the same word—'always'—with different intonation, first as a statement and then as a question posed to the analysand, which in line 404 the analysand repeats as a statement, at the same time as the analyst, who for the third time repeats this word. Their linguistic alignment emphasizes that the interlocutors agree: this behaviour is a permanent pattern in the analysand's life.

In Excerpt 7.2, a deeper layer of the relational conflict emerges: Clara recounts a past relationship where mutual love existed, but remained unknown at the time (lines 386–87). The emotional core of this moment is missed recognition, a theme that is both personal and intersubjectively co-constructed in the analytic setting.

The analyst's intervention (lines 397–406) emphasizes the repetition of this pattern ('always'), highlighting its pervasive and unconscious nature. Clara's response ('Well, this is it') suggests a partial acknowledgment, but also an affective resignation, reinforcing the intersubjective nature of self-experience: she is caught between the longing for recognition and the expectation that recognition will never be fully realized.

From a relational perspective, the dialogic structure of this moment is crucial: The analyst does not impose an external interpretation but co-constructs the meaning through repetitive linguistic mirroring ('always'). Clara's final repetition of 'always' (lines 404–05) suggests a moment of recognition—a realization of how pervasive this pattern is. This interaction exemplifies Benjamin's (1995) concept of mutual recognition: it is in the analyst's ability to hold and mirror this paradox that Clara momentarily glimpses the pattern from within rather than merely describing it from the outside.

A key characteristic of Clara's narrative style is her preference for external focalization—this narrative stance minimizes vulnerability, reflecting an unconscious defence against the anxiety of recognition. In Excerpt 7.1, Clara avoids describing her own emotions about Z's approach. In Excerpt 9.2, the realization that G loved her 'fatally' (line 387) triggers a defensive response (a long pause, followed by an impersonal statement about feeling 'bad' rather than an emotionally engaged reflection). This detachment from internal affect aligns with Bromberg's (1998) idea of dissociation as a relational phenomenon: Clara unconsciously protects herself from affective intensity by keeping emotions externalized or only fleetingly acknowledged.

This pattern also reflects Kernberg's (1975) conceptualization of splitting and affective inhibition: by maintaining relational experiences as disjointed and disconnected, Clara preserves an internal structure where intimacy remains distant and inaccessible.

A relational-intersubjective interpretation suggests that these moments are not just analytic observations but enactments occurring within the analytic dyad itself. Clara's defensive narrative shifts, her reluctance to elaborate on contradictions, and her co-construction of meaning with the analyst reveal the emotional risks involved in being recognized and understood. The analyst's non-intrusive yet persistent interventions (e.g. highlighting the contradiction in Extract 7.1, mirroring 'always' in Extract 7.2) create a holding environment (Winnicott 1971 that allows Clara to tentatively engage with her own patterns without direct confrontation. This facilitates a slow process of affect integration where Clara's fragmented relational experiences may be linked together over time. Her unconscious expectation of missed recognition can be experienced differently within the analytic relationship. The analytic dyad itself becomes a space where recognition is not a demand but a process. This aligns with Orange et al.'s (1997) intersubjective systems theory, which emphasizes that meaning and affect are not uncovered but co-constructed in the shared analytic field. Clara is not simply 'analysed'—her self-experience is actively reshaped within the analytic relationship.

Clara's narratives reflect a deeply ingrained relational pattern where mutual love and recognition exist but remain unregistered in real time. This theme is not only a past trauma but an ongoing intersubjective reality—one that unfolds within her relationships and within the analytic field itself. Through a relational-intersubjective lens, we can see how Clara's defensive externalization of emotions serves as a buffer against vulnerability. Relational coordination with the analyst reflects an unconscious attempt to work through recognition anxieties. Missed romantic encounters mirror an ongoing intersubjective enactment, which the analytic process gradually brings into awareness. The therapeutic challenge is not to simply analyse Clara's contradictions, but to participate in a process where she can begin to register her own relational experiences as real, mutual, and meaningful. In this way, the analytic dyad becomes not only a site of insight but a space for transformation—where the very wish 'to be loved and understood' is gradually lived rather than merely spoken.

After a discussion of the analysand's recognition of her relationship behaviour patterns, the analysand and analyst agree on the discussion of one example of such behaviour in the case of Z, which was the latest manifestation of the analysand's avoidant behaviour in relationships. In Z's case Clara and the analyst discuss (Excerpt 7.3) the potential causes of the analysand's reaction to him:

Excerpt 7.3 (session 6, L23)

492TER:	öö +	eeer+
493TER:	egy lehetséges, de csak egy lehetséges magyarázat.	one possible, but only a possible explanation.
494PAT:	lehet hogy én nem akarom, hogy válaszoljon?	is it possible that I don't want him to answer?
495TER:	hát ööö+..	well eeer+…
496TER:	igen.	yes.
497PAT:	valamilyen valamilyen félelem miatt.	because of some some fear.
598TER:	nem hinném, hogy +..	I don't think that+…
599TER:	hogy ez ez tudatos.	that this is this is conscious.
500PAT:	persze hogy nem.	of course not.

Looking at the discourse level in Excerpt 7.3 we see that both the analysand and the analyst are using the therapeutic here and now, which level is suitable for discussing emotions and thoughts arising at the session. In line 493 the analyst initiates this perspective and, in turn, the analysand also shifts into this perspective in line 494, exhibiting the coordination of perspectives. In cooperation with the analyst, she elaborates further the potential causes of her behaviour with Z. Clara recognizes her own fear and accepts the analyst's interpretation (lines 498–99) of the nature of this anxiety in line 500. Following Clara's acceptance, the therapist continues her interpretation (Excerpt 7.4):

Excerpt 7.4 (L23)

501TER:	vagyis a tudatos része az,	well what is conscious is that,
502TER:	hogy ő nem fog válaszolni.	he will not answer.
503TER:	de talán a a a rejtett érzés,	but perhaps the the the hidden emotion,
504TER:	ami ami itt lehet, az hogy,	that that may be here is that,
505TER:	ha válaszolna akkor bonyodalmak keletkeznének.	if he would have answered then there would be complications.
506TER:	és akkor szoronganék.	and then I would be anxious.
507TER:	és ö+..	and eer+...
508TER:	egy idő után megint úgy érezném,	after a while I would again feel,
509TER:	hogy visszautasítanak.	that I am being rejected.
510PAT:	ez biztos.	this is for sure.

In Excerpt 7.4 the analyst begins in line 501 a long interpretation. She uses the present tense, hetero-diegesis until line 505, and shifts into pseudo-diegesis in lines 506–10. She uses the first-person singular, talking in the name of the analysand, expressing her identification with her, as well as her empathy, taking the analysand's role in the dialogue. So, in this position, the analyst demonstrates the emotions that the analysand would live through in such a hypothetical situation, in other words where a relationship began between Clara and her love interest. The analyst uses the present tense, creating an 'as if' potential space for the analysand to imagine and identify with her possible self. The analysand—perhaps partly due to the intense attunement with the analyst—expresses her agreement in line 510. It is important to note that the analyst here does not merely interpret the analysand's unconscious feelings and emotions underlying her behaviour, but also creates a climate for the analysand to accept these threatening emotions by her perspective shifts, specifically her use of pseudo-diegesis.

The analyst's use of perspective shifts also includes her use of agency. In her pseudo-diegetic interpretation of the analysand's emotions (analyst narrator = analysand), she uses self-agency, thus demonstrating for the analysand a potential agentic attitude towards her own emotional reactions. The analyst demonstrates to the analysand how she can experience threatening emotions while not losing control over the situation. In other words, we can say that the analyst is able to contain the analysand's emotions in such a way that she makes Clara experience that she herself is able to do the same. This is achieved by using the pseudo-diegetic perspective.

From a relational and intersubjective psychoanalytic perspective, Clara's dialogues in these excerpts illuminate the co-constructed nature of meaning-making in the analytic dyad and how implicit relational knowing (Lyons-Ruth et al. 1998) shapes her emotional experience. Additionally, by incorporating Tronick's (2003) ideas on dyadic emotional regulation and the Boston Change Process Study Group's (BCPSG) findings on implicit relational processes, we can further understand how attunement, rupture, and repair unfold in this interaction and contribute to Clara's emerging capacity for self-agency in relationships.

In Excerpt 7.3, we see Clara and the analyst working together to uncover the deeper emotional underpinnings of her relational avoidant behaviour. The analyst introduces an interpretive space (line 493: 'one possible explanation'), and Clara immediately joins the meaning-making process (line 494: 'Is it possible that I don't want him to answer?'). This marks a shift into the therapeutic here and now, a moment where implicit relational knowing becomes explicit and Clara begins engaging in self-reflection.

The relational-intersubjective framework (Stolorow et al. 2002) emphasizes how meaning and affect regulation occur within a shared intersubjective field, and Excerpt 7.3 is an example of such a process. The analyst does not impose an interpretation; instead, she co-creates meaning with Clara, following her lead. This exemplifies attunement and coordination, key concepts in Tronick's mutual regulation model, where the analyst's affective stance provides a scaffold for Clara to access and tolerate her unconscious fears.

Coordination of perspectives occurs in lines 493–500, where Clara and the analyst dynamically exchange ideas, allowing Clara to safely engage with difficult emotional content. Clara's question in line 494 suggests that she is tentatively trying on the analyst's interpretation, engaging in a process of affective and cognitive exploration within the analytic space. In line 497, she names 'some fear' as a possible cause, indicating a nascent ability to symbolize her emotions—a crucial developmental shift. The analyst's next response (lines 498–99: 'I don't think this is conscious') functions as a containment mechanism (Bion 1962a), reassuring Clara that her defensive reaction is not a conscious choice but a deeper, structural pattern. Clara immediately affirms this in line 500 ('Of course not'), reinforcing the idea that this implicit pattern is becoming explicit within the dyad.

In Excerpt 7.4, the analyst takes a more active role in emotional mirroring and containment, shifting from hetero-diegesis (external narration) to pseudo-diegesis (speaking in the voice of the analysand). This shift is not simply an interpretive move but an intersubjective enactment, where the therapist embodies Clara's internal experience to help her tolerate and integrate difficult emotions. The use of pseudo-diegesis may help create an 'as-if' potential space (Ogden 2018) in which Clara can imagine experiencing the emotions without fully merging with them. This manoeuvre (1) externalizes the anxiety by initially locating it in the analyst's voice, giving her greater psychological distance; and (2) establishes a transitional affective space in which she can safely engage with feelings that might otherwise be overwhelming.

This moment aligns with Tronick's (2003) view of dyadic affect regulation, where the analyst temporarily 'holds' an unprocessed affective state for the analysand, modelling how it can be named, tolerated, and integrated. The analyst's voice functions as a regulatory mechanism, translating an implicit, dissociated affect into an explicit, symbolized narrative. The analyst is not merely 'naming' Clara's emotions but is demonstrating a way to process and regulate them. This dynamic mirrors the interactive process of infant–care-giver dyads, as described by the Boston Change Process Study Group (2005), where affective mismatches and repairs create new modes of relational experiencing. Clara's immediate affirmation in line 510 ('This is for sure') suggests that she is beginning to integrate this new emotional understanding within herself.

The analyst's use of perspective shifts contribute to the further development of self-agency. One of the most significant elements of the analyst's intervention is how she demonstrates an agentic stance towards emotions. The analyst does not describe emotions as external facts but as lived experiences, reinforcing the idea that Clara can actively engage with her affective states instead of being passively overwhelmed by them. This also aligns with BCPSG's concept of 'moving along' moments, where therapeutic change does not happen through insight alone, but through experiential, embodied shifts within the dyad. Clara's recognition in line 510 signals that a new self-state is being integrated, where she can begin to recognize her avoidant relational patterns without fully identifying with them.

The process of therapeutic change in that section moves from implicit patterns to explicit meaning. By examining Clara's process through a relational-intersubjective lens, we can see that her change is not occurring through direct confrontation or interpretation alone, but through a co-regulated, affective process within the analytic dyad. The oscillation between implicit and explicit knowing (Lyons-Ruth et al. 1998) is a key mechanism at work. Through pseudo-diegesis, affective containment, and self-agency modelling, the analyst creates a transitional space where new relational possibilities emerge.

Tronick's mutual regulation model highlights how affective ruptures (e.g. Clara's avoidance) and repairs (e.g. the analyst's attunement and scaffolding) create new implicit relational templates. Ultimately, the analyst's perspective shifts do not just serve an interpretative function but facilitate Clara's gradual movement towards a more integrated relational experience. In doing so, the analyst embodies a different way of relating to emotions and relationships, allowing Clara to begin internalizing this stance for herself.

We can conclude that affective change at this session happened through the changes in the intersubjective field. Clara's therapeutic journey in these excerpts reflects a process where intersubjective attunement, co-regulation, and perspective shifting allow for the emergence of a more integrated and agentic self-experience. What we have seen in this process is attunement and coordination. The analyst does not impose meaning but co-constructs it, allowing Clara to engage at her own pace. The second therapeutic process is containment through pseudo-diegesis: the analyst momentarily 'holds' difficult affective states, allowing Clara to process them with distance. This also includes the modelling of self-agency: the analyst demonstrates a way to tolerate and integrate emotions, which Clara begins to internalize. It represents moving along moments (BCPSG): instead of a single interpretive breakthrough, therapeutic change happens through the embodied, affective experience of co-regulation and repair. By integrating Tronick's mutual regulation model, BCPSG's process-oriented framework, and relational-intersubjective psychoanalysis, we can see that Clara is not just learning about her emotions—she is learning how to live within them, tolerate them, and relate to them differently within an emerging intersubjective space.

At the end of the discussion at the session, the analysand and analyst discussed some more situations in which Clara rejected potential love interests and her reasons for avoidant behaviour, which constitutes a turning point in the psychoanalysis of Clara, because this is the point she recognizes not only her repetitive behaviour pattern with others from whom she expects love and understanding but, further, her underlying emotions, and reasons for avoiding intimacy and love. So, despite her most frequent wish 'to be loved and understood'—expressed more clearly as increasing time spent in psychotherapy—she undermined her own relationships with potential and actual romantic partners. The analysand recognized this, and drew the adequate conclusions at this session.

Reactions of others

As we mentioned, a constituent of relational episodes is the reaction of others—not so much as it takes place in reality, but as it is filtered through the perspective of the analysand—namely, how she sees others reacting to her own wishes and expectations. Table 7.11 contains the distribution of others' reactions in terms of the standard clusters described by Luborsky and colleagues (Barber et al. 1990).

As we can see in Table 7.11, others' reactions to the analysand's wishes was found to be 'rejecting and opposing' (27.8%) in the greatest proportion. The second greatest proportion was others being 'helpful' (22.3%), and the third was others being 'understanding' (15.9%). These results are somewhat contradictory, since the positive reactions—being 'helpful' and 'understanding'—taken together (38.2%) outweigh the negative reaction of 'rejecting and opposing' (27.8%). So, we can say that, looking at the negative and positive reactions from others, positive reactions are more pronounced among the most important reactions, despite the fact that the reaction in the greatest proportion is a negative one, which means that the analysand experienced others' reactions in a diverse, somewhat ambivalent way.

There is a significant change between the three observed phases of psychotherapy in the proportion of response from others, $\chi2(14, 327) = 57.13$ $p < .001$ $\varphi = .42$. The following analysis contains an examination of the changes regarding the proportion of responses from others. We will compute a series of $\chi2$ tests, examining all response categories separately. The multiple testing increases the chances of type one error; therefore, using the Holm procedure, we decreased the acceptable level of significance to 0.008. So, the results will only be significant if they are below this level. If a response category is significant, there is no need

Table 7.11 Reactions of others

	First phase	Second phase	Third phase	Total
strong	4.1%	0%	0%	**1.5%**
controlling	13.0%	5.4%	9.7%	**9.5%**
upset	18.7%	9.9%	2.2%	**11.0%**
bad	8.9%	7.2%	1.1%	**6.1%**
rejecting and opposing	22.0%	33.3%	29.0%	**27.8%**
helpful	17.9%	22.5%	28.0%	**22.3%**
likes me	8.1%	7.2%	1.1%	**5.8%**
understanding	7.3%	14.4%	29.0%	**15.9%**

for further correction; thus we can use the original, α = .05, significance level in further computations.

The proportion of the category of 'strong' is very low, and does not show significant change during the observation period, $\chi 2(2, 327) = 8.42$ $p = .015$ $\varphi = .160$. The category of 'controlling' does not show significant change either, $\chi 2(2, 327) = 3.94$ $p = .140$ $\varphi = .11$. The proportion of the category of 'upset' shows a significant change during the observation period, $\chi 2(2, 327) = 15.01$ $p = .001$ $\varphi = .21$. The difference between the first and second phases is not significant, $\chi 2(1, 234) = 3.63$ $p = .057$ $\varphi = .13$. Between the second and third phases the decrease is significant, but weak, $\chi 2(1\ 204) = 5.11$ $p = .024$ $\varphi = .16$. The decrease between the first and third phases is significant, and moderate, $\chi 2(1, 216) = 14.17$ $p < .001$ $\varphi = .26$. It is worth noting that in the first phase there is only one session (the second). The proportion of the category of 'bad' does not show a significant change during the observation period, $\chi 2(2, 327) = 6.06$ $p = .048$ $\varphi = .14$. The proportion of the category of 'rejecting and opposing' is high, but it does not show a significant change during the observation period, $\chi 2(2, 327) = 3{,}86$ $p = .145$ $\varphi = .11$. The proportion of the category of 'helpful' is high, and it does not show significant change during the observation period, $\chi 2(2, 327) = 3.10$ $p = .212$ $\varphi = .10$. The category of 'likes me' does not show significant change during the observation period, $\chi 2(2, 327) = 5.42$ $p = .067$, $\varphi = .13$. The proportion of the category of 'understanding' shows a significant change during the observation period, $\chi 2(2, 327) = 18.95$ $p < .001$ $\varphi = .24$. The difference between the first and second phase is not significant, $\chi 2(1, 234) = 3.08$ $p = .079$ $\varphi = .12$. The increase between the second and third phase is significant, and weak $\chi 2(1\ 204) = 6.50$ $p = .011$ $\varphi = .18$. The difference between the first and the third phase is significant, and moderate $\chi 2(1, 216) = 17.98$ $p < .001$ $\varphi = .29$.

To summarize, among the reactions of others, the category of being 'upset' (11%) and of being 'understanding' (approximately 16%) show a significant change during the observation period. We will now discuss these results in more detail.

The reaction of others being 'upset' refers to the standard categories of others being 'hurt', 'dependent', 'anxious', 'angry', and 'out of control'. More specifically, in Luborsky's category system others being 'hurt' means that they are pained, injured, and wounded (emotionally); others being 'dependent' means that they are influenced by the self, and they are submissive; others being 'anxious' means that they are being scared, worried, and nervous; others being 'angry' means that they are irritable, resentful, and frustrated; and others being 'out of control' means that they are unreliable, are not dependable, and are irresponsible (Barber et al. 1990).

So, our results show that Clara feels that she upsets others, but this feeling diminishes by the end of the observation period to a relatively low level, approximately 2%. The analysand's initial feeling that she upsets others during the beginning phase of therapy (approximately18%) suggests that she is concerned about hurting others, or making them angry and frustrated. This might be explained in psychoanalytic terms as the self being overly dependent on other's approval, and on others being accepting towards the self.

Based on the same category system (Barber et al. 1990), others' 'understanding' reaction refers to the standard categories of others being 'open', 'understanding', and 'accepting'. More specifically, others being 'open' refers to others being expressive, disclosing, and available; being 'understanding' refers to being empathetic, sympathetic, and seeing the self accurately; being 'accepting' refers to others do not rejecting the self, approving and including the self. Others' understanding response increases from approximately 7% in the beginning phase of psychotherapy to approximately 16% in the working phase of therapy, by the third phase of the observation period. This increase is congruent with therapeutic goals, since the analysand experiences her interpersonal relationships as more in line with her own positive expectations as psychoanalysis progresses. As we discussed above, Clara's major wish (expectation) towards others is 'to be loved and to be understood'. So, the fact that she experiences others as being increasingly more 'understanding' represents an affirmative response from others in her case.

As we can see in Figure 7.3, the response 'understanding' from others is highest in session 8. This session has already been mentioned as the session in

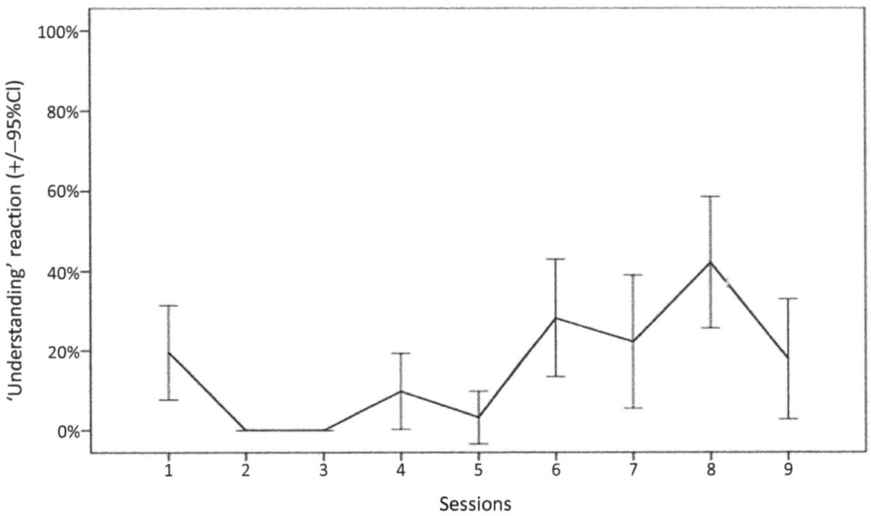

Figure 7.3 Changes of 'Understanding' reaction from others during the observation period

which the analysand's desire 'to be loved and understood' also hit a high point. We will discuss this session in more detail below, using qualitative analysis of NP shifting behaviour at the session. Before turning to that discussion, however, we will describe who those 'others' are, who react to the analysand—according the analysand's recounting of relationship episodes during the observation period.

As we can see in Table 7.12, the response of 'rejecting and opposing' from others is more than one-quarter of all reactions to the analysand's wishes, and is present in great proportion in all three phases of the observation period. There is a tendency on the part of the self to be experienced as rejecting and opposing by the analysand—in analytic terms this could be an overly strict super-ego, or strong aggressive or sexual drives, which the ego can only partially tame, and with difficulty. We can see tendencies of 'rejecting and opposing' also on the part of the mother, the partner, and female authority figures. It is interesting to see that, from the analyst, the analysand does not express such an experience to a substantial degree, which may be due to positive transference. We must

Table 7.12 Reactions from others: rejecting and opposing

		First phase	**Second phase**	**Third phase**	Total
Rejecting and opposing	N	27	37	27	91
	Percent	22.0%	33.3%	29.0%	27,8%
		First phase	**Second phase**	**Third phase**	Total
Self		**29.6%**	**10.8%**	**33.3%**	**23.1%**
Analyst		7.4%	2.7%	0.0%	3.3%
Mother		**14.8%**	**24.3%**	**11.1%**	**17.6%**
Father		0.0%	5.4%	0.0%	2.2%
Sibling		**22.2%**	0.0%	0.0%	6.6%
Children		0.0%	0.0%	0.0%	0.0%
Partner		7.4%	0.0%	**44.4%**	**15.4%**
Male authority figures		7.4%	10.8%	3.7%	7.7%
Female authority figures		0.0%	**27.0%**	3.7%	**12.1%**
Male friends		0.0%	8.1%	0.0%	3.3%
Female friends		11.1%	8.1%	0.0%	6.6%
Other		0.0%	2.7%	3.7%	2.2%

Table 7.13 Reactions from others: helpful

		First phase	**Second phase**	**Third phase**	Total
Helpful	N	22	25	26	73
	Percent	17.9%	22.5%	28.0%	22.3%
		First phase	**Second phase**	**Third phase**	Total
Self		18.2%	12.0%	0.0%	9.6%
Analyst		**36.4%**	**72.0%**	**57.7%**	**56.2%**
Mother		4.5%	4.0%	15.4%	8,2%
Father		0.0%	0.0%	3.8%	1.4%
Sibling		13.6%	4.0%	0.0%	5.5%
Children		0.0%	0.0%	0.0%	0.0%
Partner		0.0%	0.0%	7.7%	2.7%
Male authority figures		4.5%	4.0%	7.7%	5.5%
Female authority figures		9.1%	0.0%	7.7%	5.5%
Male friends		0%	0.0%	0.0%	0.0%
Female friends		9.1%	0.0%	0.0%	2.7%
Other		4.5%	4.0%	0.0%	2.7%

emphasize, however, that the mentioned differences are only tendencies, because due to the low amount of data, we could not calculate any statistical tests.

As we can see in Table 7.13, the 'helpful' response from others is described in a great proportion of relationship episodes, in all three phases of psychotherapy. We can see a tendency that it is the analyst whom the analysand experiences as helpful in the greatest proportion—more than half of the occurrences of this response. This result is in harmony with the previously described 'rejecting and opposing' response, where the analyst had a very low proportion of such responses. So, these two antagonistic responses in the case of the analyst may be said to verify each other. These results also lend support to the idea that the working alliance in the case of this dyad is well developed by the end of the observation period, 1.5 years into psychoanalysis.

In the case of the next response from others, 'upset', we can only interpret results for two phases of the observation period, due to a low level of occurrence in the third phase. However, there is a significant decrease by the third phase, as we described above.

Table 7.14 Reactions from others: upset

	First phase	**Second phase**
Self	**30.4%**	9.1%
Analyst	0.0%	0.0%
Father	0.0%	0.0%
Mother	0.0%	**45.5%**
Sibling	0.0%	0.0%
Children	0.0%	0.0%
Partner	0.0%	0.0%
Male authority figures	0.0%	9.1%
Female authority figures	8.7%	**18.2%**
Male friends	**47.8%**	9.1%
Female friends	8.7%	9.1%
Other	4.3%	0.0%

As we can see in Table 7.14 there is a high tendency of giving the response 'upset' by male friends in the first phase of therapy, as well as by the self; whereas in the second phase, this response was given by the mother, as well as female authority figures, in a greater proportion of cases. These results suggest that the analysand was concerned about her own emotional responses to events and wishes, as well as about other important loved ones, such as the mother. The fact that she mentioned this reaction as coming from male friends points to the conflictual nature of her relationship with men in general and with potential love interests.

Finally, another important reaction we discussed above is others being perceived as 'understanding' by the analysand.

As we can see in Table 7.15, there is a tendency for the analyst to be perceived as reacting to the analysand with understanding—approximately 62% of all such responses. This again, supports the idea that the analyst is being perceived by the analysand as responding adequately to her needs, and in turn suggests that the working alliance must be well developed and strong between the participants. Other people who are perceived as reacting with understanding to the analysand's needs—although to a much lesser extent—are male friends (approximately 17%), and the analysand's partner. The latter reaction is more pronounced in the third phase of the observation period (approximately 19%).

From a relational-intersubjective perspective, the analysand's experience of how others react to her desires and expectations is co-constructed within the

Table 7.15 Reactions from others: understanding

		First phase	Second phase	Third phase	Total
understanding	N	9	16	27	**52**
	Percent	7.3%	14.4%	29.0%	**15.9%**

	First phase	Second phase	Third phase	Total
Self	0.0%	6.3%	0.0%	**1.9%**
Analyst	**77.8%**	**31.3%**	**74.1%**	**61.5%**
Mother	0.0%	12.5%	0.0%	**3.8%**
Father	0.0%	6.3%	0.0%	**1.9%**
Sibling	0.0%	0.0%	0.0%	**0.0%**
Children	0.0%	0.0%	0.0%	**0.0%**
Partner	0.0%	0.0%	**18.5%**	**9.6%**
Male authority figures	0.0%	0.0%	3.7%	**1.9%**
Female authority figures	0.0%	0.0%	0.0%	**0.0%**
Male friends	**22.2%**	**43.8%**	0.0%	**17.3%**
Female friends	0.0%	0.0%	0.0%	**0.0%**
Other	0.0%	0.0%	3.7%	**1.9%**

analytic relationship and shaped by implicit relational patterns (Stolorow et al. 2002). Drawing from Tronick's (2003) mutual regulation model and the Boston Change Process Study Group (BCPSG 2010), our analysis focuses on how perceived interpersonal reactions evolve over time and how the therapeutic relationship facilitates implicit relational shifts and affect integration.

Clara's experience of how others respond to her is not simply an objective recollection of social interactions, but a dynamic, emotionally filtered reconstruction of past and present relational experiences. The data suggests an ambivalent perception of others, where the most frequent reaction is 'rejecting and opposing' (27.8%); yet overall positive responses ('helpful' and 'understanding') outweigh the negative ones. This contradiction signals a split in Clara's relational experience, in which both acceptance and rejection co-exist, yet rejection remains the dominant response.

The consistently high percentage of 'rejecting and opposing' suggests the presence of a rigid internal relational schema in which Clara anticipates being opposed, dismissed, or rejected, particularly by authority figures and close relational partners. The increase in 'understanding' responses over time (from 7.3% to 29%) reflects a therapeutic shift, where Clara begins to perceive others (particularly the analyst) as more accepting and attuned. The decrease in 'upset' responses suggests a diminishing fear that her presence or actions cause distress in others, indicating a gradual reduction in self-blame and excessive concern for others' emotional states. These shifts align with BCPSG's concept of relational knowing (Lyons-Ruth et al. 1998), wherein implicit expectations of relationships—formed through past experiences—gradually change within the therapeutic dyad as new relational experiences unfold. A critical aspect of Clara's transformation occurs within the therapeutic relationship in Excerpt 7.4. The strong working alliance with the analyst, evidenced by the high proportion of 'helpful' (56.2%) and 'understanding' (61.5%) responses attributed to her, plays a pivotal role in shaping Clara's new relational experiences.

Tronick's mutual regulation model (2003) emphasizes that emotional development is shaped through dyadic interactions, where affective states are continuously regulated through cycles of attunement, rupture, and repair. Clara's early experiences of being 'upset' (18.7%) or causing distress in others suggest an internalized mismatch–repair cycle that remained unresolved in past relationships. As therapy progresses, the increasingly 'understanding' response from the analyst provides a new relational template, wherein distress can be held, processed, and transformed rather than avoided or dismissed. This attuned therapeutic environment allows Clara to reconstruct her perception of others and re-examine her relational patterns in real-time interactions with the analyst.

As we have mentioned earlier, the greatest proportion of the 'understanding' response was found at session 8, directed towards the analysand's boyfriend. Now we will discuss that session in more detail, specifically looking at NP shifting behaviour at relevant moments of the session.

Session 8 (L3.2), examining the complexity of 'understanding' reaction of others

At session 8 of the female analysand–female analyst dyad the interlocutors discuss issues related to compromises in (romantic) relationships, and in connection to the issue of integrating positive and negative aspects of people, situations, and the analysand's swiftly changing ambivalent feelings and judgments of these positive and negative aspects of events and persons. Further, they discuss issues related to the analysand's self-view, which is also very unstable, and relating to her own self is prone to undergo similar processes as the analysand's relationship with others. In psychoanalytic terms, these would be processes of splitting both objects and the self, and being unable to integrate positive and negative feelings related to them. We will discuss three excerpts from this session.

At the beginning of the session (Excerpt 7.5), the analysand and analyst talk about relationship problems with the analysand's boyfriend, L., with whom the analysand got into an argument over where to sleep at the weekend. L. wanted them to sleep at his place, while the analysand resented this.

Excerpt 7.5 (session 8, L32)

65PAT:	hogy mer hogy én nem tudok ott aludni.	so because I cannot sleep there.
66PAT:	mer minden tele van macskaszőrrel,	because everything is full of cat hair,
67PAT:	és hogy iszonyú alergiás vagyok macskaszőrre.	and that I am terribly allergic to cat hair.
68PAT:	és az nekem nem+/	and for me that is not+/
69PAT:	egyszerűen nem tudok ott aludni.	I am simply unable to sleep there.
70PAT:	és ö és iszonyú ingerült volt a telefonba,	and uh he was terribly irritated on the phone,
71PAT:	de aztán így azt mondta,	but then he said like,
72PAT:	hogy jó,	that it was ok,
73PAT:	akkor menjek oda,	that I should go there,
74PAT:	és akkor elmegyünk az ő cuccáért,	and then we'll go to pick up his stuff,
75PAT:	aztán meg majd,	and then later,
76PAT:	este meg majd nálunk alszunk.	at night we should sleep at my place.
77PAT:	és én iszonyú rosszul éreztem magamat ettől,	and I felt terribly bad because of this,
78PAT:	de nagyon,	but very much so,

In the story in Excerpt 7.5 the analysand recollects a recent discussion with her boyfriend, when, after a compromise reached with him on the issue of where to sleep that night, she did not feel satisfied; instead, she felt 'terribly bad'. The analyst does not intervene during the recollection. In lines 65–69 the analysand uses the present tense, homo-diegesis, first-person singular—creating tension, and involvement at the beginning of her story, clearly signalling that she is very emotional or even upset while recollecting the cause of the conflict between her and her boyfriend, regarding cat hair. She shifts into hetero-diegesis in line 70, when she begins to talk about her boyfriend's behaviour on the phone, shifting into the past tense—thus creating more emotional distance between herself and the characters in her story. The compromised solution of where to sleep is described indirectly quoting the boyfriend, L., in lines 71–76, using the same perspective as before. So, here the analysand takes on the boyfriend's perspective, while describing the conversation from his point of view. Next, the analysand draws her conclusion in lines 77–78 remaining in the past tense, in the first-person singular: 'I felt terribly bad', despite winning the argument.

Session 8 provides a key example of how Clara struggles to integrate conflicting aspects of relationships. The discussion about her boyfriend highlights a pattern of relational ambivalence and splitting, where positive and negative emotions cannot be held simultaneously. We can observe a splitting and the inability to integrate positive and negative aspects of others. In her account of the argument over sleeping arrangements, Clara exhibits significant shifts in narrative perspective that reflect her difficulty in maintaining a coherent emotional stance: The inability to maintain positive relational moments suggests a dominance of negative affective expectations, consistent with an internalized relational schema shaped by past experiences of rejection. This aligns with object relations theory (Kernberg 1975), where early relational patterns lead to difficulty integrating love and aggression, resulting in unstable interpersonal experiences.

By refraining from immediate interpretation or confrontation, the analyst allows Clara to sit with her ambivalence, facilitating a gradual process of self-reflection rather than defensive splitting. This aligns with BCPSG's (2005) 'something more than interpretation' approach, where therapeutic change is facilitated not just through cognitive insight but through relationally co-constructed affective experiences. The analyst's consistent understanding stance provides Clara with a stable relational environment where emotions can be explored rather than reacted to impulsively.

Across therapy, Clara's shifting perceptions of others' reactions suggest a gradual restructuring of her implicit relational knowing. This transformation is not merely an intellectual insight but an experiential shift in emotional regulation and self–other expectations. The beginning phase is characterized by the high prevalence of 'rejecting and opposing' responses, which suggests an internalized expectation of being dismissed or misunderstood. In the second phase, increasing 'understanding' responses (14.4%) reflect a growing capacity to register acceptance and attunement from others. During the third phase 'understanding' responses peak at 29%, suggesting a more stable internalized sense of being recognized and valued. These shifts align with Tronick's dyadic expansion of consciousness model, wherein successful mutual regulation in the therapeutic dyad leads to increased self-agency and relational flexibility. Clara moves from rigid, conflictual relational expectations to a more nuanced, integrated experience of interpersonal relationships.

Clara's journey in psychoanalysis demonstrates how implicit relational expectations can shift within a stable, attuned analytic relationship. Through affective co-regulation, containment, and attunement, the analyst provides a relational space where past relational patterns are re-experienced, examined, and transformed. Ambivalence in relational experiences is co-constructed at the session, where the analyst serves as both a recipient and regulator of Clara's projected expectations. Therapeutic change occurs through implicit relational shifts, where Clara moves from an expectation of rejection to an increasing capacity to perceive understanding and attunement. The integration of conflicting relational experiences is supported by the analyst's ability to hold and mirror both negative and positive aspects of relationships without reinforcing splitting defences. By integrating relational-intersubjective psychoanalysis, Tronick's mutual regulation model, and BCPSG's developmental perspective, Clara's progress in therapy can be seen as a transformation of relational knowing, where she experientially reconstructs a more stable, accepting, and integrated sense of self in relation to others.

After describing the central conflict between her boyfriend and herself in Excerpt 7.5, the analysand continues (in Excerpt 7.6) to describe events—various complications—of the story: she shows up to meet her boyfriend but, by that time, she decides to avoid the conflict by agreeing to sleep at his place. He, however, becomes upset, because she changed her mind again—and, as the analysand describes, it turns out that he has not even been irritated before, over his having to sleep at the analysand's place. This incident illustrates one of the major interpersonal problems of the analysand, which is the assertion of the self with attachment persons, and this problem is related to her problem with boundaries with others. She is not able to defend her own boundaries, and is puzzled by her boyfriend's defending his. In Excerpt 7.6 the analysand and the analyst continue the discussion of the interaction between Clara and her partner in Excerpt 7.5.

Excerpt 7.6 (session 8, L32)

151PAT:	van egy másik érzés,	there is another emotion,
152PAT:	amit nyilván kifejezett,	he definitely expressed,
153PAT:	és nem csak a kedvességet,	and not merely kindness,
154PAT:	akkor én már nem tudom végigvinni,	then I am unable to carry out,
155PAT:	amit szeretnék.	what I want.

156PAT:	és hogy még igazából persze végigvittem,	and that I have carried it out in reality, off course,
157PAT:	csak mm+...	but mm+...
158PAT:	igen nagy kerülőkkel.	in really great roundabout ways.
159PAT:	nem tudom olyan furcsa volt.	I don't know, it was really strange.
160TER:	nem egészen értem.	I don't really understand it.
161TER:	talán.	maybe.
162TER:	hogy más is benne van mint kedvesség,	there is something else in it, other than kindness,
163TER:	jól é+/	correctly+/
164TER:	jól hallottam?	did I hear it correctly?
165TER:	hogy valami ilyesmit mondott?	that you have said something like this?
166TER:	de nem egészen értem.	but I don't understand exactly.
167TER:	miről van szó.	what is meant by that.
168PAT:	tehát arról van szó,	well, what is meant by that,
169PAT:	hogy ő nem örült annak amit én mondtam.	is that he was not happy about what I said.

In Excerpt 7.6 the analysand describes her emotions when asserting the self. She may feel unconscious/conscious guilt about her actions. In lines 151–59 she uses the narrator level, present tense to discuss her emotions related to her boyfriend's behaviour in general terms. The analyst asks for clarification in lines 160–67, using the level of therapeutic here and now, and the present tense first-person singular, homo-diegesis in lines 160–61, then shifts to the past tense, but stays in the first-person singular, homo-diegesis in line 162. These perspectives show a high level of affective involvement on the part of the analyst. Instead of looking at the story from the outside point of view, she describes her own uncertainties related to what is happening at a given moment at the session. The analysand answers in lines 168–69, repeating the analyst's words ('what is meant by that'), and hence taking on the analyst's perspective at the level of the here and now of the session—perhaps also expressing some irony. However, due to this, in line 169 the analysand is finally able to summarize the situation, and describe her boyfriend's emotional reaction more precisely, using internal focalization: 'he was not happy about what I said'. So, in Excerpt 7.6, the analyst's patience and curiosity about the exact nuances of the analysand's emotions help Clara to clarify the problem of understanding and accepting her boyfriend's emotional reactions to her wishes, as well as her own emotional reactions to her boyfriend's reactions.

Building on the previous relational-intersubjective analysis, we now examine Clara's difficulty in asserting herself in relationships through the lens of mentalization theory (Fonagy et al. 2002; Fonagy & Allison 2013), Tronick's mutual regulation model (2007), and the Boston Change Process Study Group's (BCPSG) conceptualization of implicit relational knowing (2005, 2010).

Excerpt 7.6 provides a critical moment in the therapy, where Clara struggles with the assertion of self and boundary-setting with her boyfriend, yet through the attuned intervention of the analyst she is able to articulate a more nuanced understanding of her interpersonal conflict.

According to Fonagy et al's model of mentalization, individuals with unstable attachment histories often experience difficulties in accurately representing their own emotions and the emotions of others. In these cases, mentalization failures can take different forms: 1) psychic equivalence mode: The inner world is equated with external reality (e.g. 'If I feel rejected, it means I truly am unwanted'); 2) pretend mode: Emotional states feel disconnected from external interactions (e.g. 'I talk about my emotions, but I don't really feel them'). 3) hypermentalization: Over-attributing motives and intentions to others in a way that is not grounded in reality.

In Excerpt 7.6, Clara's difficulty asserting the self in relationships can be linked to mentalization failures, where she struggles to differentiate between her emotions, her boyfriend's emotions, and their interactive dynamic. In lines 151–59, Clara expresses internal confusion about her emotions when asserting herself. She recognizes her actions ('I carried it out'), yet simultaneously diminishes their legitimacy ('in really great roundabout ways'), revealing a lack of agency and self-assertion. Her statement in line 159 ('I don't know, it was really strange') suggests a breakdown in reflective function, where she struggles to articulate a clear cause-and-effect understanding of her emotional responses. These struggles align with Fonagy et al's (2002) conceptualization of low reflective function, where the individual feels emotions but cannot symbolize them effectively, leading to internal fragmentation and difficulty regulating affect. Also, Clara misinterprets her boyfriend's initial reaction—she assumes he was irritated about her request when, in reality, she later realizes that he was not even upset to begin with. This reflects hypermentalization, where Clara over-attributes negative emotions to her boyfriend, reinforcing a pre-existing relational schema of rejection and disapproval.

From a relational-intersubjective perspective, Clara experiences others through the filter of past relational traumas, which leads to misattuned interpretations of their emotions and reactions. The analytic process, then, becomes a space where these distorted representations can be examined, reworked, and corrected through an attuned relational dialogue.

The analyst's use of the first-person singular (lines 160–67, 'I don't really understand it' / 'Did I hear it correctly?') is a key mentalization-facilitating intervention. By expressing her own uncertainty, the analyst models mentalization, demonstrating that it is possible to tolerate ambiguity and not immediately jump to conclusions. This technique mirrors the process of secure attachment interactions, where a care-giver helps the child differentiate between their emotions and external reality. This interactive mentalization scaffolding aligns with Tronick's (2007) mutual regulation model, which highlights how affect regulation is co-constructed within dyadic interactions. The analyst is not just interpreting—she is actively shaping Clara's capacity to reflect on and process emotions.

The analyst shifts from past narrative (hetero-diegesis) to present interactive experience (homo-diegesis), engaging Clara in a real-time process of emotion clarification. This shift encourages Clara to move beyond a disconnected recounting of events and into a live experience of affect exploration. The repetition of 'Did I hear it correctly?' and 'What is meant by that?' in lines 162–67 forces Clara to re-engage with her experience rather than defensively dissociate from it. These interventions exemplify BCPSG's model of implicit relational knowing (2005, 2010), where therapeutic change occurs not just through insight but through the embodied, interactive experience of affective shifts within the therapeutic dyad.

At the start of Excerpt 7.6, Clara's description of her boyfriend's reaction is framed externally. She experiences his emotions as external obstacles that she must navigate rather than as expressions of an intersubjective dynamic. She assumes his emotions dictate her actions, reinforcing a passive relational stance where she struggles to hold onto her own needs. As the dialogue progresses, the analyst's patience and careful questioning lead Clara to acknowledge the complexity of the interaction, shifting from a purely external attribution of blame to an internal exploration of her emotional process. This transition reflects an expansion in Clara's mentalization capacity, allowing her to hold multiple perspectives simultaneously rather than collapsing into rigid interpretations.

In line 169, Clara finally articulates a more precise understanding of her boyfriend's emotional state: 'He was not happy about what I said'. This shift signifies a movement from an unmentalized, affect-driven reaction to a mentalized, differentiated understanding of relational dynamics. Notably, she uses internal focalization, signalling a greater capacity to register and reflect on her partner's emotions rather than reacting defensively. From Fonagy and colleague's perspective, this shift represents an increase in reflective function, allowing

Clara to move from emotionally enmeshed, reactive states to a more flexible, reflective mode of relating.

Clara's difficulties with self-assertion and boundary negotiation are linked to mentalization failures, where emotions remain undifferentiated and relationships are misinterpreted through past relational expectations. The analyst's use of perspective-taking and first-person engagement facilitates a mentalization process, modelling how to explore emotions with curiosity rather than rigid assumptions. Clara's shift from externalized blame to internal reflection represents a breakthrough in mentalization capacity.

As her analysis progresses, Clara can increasingly integrate affective complexity, leading to a more stable sense of self in relationships. By fostering a reflective space rather than pushing interpretations, the analyst enables Clara to construct her own meaning, reinforcing a newfound sense of agency. The therapeutic dyad itself serves as a corrective emotional experience, where Clara experiences relational attunement in real time, challenging her habitual expectations of rejection and conflict.

While Fonagy et al. emphasize affect regulation via reflective functioning, Tronick's mutual regulation model and the BCPSG's implicit relational knowing highlight that therapeutic change is not merely cognitive but embodied and interactional, unfolding in the live intersubjective moment between analyst and analysand. This integration of mentalization theory, relational-intersubjective psychoanalysis, and dyadic affect regulation models provides a comprehensive understanding of Clara's evolving therapeutic process and the mechanisms by which psychoanalysis facilitates relational transformation.

In Excerpt 7.7, the analysand discusses her feelings about her boyfriend, who—she feels—does not understand her emotions, what she wants to say, and, in general, 'moves on a different plane' than she does. However, at the same time she claims that she knows that he does understand her.

Excerpt 7.7 (session 8, L32)

523PAT:	meg hogy valahogy az is+/	and somehow also+/
524PAT:	tehát hogy olyan érzésem is van,	well that I also have the feeling,
525PAT:	mint hogyha nem is akarnám, hogy megértse.	as if I did not want him to understand.
526PAT:	sokszor.	often.
527TER:	ez érdekes kérdés.	this is an interesting question.
528TER:	miért?	why?
529PAT:	nem tudom.	I don't know.
530PAT:	nem tudom.	I don't know.

531PAT:	többször észrevettem saját magamon,	I have noticed myself many times,
532PAT:	hogy egyszerűen nem is akarom hogy megértse.	that I simply don't even want him to understand.
533PAT:	miközben persze akarom,	while at the same time I do off course,
534PAT:	csak hogy +…	however+…
535%com:	pat laughs	
536PAT:	azon belül meg valahogy nem.	within that I somehow don't.
537TER:	érdekes.	interesting.
538TER:	ezzel mintha azt mondta volna az előbb,	as if you would have been saying with this before,
539TER:	hogy úgysem érti meg.	that he does not understand it anyhow.
540TER:	tehát hogy valahogy mintha ha ezzel leértékelné őt.	as if somehow you would underestimate him by this.
541TER:	minek beszéljek egy olyan embernek,	why should I talk to such a person,
542TER:	aki úgysem érti meg.	who does not understand it anyhow.
543TER:	más síkon mozog mint én.	who moves on a different plane than I do.
544TER:	ilyesmit mondott.	you have said something like this.
546PAT:	igen.	yes.
547PAT:	de hogy+/	but that+/
548PAT:	tehát hogy,	well that,
549PAT:	igen,	yes,
550PAT:	de hogy közben meg tudom hogy megérti.	but that at the same time I know that he understands.

Using internal focalization, narrator-level, present tense in lines 523–6 the analysand describes her emotions related to her boyfriend's understanding of her. She expresses her ambivalence about being understood by him. In line 527 the analyst intervenes, shifting to the here-and-now level of the session. She enquires about why it is that she feels as if she does not want her boyfriend to understand her really. The analysand, shifting to the same perspective as the analyst, stays in the here-and-now level of the session in lines 529–30. So, here she steps out of her story and tries to reflect on the analyst's question. From line 531 she indicates reasons why she thinks she does not want her boyfriend to understand her, using internal focalization to describe her thought process. however, instead of giving a real explanation, she just states that, on some occasions, she noticed that she does not want him to understand her, while at the same time she still wants him to understand.

In line 537 the analyst reacts, shifting into the past tense, reminding the analysand of her previous statements at the session, and in line 540 shifts back into the present tense, using hetero-diegesis, thus staying outside the story while interpreting the analysand's previous statements. However, in the next line she shifts into pseudo-diegesis, using a direct quote from the analysand's imagined way of reasoning, using the first-person singular: 'why should I talk to such a person, who does not understand it anyhow'. The analyst stays in this perspective until line 543. By using a direct quote from what might be the analysand's imagined inside monologue, based on what she has said before, the analyst shifts into Clara's perspective. She describes to the analysand how she may feel towards her boyfriend. The analyst does not merely explain to the analysand in her lines 538–40 interpretation what her way of thinking about her boyfriend means—namely that she devaluates him—but also illustrates this view by shifting into the analysand's perspective. So, the analyst's message is delivered in two different ways to convince the analysand about her way of responding to her boyfriend.

In line 544 the analyst shifts back to the therapeutic here and now, to hetero-diegesis, putting the analysand into the agent's position. By this perspective, the analyst invites the analysand to share her own thoughts at the level of the here and now. The analysand replies in line 546 by agreeing, accepting the analyst's view, and shifting into the therapeutic here and now as well. At the same time, she adds in lines 547–50 that she knows that her boyfriend understands her, using the present tense, first-person singular, thus expressing a high level of self-involvement with this perspective.

In Excerpt 7.7, Clara expresses a central relational conflict: her ambivalence towards being understood by her boyfriend. This dynamic can be examined through relational-intersubjective psychoanalysis (Stolorow et al. 2002), Tronick's mutual regulation model (2007), the Boston Change Process Study Group's (BCPSG) research on implicit relational knowing (2005, 2010), and Fonagy et al's mentalization-based model (2002, 2011).

Excerpt 7.7 highlights Clara's struggle with being understood, which reflects underlying attachment and self–other regulation difficulties. The role of the analyst is scaffolding Clara's mentalization process, helping her move from implicit relational knowing to explicit reflective awareness. We showed the intersubjective process of co-constructing meaning, where the analyst's use of pseudo-diegesis plays a key role in deepening Clara's self-reflection.

Clara's statements in lines 523–26 suggest a mentalization breakdown, where she struggles coherently to integrate her conflicting desires. She simultaneously wants and does not want to be understood. This contradiction is not fully symbolized, leaving her in a state of affective and cognitive dissonance. According to Fonagy et al. (2002), individuals with insecure attachment histories often develop defensive mentalization strategies, where they diminish the emotional significance of being understood to protect against potential disappointment (defensive detachment), and anticipate misunderstanding or misattunement, reinforcing past relational schemas of not being seen. Clara's ambivalence may stem from a fear of vulnerability—if she allows herself to be fully understood, she might become too dependent or exposed in the relationship.

Clara's difficulty articulating why she does not want to be understood (lines 529–30, repeated 'I don't know') suggests that this is an implicit, procedural relational pattern rather than a consciously reflected-upon belief. According to BCPSG (2005), implicit relational knowing consists of unconscious, embodied patterns of relating that emerge in interactions but are not yet verbalized or symbolized. Clara's inability to give a reason for her ambivalence indicates that this is not just a cognitive dilemma but an affective, relational expectation shaped by past experiences. Her laugh in line 535 may signal affective tension, as she struggles to engage in reflective processing of an emotionally charged realization.

The analyst intervenes at a critical moment (lines 527–28), posing the direct question, 'Why?' This shifts the discourse to the therapeutic here and now, inviting Clara to step out of her habitual pattern and reflect on her own thought process. Clara's immediate response ('I don't know') signals an initial mentalization failure, but her later attempts (lines 531–36) suggest that the analyst's question has activated a reflective process.

A key intervention occurs in lines 538–43, when the analyst shifts into pseudo-diegesis, momentarily adopting Clara's imagined thought process: 'Why should I talk to such a person, who does not understand it anyhow?' (line 541). This technique mirrors Fonagy's concept of 'marked mirroring' (Fonagy et al. 2002)—the analyst temporarily steps into Clara's perspective, giving voice to an unconscious belief that Clara has not yet verbalized. This strategy externalizes Clara's implicit assumptions, helping her see her own thoughts from a distance, a process critical to strengthening the reflective function.

The analyst's shift back to hetero-diegesis in line 544 invites Clara to actively engage in reinterpreting her experience. Clara's response in line 546 ('Yes') suggests an initial moment of agreement, but she immediately adds nuance in lines 547–50: 'But at the same time, I know that he understands.' This marks a shift from absolute thinking to a more complex, integrated view of her relationship. This process reflects a core goal of mentalization-based therapy (MBT) (Bateman & Fonagy 2016), which is moving from rigid, implicit relational patterns ('He does not understand me') to a more flexible, reflective stance ('Sometimes I feel he doesn't, but I also know he does').

This analysis demonstrates how psychoanalysis fosters relational transformation through attuned interaction, perspective-taking, and scaffolding mentalization capacity, ultimately allowing Clara to develop a more integrated and flexible understanding of relationships. So, we can say that by discourse analysing shifts in perspective during session 8, we can better understand the psychotherapeutic processes behind others' 'understanding' reactions—especially the 'understanding' reaction of the analysand and the boyfriend, which takes up a major part of the discussion at session 8. This 'understanding' reaction is described in a very complex and ambivalent way by the analysand, since she wants to be understood while at the same time she does not want to be. She thinks her boyfriend moves on a different plane and does not understand her, while at the same time she knows he understands. This double contradiction or ambivalence in the analysand's relating to her intimate partner and interpreting his 'understanding' reaction towards her self is revealing also of the underlying emotional complexity of her desire 'to be loved and understood', which also reaches statistically high proportions in this session, as we have mentioned above. The ambivalence of this desire is evident in our analysis of how the analysand wants two opposing things at the same time (to be understood and not to be understood), and she becoming aware of these contradicting emotions and wishes at the session, thus gaining insight. The confirming reaction of others to this wish—in this case from the partner—is 'understanding'. This understanding response, however, in the analysand's interpretation is also filtered through her own ambivalent feelings of whether her partner is able to understand her in the first place.

Clara's ambivalence about being understood reflects underlying attachment anxieties and defensive mentalization strategies. The analyst's scaffolding techniques, particularly pseudo-diegesis and perspective-taking, help Clara move from implicit relational knowing to explicit reflection. This moment represents a shift in Clara's ability to hold multiple perspectives simultaneously, a crucial marker of increasing mentalization capacity. This transformation is not just an intellectual insight but an intersubjective, embodied experience, facilitated through dyadic affect regulation and perspective alignment. Through this process, the analytic dyad co-constructs new relational meanings, allowing Clara to gradually reshape her expectations in relationships and increase her tolerance for intimacy and mutual understanding.

Responses of the self to others' reactions

So far we have discussed two elements of Luborsky's schema for relationship episodes: the narrator's wishes and expectations from others, as well as others' reactions to these expectations. Luborsky's schema includes a third element, namely the self's response to others' reactions. Table 7.16 contains the distribution of the self's responses to others' reactions in terms of the standard clusters described by Luborsky and colleagues (Barber et al. 1990).

As we can see from Table 7.16, the most frequent response of the self to others' reactions is being 'helpless' (24%). According to Luborsky's category system, the response cluster of being 'helpless' is composed of the standard categories of being 'out of control', 'helpless', 'uncertain', and 'dependent'. Being 'out of control' means being irresponsible, impulsive, and unreliable. Being 'helpless' means being incompetent and inadequate. Being 'uncertain' means feeling torn, ambivalent, and conflicted, and being 'dependent' means being submissive and passive (Barber et al. 1990).

The second most frequent response of the self is being 'anxious and ashamed' (19.8%). According to Luborsky, the response cluster of being 'anxious and ashamed' is composed of the standard categories of being 'anxious', 'ashamed', and 'feeling guilty'. Being 'anxious' means feeling scared, worried, and nervous.

Table 7.16 Responses of the self to others' reactions

	First phase	**Second phase**	**Third phase**	Total
Helpful	14.9%	16.9%	12.0%	**14.8%**
Unreceptive	3.5%	16.9%	10.0%	**9.7%**
Respected and accepted	5.0%	6.8%	8.0%	**6.4%**
Oppose and hurt others	12.8%	2.5%	7.0%	**7.8%**
Self-controlled and self-confident	4.3%	6.8%	4.0%	**5.0%**
Helpless	22.0%	20.3%	31.0%	**24.0%**
Disappointed and depressed	9.9%	13.6%	15.0%	**12.5%**
Anxious and ashamed	27.7%	16.1%	13.0%	**19.8%**

Being 'ashamed' means feeling embarrassed and abashed. 'Feeling guilty' means blaming the self, feeling wrong, and at fault (Barber et al. 1990).

The third most frequent response of the self is being 'helpful' (14.8%). According to Luborsky's system, the cluster 'helpful' consists of the standard categories of being 'open', 'understanding', and 'helpful'. Being 'open' means expressing oneself. Being 'understanding' means comprehending, realizing, and seeing another accurately. Being 'helpful' means being supportive, trying to please others and being giving (Barber et al. 1990).

The results in Table 7.16 show that negative responses from the self (being helpless, anxious, and ashamed, 43.8% in total) outnumber the positive reactions (helpful, 14.8%). This is a surprising result if we consider that others' reactions were more positive than negative in valence when we looked at the most frequent reactions: others' reactions of being helpful and understanding, taken together (38.2%), outnumbered the negative reactions of rejecting and opposing (27.8%). However, looking at the most frequent reactions of others and responses of the self, we can see that there is a tendency on the part of the analysand to react negatively in greatest proportion to what she sees as others' positive reactions in greatest proportion. This might be explained by the analysand's relating to important others in an ambivalent way, disregarding the valence of others' reactions, or others' intentions—evidence of which we have encountered while discussing excerpts from session 8, and to which point we shall return below.

The change in the proportion of self-responses between the three phases of the observation period was significant $\chi2(14, 359) = 23.30$ $p < .001$ $\varphi = .314$. The following analysis contains an examination of the changes regarding the proportion of responses from others. This means that we will compute a series of $\chi2$ tests, examining all response categories separately. The multiple testing increases the chances of type one error; therefore, using the Holm procedure, we decreased the acceptable level of significance to 0.007. So, the results will only be significant if they are below this level. If a response category is significant, there is no need for further correction; thus we can use the original, $\alpha = .05$, significance level.

The response of the self being 'helpful' did not show significant change during the observation period, $\chi^2(2, 359) = 1.06$ $p = .590$ $\varphi = .05$. The response of being 'unreceptive', however, showed significant change, $\chi2(2, 359) = 13.13$ $p = .001$ $\varphi = .19$. This was based on the significant increase between the first and second phases of the observation period, $\chi2(1, 259) = 13.23$ $p < .001$ $\varphi = .23$). Between the second and third phases there was no significant difference $\chi2(1, 218) = 2.20$ $p = .138$ $\varphi = .10$, whereas the increase between the first and third phase was significant, but small $\chi2(1, 241) = 4.18$ $p = .041$ $\varphi = .13$. The response of the self being 'respected and accepted' showed no significant difference during the observation period: $\chi2(2, 359) = 0.94$ $p = .625$ $\varphi = .05$, nor did the response 'oppose and hurt others', $\chi2(2, 359) = 9.46$ $p = .009$ $\varphi = .16$. The response 'self-controlled and self-confident' did not show significant changes during the observation period either: $\chi2(2, 359) = 1.16$ $p = .560$ $\varphi = .06$, neither did the response 'helpless', $\chi2(2, 359) = 3.87$ $p = .144$ $\varphi = .10$; nor did the response 'disappointed and depressed', $\chi2(2, 359) = 1.54$ $p = .463$ $\varphi = .07$, and 'anxious and ashamed', $\chi2(2, 359) = 9.42$ $p = .009$ $\varphi = .16$.

In summary, we can say that, out of all responses of the self to the reaction of others categories, only the response of being 'unreceptive' showed significant change (increase) in occurrence during the observation period. According to Luborsky's category system, the response cluster 'unreceptive' is composed of the standard categories of 'not understanding', 'not being open', and 'disliking others' (Barber et al. 1990). 'Not understanding' means being confused, being surprised, having poor self-understanding. 'Not being open' means being inhibited, not being expressive, and being distant. 'Disliking others' means hating others (Barber et al. 1990).

Aside from 'unreceptive' all the rest of the response categories were stable throughout the three phases, including the most frequent responses of 'helpless', 'anxious and ashamed', and 'helpful'. This suggests that the analysand's responses to other's reactions show a relatively stable pattern, which, again, suggests that she may not adequately differentiate her responses to others' reactions, and this remains unchanged during the observation period.

We will now examine the target person of the analysand's responses, in other words towards whom the analysand showed some of these responses based on the high frequency of the response, or the change of the response during the observation period.

As we can see in Table 7.17, the response of the self being 'helpless' occurs in relatively high proportion in all three phases of the observation period.

Table 7.17 shows that the two main targets of the response of the self being 'helpless' are the self itself (approximately 19%) and the sexual partner (approximately17%). Regarding the self, the highest proportion of 'helpless' response occurs in the first and third phases. Such high proportions of this response suggest that the analysand feels unable to tackle her strong internal impulses. She feels out of control, defeated, unable to act; but she also feels uncertain about her goals and identity, and uncertain about her relationships as well, while remaining dependent on others. The feeling of helplessness in case of the partner occurred in greatest proportion in the third phase (approximately 45%). Such high occurrence suggests that the analysand finds her sexual and love relationships

Table 7.17 Response of the self: Helpless

	First phase	Second phase	Third phase	Total
Helpless	22.0%	20.3%	31.0%	**24,0%**
	First phase	**Second phase**	**Third phase**	Total
Self	22.6%	8.3%	22.6%	**18.6%**
Analyst	3.2%	12.5%	9.7%	**8.1%**
Mother	6.5%	20.8%	9.7%	**11.6%**
Father	0.0%	0.0%	3.2%	**1.2%**
Sibling	9.7%	0.0%	0.0%	**3.5%**
Children	0.0%	0.0%	0.0%	**0.0%**
Partner	3.2%	0.0%	45.2%	**17.4%**
Male authority figures	0.0%	25.0%	6.5%	**9.3%**
Female authority figures	12.9%	20.8%	0.0%	**10.5%**
Male friends	29.0%	12.5%	0.0%	**14.0%**
Female friends	12.9%	0.0%	0.0%	**4.7%**
Others	0.0%	0.0%	3.2%	**1.2%**

problematic, and is incapable of dealing with such problems effectively. The third highest proportion of the 'helpless' response on the part of the self occurred in the case of male friends. Male friends refer in the transcribed texts mainly to the analysand's male friends and potential love interests. The fact that the analysand feels helpless towards them underlines the importance of feeling incapable of solving various relationship problems, or confronting her male friends when the situation requires a firm response.

The next response of the self, occurring in great proportion—mainly in the first and second phases—is being 'anxious and ashamed'.

As we can see in Table 7.18, the self-response 'anxious and ashamed' was given by the analysand in the greatest proportion to male authority figures, in the second greatest proportion towards the self, and in the third greatest proportion to female authority figures. These results suggest that the analysand shows feelings of anxiety, shame, and guilt towards authority figures in general, as a result of their perceived reactions towards her. The second greatest proportion of the response 'anxious and ashamed' is directed towards the self, which occurs in the first and third phases of the observation period. These high proportions suggest

Table 7.18 Response of the self: anxious and ashamed

	First phase	**Second phase**	**Third phase**	Total
Anxious and ashamed	27.7%	16.1%	13.0%	**19.8%**
	First phase	**Second phase**	**Third phase**	Total
Self	25.6%	0.0%	23.1%	**18.3%**
Analyst	2.6%	0.0%	15.4%	**4.2%**
Mother	0.0%	26.3%	23.1%	**11.3%**
Father	0.0%	5.3%	0.0%	**1.4%**
Sibling	0.0%	0.0%	0.0%	**0.0%**
Child	0.0%	0.0%	0.0%	**0.0%**
Partner	7.7%	0.0%	7.7%	**5.6%**
Male authority figures	30.8%	10.5%	0.0%	**19.7%**
Female authority figures	7.7%	31.6%	15.4%	**15.5%**
Male friends	12.8%	15.8%	0.0%	**11.3%**
Female friends	2.6%	0.0%	0.0%	**1.4%**
Other	10.3%	10.5%	15.4%	**11.3%**

that the analysand often uses self-blaming and self-shaming as a reaction to her inner conflicts.

The next response of the self occurring in relatively large proportion is 'helpful' (14.8%), which occurs in relatively large proportions in all three phases of the observation period.

Finally, the response of the self being 'unreceptive' occurs relatively rarely. however, there is a significant change in its frequency during the three phases of the observation period. Due to its low frequency, however, the first phase cannot be interpreted, and the second and third phase can be interpreted with caution.

As we can see it in Table 7.20, the response of the self being 'unreceptive' is directed towards the analyst in the greatest proportion. It is relatively high in both the second and third phases, and, in addition, there is an increase in proportion from 30% to 60%. This response of the self, directed towards the analyst, may suggest that the analysand does not understand or agree with therapeutic interpretations and suggestions and is having a difficult time understanding herself. Also, she may not feel open towards the analyst at certain times during the session, being inexpressive, inhibited, and distant.

Table 7.19 Response of the self: helpful

	First phase	**Second phase**	**Third phase**	Total
Helpful	14.9%	16.9%	12.0%	**14.8%**
	First phase	**Second phase**	**Third phase**	Total
Self	0.0%	0.0%	0.0%	**0.0%**
Analyst	61.9%	75.0%	100.0%	**75.5%**
Mother	4.8%	0.0%	0.0%	**1.9%**
Father	0.0%	0.0%	0.0%	**0.0%**
Sibling	0.0%	0.0%	0.0%	**0.0%**
Child	0.0%	0.0%	0.0%	**0.0%**
Partner	4.8%	0.0%	0.0%	**1.9%**
Male authority figures	0.0%	0.0%	0.0%	**0.0%**
Female authority figures	4.8%	0.0%	0.0%	**5.7%**
Male friends	14.3%	10.0%	0.0%	**9.4%**
Female friends	9.5%	5.0%	0.0%	**5.7%**
Others	0.0%	0.0%	0.0%	**0.0%**

Table 7.20 Changes in occurrence of the response of the self: unreceptive

	First phase	**Second phase**	**Third phase**	**Total**
unreceptive	3.5%	16.9%	10.0%	**9.7%**
		Second phase	**Third phase**	
Self		0.0%	10.0%	
Analyst		**30.0%**	**60.0%**	
Mother		**25.0%**	0.0%	
Father		0.0%	0.0%	
Sibling		0.0%	0.0%	
Child		0.0%	0.0%	
Partner		0.0%	**30.0%**	
Male authority figures		0.0%	0.0%	
Female authority figures		0.0%	0.0%	
Male friends		**40.0%**	0.0%	
Female friends		5.0%	0.0%	
Other		0.0%	0.0%	

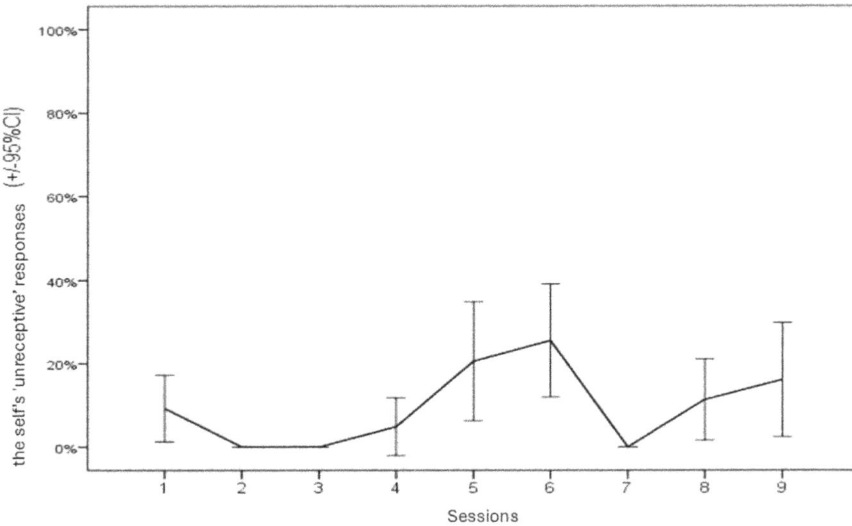

Figure 7.4 Response of the self of being 'unreceptive' by session

This response of the analysand towards the analyst may create difficulties in treatment, making it harder for the therapist to achieve progress in the working phase of the therapy.

In the second phase of the observation period, as we can see in Table 7.20, the response of being 'unreceptive' is directed towards male friends in a relatively large proportion (40%), and towards the mother in a smaller, but still substantial, proportion (25%). In the third phase, the response is also directed towards the partner (30%).

Looking at Figure 7.4 we can see that the self-response of being 'unreceptive' reaches its highest proportion at session 6. We have previously analysed the interaction at this session in terms of the NP shifting behaviour of the speakers, since this is the same session in which the whish 'to be loved and understood' reaches its high level as well. We shall discuss this in more detail below.

Examination of the self-response of being 'unreceptive' in terms of narrative interaction

Excerpt 7.8 is from session 6, during which the analyst and analysand discuss interactions with male friends and potential love interests. It is a continuation of Excerpt 7.4, in which the interlocutors discussed the case of Z., a male friend with whom the analysand keeps in touch via email, but often it is difficult for her to answer his letters. Excerpt 7.8 illustrates how the analysand becomes 'unreceptive' to potential love interests due to her own insecurities—as discussed in Excerpt 7.4.

Excerpt 7.8 (session 6, L23)

511PAT:	meg ö +..	and er+...
512PAT:	egyébként ami még érdekes,	anyway what is also interesting,
513PAT:	hogy azóta váltottunk néhány emailt,	that we have exchanged a few emails,
514PAT:	de most megint nem válaszolok neki két napja.	but I haven't answered in the past two days.
515TER:	ühüm.	uhum.
516%com:	pat laughs	
517TER:	és miért?	and why?
518PAT:	mert nem+..	because I haven't+...
519PAT:	nincs kedvem leülni neki megírni a levelet.	I don't feel like sitting down and writing him the letter.
520PAT:	nem tudom.	I don't know.

In Excerpt 7.8, Clara begins her story about the correspondence with Z. in line 513 in the past tense, first-person, homo-diegesis, using character level and external focalization. In line 514, she shifts into the present tense. Some of these perspectives suggest a high level of affective involvement on the part of the narrator—such as the present tense, the first person, and character level—whereas others suggest less involvement—such as external focalization. The analyst in line 517 interrupts the analysand's story and, using hetero-diegesis and narrator level, tries to focus the analysand's attention on the reasons behind her behaviour. By this, she turns the analysand's focus inward, which perspective the analysand adopts when she shifts into internal focalization in lines 518–20, in line 520 admitting that she does not know the reason or does not want to know and think about the real motivations of her being unreceptive towards Z. So, she even seems to be dismissive towards the analyst's suggestion of thinking about the reasons behind her rejecting Z., which is—as we have seen in previous excerpts—a typical pattern in the analysand's case regarding her potential romantic relationships, and male friends in general. In this case, however, she is being unreceptive towards the analyst as well. Being unreceptive has reached its peak in session 2.3 (6), subsiding afterwards, which suggests that such reactions fluctuated during the course of the observation period. The analysand's dismissive, unreceptive reaction to the analyst's question may be interpreted as resistance towards psychoanalysis itself. Using expressions such as 'I do not know' and resisting a more elaborate answer may slow down progress of the psychotherapeutic process. The fact that the unreceptive response of the self towards the analyst has doubled by phase three confirms this understanding of the analysand's response, and draws attention to the difficulties with the analytic process.

The analysand's unreceptiveness towards both Z. and the analyst can be understood as a defensive mentalization breakdown. Clara's avoidance of reflecting on why she does not answer Z's emails (lines 518–20) signals a temporary suspension of reflective function, a moment where she struggles to access her own emotional motivations. The 'I don't know' response (line 520) is particularly significant—it is not merely a cognitive gap but an affective block, where the analysand shuts down the reflective process, resisting the invitation to explore her internal world.

According to Bateman and Fonagy (2016), individuals with insecure attachment histories tend to show mentalization-limiting processes under relational stress. Clara's refusal to answer Z. may serve as an unconscious defence against intimacy, as engaging with him might activate fears of rejection or dependency. Her resistance to the analyst's questioning (line 517) suggests a reluctance to engage with potentially painful emotional material—perhaps to avoid confronting feelings of inadequacy, fear of closeness, or past relational disappointments. By shutting down reflection, Clara momentarily protects herself from affective discomfort but, in doing so, she also limits opportunities for insight and growth.

Tronick's Mutual Regulation Model (Tronick 2007) posits that emotion is co-regulated in relationships, including the therapeutic dyad. Clara's laugh (line 516) functions as a dysregulatory signal—a nonverbal cue that diffuses emotional intensity rather than engaging with it. The analyst's intervention (line 517, 'And why?') attempts to re-establish mentalization, but Clara remains unreceptive. This moment can be seen as an instance of temporary misattunement in the analytic dyad, where the analyst's attempt to deepen exploration is met with withdrawal rather than engagement.

According to Tronick (2007), ruptures in mutual regulation are inevitable in relationships, but their repair is essential for emotional growth. Clara's avoidance of answering Z. may parallel her avoidance of emotionally engaging with the analyst. Her unreceptiveness serves as a regulatory strategy, preventing her from experiencing emotional vulnerability in real time. Without re-engagement and repair, this pattern could reinforce detachment and relational distancing.

Relational psychoanalysis (Stolorow et al. 2002) emphasizes how past interpersonal experiences shape current relational patterns, including those within the analytic dyad. Clara's withdrawal from both Z. and the analyst suggests a deeply ingrained relational schema of avoidance and disengagement. Her dismissive reaction towards the analyst's question mirrors the same distancing she exhibits in her romantic life—suggesting that unreceptiveness may function as a defence against relational expectations in general.

The analyst's persistent questioning (lines 517–20) may inadvertently re-enact a past dynamic where Clara felt pressured to engage when she was not emotionally ready. Clara's resistance ('I don't know') can be understood as a transference reaction, where she experiences the analyst as an intrusive or demanding figure, echoing earlier relational experiences where emotional engagement felt overwhelming. This highlights the intersubjective nature of resistance—not merely an individual defence, but an emergent quality of the analytic relationship itself. Recognizing this moment as a relational re-enactment rather than a simple resistance can allow for a more nuanced therapeutic intervention—one that acknowledges the analysand's need for autonomy while gently encouraging deeper reflection.

The Boston Change Process Group (BCPSG 2005, 2010) point to a layer of relational change, which happens at the procedural, implicit level—through the micro-experiences of interaction in the analytic setting besides the changes that happen through intellectual insight. Clara's 'I don't know' response is not just a verbal statement—it is an embodied relational move, signalling non-engagement as an implicit way of being with others. The key therapeutic task is not merely to uncover why Clara avoids Z., but to offer her a different kind of relational experience where disengagement is met with curiosity and safety rather than pressure or withdrawal.

The analyst's ability to stay with Clara's avoidance without pressuring her to elaborate is crucial in offering a corrective relational experience. The therapeutic goal is not simply to interpret Clara's defences, but to create a relational space where curiosity, self-exploration, and engagement feel safe and meaningful.

Clara's unreceptiveness is not merely a resistance to therapy but a defensive strategy rooted in affect regulation difficulties and attachment fears. Her difficulty engaging with the analyst mirrors her struggle in romantic relationships, reinforcing a pattern of avoidance and disengagement. The therapeutic process must focus on rebuilding mutual regulation, ensuring that Clara's moments of withdrawal are met with attunement rather than confrontation. The BCPSG's concept of implicit relational knowing highlights that relational change occurs through the felt experience of engagement, rather than just cognitive insight.

Encouraging reflective function gently, without pressure, instead of pushing Clara to analyse why she avoids Z., the analyst might normalize relational hesitations and offer open-ended curiosity rather than direct questioning. Addressing resistance through relational attunement means that recognizing Clara's withdrawal as an affect regulation strategy rather than a mere avoidance defence can shift the therapeutic stance to one of deeper empathy. Exploring relational enactments within the analysis itself—bringing awareness to how Clara's resistance to engaging with Z. parallels her relational stance towards the analyst—could be a meaningful intervention.

Another way to enhance the analytic process is to strengthen Clara's self-agency in her relationships, helping her distinguish defensive avoidance from deliberate, thoughtful boundaries. This could empower her to make more intentional choices in relationships. This analysis illustrates how the self-response of being 'unreceptive' reflects an interplay of affect regulation, mentalization failures, and implicit relational dynamics, all of which shape the trajectory of the therapeutic process.

Conclusions

In summary of the discussion of interpersonal relationships in this chapter, we can say that the analysand's most frequent wish towards others was 'to be loved and understood', to which others most frequently reacted by 'rejecting and opposing', to which, in turn, the analysand responded by being 'helpless'. In Table 7.21 we can see the most frequent patterns of the three components of the relationship episodes with important others.

As we can see from Table 7.21 the analysand's core conflict in relating to others was that she expected to be loved and understood by others. however, except for the analyst, important others, such as the mother and her love interest(s), reacted to her wishes by rejecting and opposing—as she has perceived it. One

Table 7.21 Wishes, reaction of others, and responses of the self in important relationships

	Analysand's wish, expectation from others	**Others' reactions**	**Response of the self to others**
Analyst	To be loved and understood	Helpful	Helpful
Self	To achieve and help others	Rejecting and opposing	Helpless
Mother	To be loved and understood	Rejecting and opposing	Helpless; disappointed and depressed
Partner	To be loved and understood	Rejecting and opposing	Helpless
Male friends	To be loved and understood	Understanding	Helpless

interesting result was that male friends reacted to her by being understanding. Towards the self she had a different wish—to achieve and help others—but even this wish on the part of the self was met with rejection and opposition. The one important exception from this trend was the analyst, who reacted to the analysand's wishes by being helpful. Others' reactions as perceived by the analysand resulted in the analysand's response of being helpless. The exception from this is again the analyst, towards whom the analysand expresses helpful behaviour.

Besides these dominating patterns, we also have shown important changes during the three phases of the observation period in terms of the structure of relationship episodes—thus supporting our main hypothesis, according to which there are changes in the way of interpersonal relating during the course of psychoanalysis, regarding the narrative structure of relating as described by Luborsky. These long-term changes suggest that the analysand's way of relating to others, as perceived and described by her at the sessions, has changed during psychoanalysis, which signals the success of the analytic work, and a change and development of the analysand's narrative self.

These substantial aspects of changes in relating included changes in wishes and expectations from others, such as 'to oppose, hurt and control others' (decrease); 'to be controlled, hurt and not be responsible' (increase); and 'to be loved and understood' (increase). This latter, the analysand's most important wish, was shown to be a complex one, undermined by ambivalent emotions, based on our discourse analysis of session 6 and 8 where this wish reached its highest proportions. The reasons for her ambivalent behaviour—longing for love and understanding and at the same time avoiding it—is fear of rejection, as the analyst pointed out. So, our analysis of NP shifting behaviour revealed how joint construction of narrative contributed to the psychotherapy process in the case of wishes or expectations from others, and in the changing of interpersonal relating during psychoanalysis.

In connection to wishes, we have also shown change in others' reactions as perceived by the analysand, such as in the category of 'upset' (decrease) and of being 'understanding' (increase). This latter reaction of others, and its increase during the course of analysis, implies that the analysand's most important wish was increasingly confirmed in the course of psychoanalysis. However, as shown by our discourse analysis of session 8—where this reaction from others has reached its highest proportion—she perceives and experiences others' understanding in a complex way. Her wish for her partner to understand her is, again, an ambivalent one, and her experience of being understood is also uncertain. With the analyst's helpful interpretations, she gains insight into her own ambivalence at the examined session. Our analysis of NP shifting behaviour again revealed how joint narrative construction contributes to the psychotherapy process.

Finally, the third aspect of relating to others we have examined is the response of the self to others' reactions. Only the response of being 'unreceptive' showed a significant change in occurrence (increase), which suggests that other aspects of the analysand's responses to others remained stable during the observation period. Being unreceptive was shown to be important in the analysand's relating to the analyst, showed by our discourse analysis of session 6, signalling that the analysand has some issues with resistance in her analytic work, which is an important implication for the psychotherapy process of the female analysand.

Our discourse analysis also illuminates the analysand's implicit relational expectations—particularly her tendency to feel helpless in response to rejection, her struggle with self-agency, and the role of psychoanalysis in reshaping her capacity for emotional regulation and relational understanding. Strengthening Clara's ability to hold both positive and negative aspects of relationships simultaneously could reduce her all-or-nothing responses (helplessness or rejection anticipation). Enhancing her capacity to mentalize would allow her to recognize that others' behaviours are not always reflections of her self-worth but are shaped by their own emotional states and histories. Addressing resistance through gentle exploration rather than confrontation may help reduce the analysand's tendency towards unreceptiveness and increase engagement in therapy.

Limitations of our study

Our two-step analysis combining quantitative and qualitative methodology has proven to be a useful tool for an in-depth understanding of how, in what ways, and why the analysand's interpersonal relating changed in the course of the psychoanalytic process during the observation period, and in what ways joint construction of narratives contributed to these long-term changes. We must note, however, that our observation period did not include the final phase of psychoanalysis, only the working phase, which continued after we concluded our study. Therefore, we cannot state that these were the only longitudinal changes or tendencies taking place during the course of the entire analysis with the female analysand. It is possible, or probable, that aspects of interpersonal relating continued to alter following our observation period during the course of psychoanalysis. Thus it would be useful to continue studying changes in interpersonal relating using our method in other cases of analysands, and in full-length therapies as well.

8 Long-term changes in expressing agency

This chapter focuses on the question of how long-term changes in the sense of agency in psychotherapy occur, and the problem of how to detect and assess such changes in self-narratives, which we discuss in connection to a longitudinal analysis of the Budapest Psychotherapy data. First, we describe the theoretical background of why it is an important priority in psychotherapy and, within this, psychoanalysis to develop the analysand's balanced sense of agency. In doing so we lean on Bandura's definition of agency and on the theory of Gorlin and Békés (2021), as well as Williams and Levitt (2007), of the interconnection between agency and awareness in psychotherapeutic practice.

Following this, we describe McAdams's theory (2001) of narrative expression of agency, which defines sense of agency by four themes occurring in self-narratives: 1) self-mastery, 2) status gain or victory in competitive situations, 3) achievement of goals and responsibility for others, and 4) empowerment by a greater 'agent' such as god or nature (McAdams et al. 1996). In order to capture the negative dimensions of agency themes we have complemented McAdams's four themes with four themes of patiency, the sense of passivity and vulnerability: 1) loss of self-control, 2) failure/loss of status, 3) failure/avoiding responsibility, and 4) disempowerment.

Following these theoretical discussions we turn to the analysis of psychoanalytic discourse based on the Budapest Psychotherapy Database. We use a quantitative analysis to establish long-term patterns of change in agency and patiency. First, we describe the methodology used in the analysis of agency and patiency, followed by a description of the long-term patterns characterizing the female analysand. In our analysis we identify sessions where salient changes in agency and patiency occurred, and examine the use of narrative perspective in the talk of both speakers in order to illustrate how changes in agency occur in self-narratives and what role the psychoanalyst's interventions play in such changes. Following this analysis we also examine the sessions of the male analysand–male analyst dyad using the same methodology. Based on our longitudinal quantitative and qualitative analysis of the Budapest Psychotherapy Data, we argue that—as our results suggest—sense of agency and patiency change with time in a non-linear fashion, and these processes may be influenced by the nature of specific problems worked through during a given session or time period. We also argue that in-session joint construction of narratives contributes to the process of change in agency and patiency.

The concept of agency

Albert Bandura, the late professor of Stanford University, developed a detailed evolutionary theory of human agency, which we shall summarize here briefly. According to Bandura (2006): 'To be an agent is to influence intentionally one's functioning and life circumstances. In this view, personal influence is part of the causal structure. People are self-organizing, pro-active, self-regulating and self-reflecting'. (2006: 164). So, according to Bandura, human agency has four basic components: 1) intentionality, 2) forethought, 3) self-reactiveness, and 4) self-reflectiveness.

Intentionality of agency means that people form action plans and work out various strategies for carrying them out either on their own, or as a group endeavour, with other humans. In this latter case, we talk about collective intentionality. Forethought of agency involves future directed planning, setting goals, and anticipating potential outcomes. Forethought as a representation of future scenarios may serve as a guide of, or motivation for, current behaviour. According to Bandura, forethoughtful perspective also provides 'direction, coherence, and meaning to one's life' (2006: 165). Self-reactiveness of agency is the construction of courses of action, and their motivation and regulation, whereas self-reflectiveness—the most distinctively human characteristic of agency according to Bandura—is the metacognitive ability to reflect on one's actions and thoughts.

Bandura describes agency as an outcome of the interplay among intrapersonal, behavioural and environmental factors. He states that 'acting as an agent, an individual makes causal contributions to the course of events' (2006: 165). Since human behaviour is embedded in social contexts, argues Bandura, a given action can be influenced by agency, or it may be a response to others' behaviour, or an environmental outcome. Human agency is also a manifestation of freedom as far as it exercises self-influence in order to reach desired goals and outcomes (Bandura 2006).

Bandura emphasizes that acting as an agent is not necessarily reduced to the level of the individual. He describes three modes of human agency: 1) individual, 2) proxy, and 3) collective. In the case of individual agency, we distinguish activities under personal control, whereas in the case of collective agency we talk about humans acting together as a group. In the case of agency by proxy Bandura describes situations in which people do not have control over social practices and institutions. In such cases they exercise their agency by influencing others, who have the means and knowledge to effect such situations. Successful functioning involves an 'agency mix' relying on all three modes of agency (Bandura 2006).

According to Bandura, a central element of one's sense of agency is the belief of personal efficacy:

> Unless people believe they can produce desired effects in their actions, they have little incentive to act, or to persevere in the face of difficulties. Whatever other factors serve as guides and motivators, they are rooted in the core belief that one has the power to effect changes by one's own actions . .. Efficacy beliefs affect whether individuals think optimistically or pessimistically, in self-enhancing or self-debilitating ways. (2006: 170)

Bandura argues that efficacy beliefs determine people's expectations about their efforts and the outcomes of those efforts, thus contributing to performance and achievement. Those with low efficacy beliefs are prone to give up their efforts towards reaching a goal. In contrast, those with high efficacy beliefs think that they are able to reach their goals by persevering. In addition, efficacy beliefs also contribute to vulnerability to stress and depression, as well as overall well-being (Bandura 2006).

The role of agency in psychotherapy

Based on Bandura's concept of agency, Gorlin and Békés, developed their theory of the role of agency via awareness as a meta-process in psychotherapy (2021). They further differentiate between the mental and physical agency of the client in psychotherapy. Mental agency refers to the client's ability to intentionally manage mental processes, for example what they choose to attend to, reflect on, or remember, whereas physical agency refers to the client's ability to intentionally manage their external environment, for example to choose goals and take action.

Gorlin and Békés argue that enhancing the client's agency is a major focus in various types of psychotherapies. They suggest that agency is linked to better therapeutic outcomes, treatment efficacy, stronger therapeutic alliance, and improvement in mental health. They further argue that an increase in the sense of agency by the self is achieved through an increase in awareness. By awareness they mean the 'grasp of whatever knowledge or understanding about oneself and the world is relevant to managing one's life' (2021: 3). They mention, for example, being aware of 'activities, experiences, risks, rewards, skills and challenges' that would be involved in trying to bring about changes in one's life, or realizing certain goals regarding one's career development or personal relationships, or articulating the nature and adaptability of 'emotions, beliefs, motivations, and habits' (2021: 3). According to Gorlin and Békés, in psychotherapy one's awareness may increase in various contexts. They mention, for example, 'encountering new knowledge', or 'bringing previous knowledge back into consciousness', 'making new connections', 'testing and internalizing new knowledge by applying it to action', and 'consciously engaging with previously avoided knowledge' (2021: 3–4).

So, the authors suggest that the deeper our awareness about the world and the environment we live in, the more effectively we will be able operate in it. Hence, an increase in our knowledge of the various aspects of our inner and outer spheres leads to an increase in our agency. Furthermore, Gorlin and Békés also suggest that the various mechanisms of increasing awareness in psychotherapy are themselves 'agential processes' (2021: 4). The increase in awareness thus leads to an increase in agency and vice versa, creating a positive spiral of increase in both aspects of the operation of the self:

> So, agency and awareness often go hand-in-hand in the therapy process, as they are inextricably connected. Exploring, attending to, reflecting on, and pursuing new experiences is often itself effortful work requiring either (and more often both) mental or physical agency. (2021: 5)

Gorlin and Békés's argument on increasing agency via awareness is in line with Williams and Levitt's research on the role of agency in the psychotherapeutic change process. In their excellent study, Williams and Levitt (2007) interviewed fourteen eminent psychotherapists from various therapeutic traditions (e.g. humanist, feminist psychodynamic, cognitive, etc.) asking questions about how they help clients to develop an agentic orientation to a given problem. The answers fell into the following three categories: 1) increasing self-determination 'as a process of skill and information building or introspection'; 2) 'exploring what is and what is not changeable to develop personal perspective and responsibility'; 3) 'working through obstructions by increasing awareness, exploring, and integrating clients' concerns' (2007: 71). Another question they explored was a holistic approach to facilitate agency by using both medication and psychotherapy. Responses to this fell into the following two categories: 1) 'medication may be necessary or helpful, but is limited by potential addiction, removal of motivation, and inability to teach necessary skills'; 2) 'tension between biological and psychological explanation: the need for a holistic approach' (2007: 75).

Based on their qualitative data, the authors developed principles that guided therapeutic work across various types of psychotherapies helping therapists to make decisions on how to facilitate their clients' change process. Regarding the first concern, developing agentic orientation towards a problem, therapists had to decide on how to structure the therapeutic hour: to foster clients to introspect and search for possible action plans, and to be reflective, or to help them learn new skills and educate them to further develop their problem-solving skills. Another principle related to the first concern is to help clients to consider the internal and external limitations and constraints to their potential actions. Furthermore, therapists helped to direct clients' attention to avoided aspects of experience when it was noticed that clients were not making progress in therapy, helping them to articulate the nature of their difficulty, and encouraging them to examine their hidden motivations for hindering change. Regarding the second concern, the use of both medication and psychotherapy in treatment, psychotherapists thought that medication could be useful in helping clients to better engage in the therapeutic process; however, medication was not considered useful when it interfered with the client's agentive processes.

Based on their study, Williams and Levitt (2007) concluded that it would be important to develop tools that measure client's progress in agency during or following psychotherapy. Indeed, there have been various measures developed that have attempted to capture agency and related concepts during psychotherapy (for a review, see Coleman & Neimeyer 2015); for example, Psychotherapy Expectations Inventory (Rickers-Ovsiankina et al. 1971), Expectations About Counselling (Tinsley et al. 1980), the Self-efficacy for Client Behaviors Scale (Longo et al. 1992), the Agnew-Davies Relationship Measure (Agnew-Davies et al. 1998), the Role Behavior Expectancy Ratings Measure (Joyce et al. 2000), etc. Most measures, however, have been based on the self-evaluation of the client or the therapist.

Another approach to the problem of agency is through the study of agency expressed in the client's self-narratives. One such study was carried out by Jonathan M. Adler (2012), who measured agency in written narratives completed during the period of psychotherapeutic treatment, using McAdams's method of coding agency in self-narratives. Before we turn to a discussion of that study, we will discuss McAdam's method of studying narrative themes of agency.

The study of motivational themes in self-narratives: agency and patiency

The study of motivational themes in self-narratives was first highlighted by Dan McAdams (McAdams 1980, 1982; McAdams et al. 1996), who examined agency and communion in important narrative episodes of the life story, also including what is termed self-defining memories (Singer & Salovey 1993). McAdams defines agency based on Bakan (1966, cited by McAdams et al1996), according to whom it expresses the 'existence of the organism as an individual', whereas communion, as a counterpart of agency, is 'the participation of the individual in some larger organism of which the individual is a part' (Bakan 1966: 15, quoted by McAdams et al. 1996). Agency in narratives involves the expression of 'strength, power, expansion, mastery, control, dominance, achievement, separation and independence' (McAdams et al. 1996: 346), whereas communion in narratives is the expression of interpersonal connection, 'love, friendship, intimacy, sharing, belonging, affiliation, merger, union, care and nurturance' (McAdams et al. 1996: 348). McAdams and his colleagues further differentiate four narrative themes of both agency and communion. For agency these are 1) self-mastery, 2) status gain/victory, 3) achievement/responsibility, and 4) empowerment; whereas for communion these themes are 1) love/friendship, 2) dialogue, 3) care/help, and 4) community.

McAdams and colleagues (1996) report that narrative themes of agency and communion are positively related to motives measured by the TAT (Atkinson 1958). Agency aligns with achievement—and more modestly with power—while communion aligns with intimacy. In further studies, narrative agency in middle-aged adults was shown to be associated with a stronger sense of purpose in life (Grossbaum & Bates 2002), as well as with higher levels of generativity (Mansfield & McAdams 1996) and better mental health, but not better physical health (Adler et al. 2015). Contrary to expectations, however, Grossbaum and Bates did not find that narrative agency was related to psychological well-being (Grossbaum & Bates 2002). Narrative communion was shown to be associated with generativity in middle-aged adult samples (Grossbaum & Bates 2002; Mansfield & McAdams 1996), with positive mental health (Adler 2012; Helgeson & Palladino 2012), as well as with the trait of agreeableness on the Big Five personality measure (McAdams et al. 2004).

Since this chapter concerns the sense of agency as expressed in narratives constructed at the psychoanalytic session, we will focus on the narrative themes of agency as described by McAdams, as well as on the narrative themes of patiency, which concept we have constructed as a negative dimension of themes of agency as described by McAdams. Patiency themes express the narrator's passivity and vulnerability to other persons acting as agents, and to environmental events or natural processes. It includes a sense of ineffectiveness in action, helplessness, loss of power and control, submission, and passivity. Narrative themes of patiency are the following: 1) helplessness/loss of self-control, 2) loss of status/losing in competition, 3) failure/irresponsibility, 4) disempowerment.

Including the negative dimension of patiency in our analysis makes it possible to capture negative emotional experience that may be characteristic of analysands participating in psychoanalysis. The frequency of such negative themes in psychoanalytic narratives may present us with a more accurate picture of how psychoanalytic treatment affects the emergence of such themes longitudinally. In the present section, we will define the narrative themes of agency and patiency, which we used for the content analysis of therapeutic texts of the Budapest Psychotherapy Database.

1) The positive theme of self-mastery vs the negative theme of helplessness and loss of self-control

McAdams and coworkers state that the concept of self-mastery is rooted in the Christian tradition (1996). According to this view, a prototypical agent is able to control their environment as well as the self, while the latter is perfected—as an increasingly separate entity from the environment—until a high degree of autonomy is achieved. The theme of self-mastery implies that, 'through forceful and effective action, thought or experience, the person is able to strengthen the self and become a larger, wiser, or more powerful agent in the world' (1996: 346–47). So, the theme of self-mastery means the activity of mastering, controlling, and perfecting the self. In contrast, the theme of helplessness and loss of self-control means the act of a failed attempt of self-mastery, namely the inability to master, control, or perfect the self. For example, if a person decides to exercise three times a week and, in consequence, they go to a gym three times a week—this would fall under the category of self-mastery. However, if they decide to start an exercise regime, and are not able to go to the gym or to work out at home, we can talk about a failure of self-mastery, or loss of self-control.

2) The positive theme of status gain/victory vs the negative theme of loss of status/losing in competitive situations

According to McAdams, agency is related to the striving for dominance, status, or social position. The common themes of status/victory are 'winning the competition, attaining victory, being "number one"' (1996: 347). By definition, there is an interpersonal aspect to this theme, since there is no victory achieved without an opponent. Expressions of this theme involve taking charge, leadership, making decisions, and winning arguments. The negative dimension of this theme is the theme of losing status/losing in competitive situations. In these cases, loss of agency also occurs in interpersonal situations such as competition, carrier advancement, elevation of social status. For example, if a person applies for a job, and wins it, we can talk about status gain/victory; however, if the company choses someone else instead then we can talk about losing status/losing in competitive situations.

3) The positive theme of achievement/responsibility vs the negative theme of failure/irresponsibility

Based on Bakan (1966, cited by McAdams et al. 1996) McAdams argues that the rise of capitalism and the spread of the Protestant work ethic have led to the dissemination and wider acceptance of various related values such as 'industry, thrift, efficiency, persistence, productivity, and entrepreneurship' (1996: 347). These represent a psychological aspect of agency related to the achievement motive. A person who is characterized by a high achievement motivation, says McAdams, 'seeks to do well, be successful, and move steadily onward and upward into the future as an effective and competent agent, meeting successive challenges, accomplishing successive goals, and building on successive achievements to create a bigger and better legacy of the self' (1996: 347–48). According to McAdams, this aspect of agency is similar to Bandura's concept of efficacy, as we discussed above (Bandura 2006). This aspect of agency is somewhat similar to status gain/victory, in that it represents instrumental individual success, and achievement, as well as the assuming of responsibility; however, without the interpersonal condition to it. The negative dimension of this theme is failure/irresponsibility, which refers to the person's lack of achievement or accomplishment of a goal that he/she tried to accomplish, or unsuccessfully taking on responsibilities, which in turn they are unable to fulfil. For example, if a person decides to take a German-language course and then a German proficiency exam and they succeed in it, then we can categorize that as achievement/responsibility; however, if they fail the exam we can talk about failure/irresponsibility, because the person was unable to accomplish the task.

4) The positive theme of empowerment vs the negative theme of disempowerment

McAdams and coworkers point out that the source of power in agentic action is not always the self, but rather 'some larger or more potent outside force' (1996: 348), which by its positive influence might be enhancing the force of the individual's action. Such situations arise when the individual sees others—such as God, nature, the universe, or an authority figure (e.g. parent, teacher, pastor, therapist, or an inspiring person)—as more powerful actors, who support or help his/her cause or action. According to McAdams (McAdams et al. 1996), in autobiographies 'the theme of empowerment is manifested in accounts in which the individual is enlarged, enhanced, empowered, ennobled, built up, or made better through his/her association with an especially powerful source' (1996: 348). In contrast, such highly powerful actors may also annul or cancel the agentic power that has enhanced the individual's action, by which the individual is lessened, weakened, condemned, disgraced, his/her power is diminished, and they feel rejected. In such cases we can talk about disempowerment. For example, where a highly respected teacher praises a student's paper and encourages him/her to continue working on it, we can talk about empowerment. However, if the highly respected teacher gives negative feedback on the paper, and even humiliates the student by telling him/her how disappointed they are in the student's performance, we are talking about disempowerment.

In our study of the Budapest Psychotherapy Database, we examined these four themes of agency and patiency. We chose a longitudinal design, examining changes in agency and patiency that took place over the 1.5 years of observation period. We coded agency and patiency in the transcribed texts of the psychotherapy sessions. In our study we hypothesized that, with the advancement of treatment, the expression of agency would increase in the analysands' narratives, and that patiency agency decrease. This hypothesis was based on Adler's (2012) study, as well as on Gordin and Békés's theorizing (2021). Before we turn to the description of the methodological details of our study, we will briefly discuss Andler's findings.

In his 2012 study, forty-seven adults wrote detailed personal narratives prior to beginning psychotherapy, and after each session, over twelve psychotherapy sessions, when they also completed the Systemic Therapy Inventory of Change (STIC, Pinsof & Chambers 2009). This questionnaire measures mental health, and also relationship, current family, and child-rearing practices. The psychotherapists participating in the study used various kinds of psychotherapies: 37% have used cognitive–behavioural techniques, 25% have used psychodynamic treatment, and the rest have used integrative or other techniques with their clients enrolled in the study. Personal narratives were coded based on McAdams's methodology for coding agency, and also for coherence. The results showed that the theme of agency, but not coherence, increased over time. Furthermore, increases in agency were related to improvements in participants' mental health as measured by the STIC. Based on his results Adler concluded that an increase in agency in the course of psychotherapy has relevance to the fields of personality development, psycho-therapy process, as well as outcome research.

So, Adler's study represents a good base for our hypotheses, namely that agency would increase during the course of treatment, whereas patiency would decrease by the end of the observation period. However, since our observation period did not extend to the end of treatment, we have also entertained an alternative hypothesis, based on which agency and patiency could fluctuate according to the types of issues discussed at a given session. sometimes the analysand may show an increase in agency and a decrease in patiency if they report on problems they have successfully mastered, or results they have achieved, whereas at other times analysands may show a decrease in agency, and an increase in patiency, when reporting failures, irresponsible behaviour, etc. In our study we tested all of these hypotheses. We now turn to a description of the methodology of that study.

Methods used in the study of agency and patiency in the psychotherapy sessions of the Budapest Psychotherapy Database

Participants

The participants in the study were the female and the male analysands working with the female and male psychoanalysts, respectively, chosen from the Budapest Psychotherapy Database.

Design

In our study of agency and patiency, we used a longitudinal design, choosing the same consecutive three sessions of the Budapest Psychotherapy Database from each of the three phases of the observation period as we chose for the study of Core Conflictual Relationship Themes (Chapter 9) in case of the female analysand–female analyst dyad. We used the same randomly chosen sessions for the female analysand–female analyst dyad, and chose sessions with a similar method with the male analysand–male analyst dyad, with the exception of choosing only two sessions from the second phase of the observation period due to the lack of availability of more sessions in this phase.

Segmentation of sessions into narratives, and the coding of agency and patiency

The method for the demarcation and identification of narratives was the same as the one used in Chapter 9. Namely, one main coder segmented the text into relationship episodes as described by Luborsky and Barrett (2007), whereas two additional coders—trained psychotherapists and psychoanalysts—coded agency and patiency in relationship episodes. The sessions for coding were assigned in a random order, and coders were blind to the real order of occurrence of the sessions. Coders first coded independently each session, and then discussed disagreements in their coding, and came to a common decision in each case. This way, disagreements between coders did not affect the validity of the coding.

Agency and patiency were coded along the following categories/themes: 1) self-mastery, 2) status gain/victory, 3) achievement/responsibility, 4) empowerment, 5) helplessness/loss of self-control, 6) loss of status/losing in competition, 7) failure/irresponsibility, and 8) disempowerment, as defined above, based on the coding manual created by McAdams (2001) for the coding of agency, as well as the one created by Berán (2013) for the coding of patiency. If a given theme of agency was present in a given narrative, it received a score of 1; where it was not present, it received a score of 0. This way, both agency and patiency could receive a total score of 4 for a given narrative.

Inter-rater reliability results

The dimensions of agency and patiency are composed of four themes or subscales, but inter-rater reliability of these eight subscales cannot be interpreted on their own, because several of them occur at very low levels. So, we either cannot compute inter-rater reliability, or it will be unacceptably low. Therefore, we have computed a summary score from 0 to 4, from the four subscales for the dimensions of agency and patiency.

Agency (Coder 2)	Coder 1: 0	1	2	3	4
0	57	0	0	0	0
1	11	11	0	0	0
2	2	1	0	0	0
3	0	0	0	0	0
4	0	0	0	0	0

Kendall's tau: 0.601

Patiency (Coder2)	Coder1: 0	1	2	3	4
0	30	8	0	0	0
1	5	22	2	0	0
2	1	7	5	0	0
3	0	0	2	0	0
4	0	0	0	0	0

Kendall's tau: 0.663

Figure 8.1 Inter-rater results of agency and patiency

Table 8.1 Inter-rater results of yes-no categorical ratings of agency and patiency

Agency		Coder1	
		0	1
Coder2	0	57	0
	1	13	12

Cohen's kappa: 0.562

Patiency		Coder1	
		0	1
Coder2	0	30	8
	1	6	38

Cohen's kappa: 0.655

We can create an agency and patiency variable, which only marks whether any of the subscales have occurred or not. Using Cohen's kappa, the reliability of these subscales is acceptable, but low.

Due to these relatively low levels of inter-rater reliability, coders, after coding independently each session, discussed any differences and came to a common agreement, so as not to affect the results of the study.

Qualitative discourse analysis of NP shifting behaviour related to results of agency and patiency occurrence

Following quantitative analysis of occurrence of agency and patiency at the chosen sessions, we examined narrative interaction in terms of NP shifting behaviour at sessions chosen using theoretical sampling:

1. sessions where there was a radical shift in the amount of agency or patiency during the observation period;
2. sessions where agency and/or patiency was particularly low or high during the observation period.

Excerpts from these sessions were chosen in order to illustrate NP shifting behaviour characteristic of the session, or points of the session where salient NP shifting behaviour was observed.

The coding of NP was carried out by two independent coders and interrater agreement was calculated for each variable, as described in Chapter 4.

Results and discussion of the analysis of agency and patiency in the case of the female analysand

Occurrence of agency in self-narratives

The expression of agency occurred in 30.2% of all narratives during the observation period. Table 8.2 and Figures 8.2 and 8.3 contain all the occurrences and percentages of total agency scores, and also for the subscales (self-mastery, achievement, status gain, and empowerment).

Differences in occurrence of agency themes

Looking at the overall number of agency themes expressed in all sessions, and using the Cochran Q-test, we can see a significant difference in agency categories Q (df = 3; N = 285) = 86,201 p < ,001. Using post hoc Sign test, and correcting for multiple testing with the Holm procedure, we can state that self-mastery (average proportion 19.65%) and achievement (16.14%) were expressed in the greatest proportion of cases, and there is no significant difference between them, $p_H = .245$. Status gain has a lower proportion (5.26%, $p_H < .001$); and the occurrence of empowerment was the lowest in proportion (.35%, $p_H < .001$), significantly lower than all others. Since empowerment and status gain have a very low occurrence, under 10%, we were not able to compute differences between the sessions. We shall now turn to discussing differences between the three blocks of the observation period.

Differences in agency between session blocks

The nine examined sessions were divided into three blocks and, as we have mentioned earlier, a substantial time (six months or more) passed between these periods. Therefore, we have compared the sessions by blocks. The comparison could be made for self-mastery and achievement as well as for the total amount of agency, taking into account that the total amount of agency is composed of almost a half part of the self-mastery and a half part of the achievement categories.

The total occurrence of agency consists of 48 out of the total number of 113 narratives in the first block (42.5%), 29 out of 90 (32.2%) in the second block, and 9 out of 82 (11%) in the third block. Using a Chi-square test we can calculate the differences between the blocks. There is an overall significant difference between the blocks: $\chi^2(2, N = 285) = 22.64$ $p < .001$ Cramer's V = .28. The post hoc comparisons show that there is no significant difference between the first

Table 8.2 Agency total score and subscales in narratives by blocks and sessions

		Total number of narratives	Narratives containing Agency		Narratives containing Self-mastery		Narratives containing Achievement		Narratives containing gain		Narratives containing Empowerment	
Block	Session	N	N	%	N	%	N	%	N	%	N	%
1	1	43	14	32.6	12	27.9	5	11.6	1	2.3	0	0.0
	2	38	18	47.4	10	26.3	12	31.6	5	13.2	0	0.0
	3	32	16	50.0	6	18.8	15	46.9	4	12.5	1	3.1
2	1	37	18	48.6	11	29.7	10	27.0	2	5.4	0	0.0
	2	21	5	23.8	5	23.8	0	0.0	0	0.0	0	0.0
	3	32	6	18.8	5	15.6	1	3.1	0	0.0	0	0.0
3	1	29	1	3.4	1	3.4	0	0.0	0	0.0	0	0.0
	2	28	7	25.0	5	17.9	3	10.7	3	10.7	0	0.0
	3	25	1	4.0	1	4.0	0	0.0	0	0.0	0	0.0

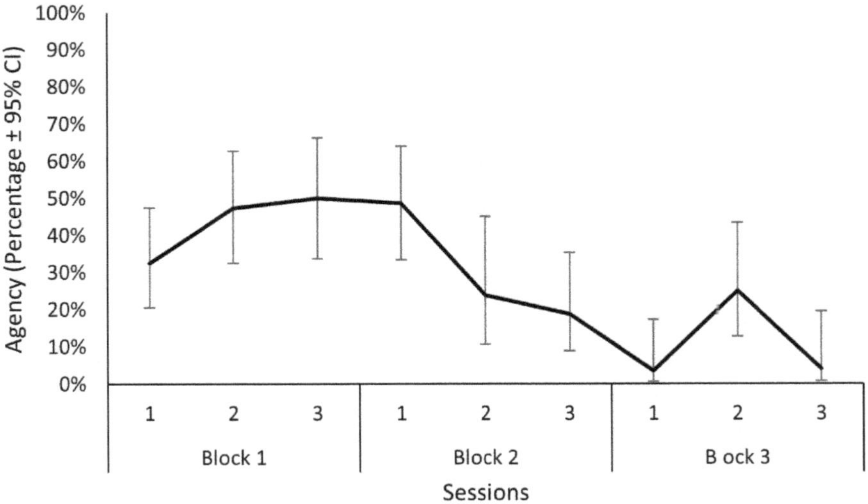

Figure 8.2 Changes in total scores of the agency in the course of the observation period

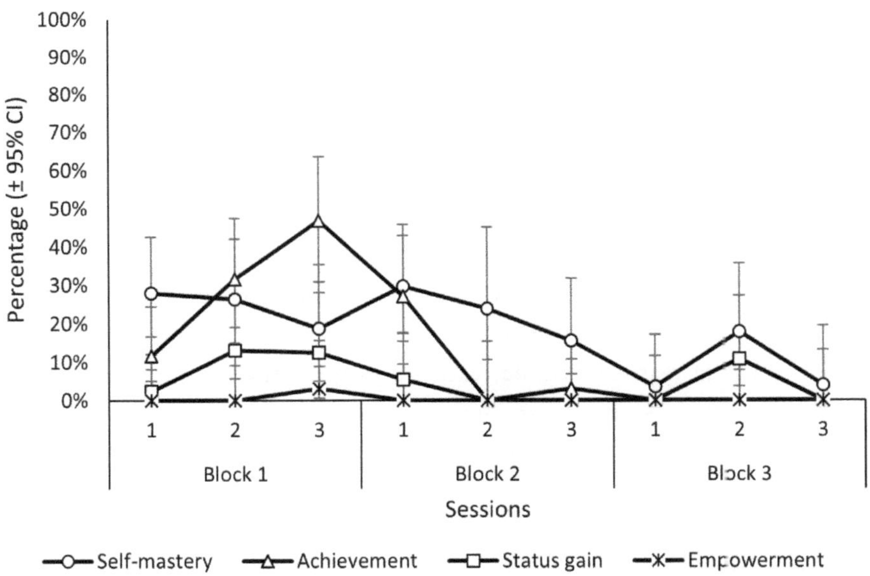

Figure 8.3 Changes in subscales of the agency in the course of the observation period

Note: On the graph we can see the percentage of appearance of Agency ± Wilson score confidence intervals for a binomial proportion

and second block: χ^2 (1 203) = 2.24 p = .135 φ = .11; however, there is a significant reduction in agency in the third block in comparison to the first block: χ^2 (1 195) = 22.80 p < .001 φ = .34, as well as in comparison to the second block: χ^2 (1, 172) = 11.25 p = .001 φ = .26. So, we can say that overall there was a decrease in agency by the end of the observation period in comparison to the beginning phase of psychotherapy, and also within two periods of the working phase. This is in contrast to our expectations based on Adler's (2012) study, as well as on Gordin and Békés's theorizing (2021).

However, looking at our alternative hypothesis, there might be some support for the idea that agency and patiency fluctuate according to the types of issues discussed at a given session. This hypothesis may be further supported by using qualitative methods: a close examination of the issues discussed at a given session where agency decreased. Looking at the third phase of the observation period (third block) we can see that, during this period, the analysand had to face serious difficulties in her life: the depression of her mother and her inability to fulfil her university requirements. These topics dominate the discussions with the analyst at the sessions, giving rise to less agency-related themes, and more patiency-related ones. The difference with Adler (2012) may also be because he examined narratives written outside the session—such narratives serving in a way as documentation of the progress of the therapy—whereas in our study we examined the texts directly from the sessions.

Returning to the differences between the three blocks, we can examine the variations in self-mastery. In the first block it occurs in 28 narratives out of 113 (24.8%), in the second block in 21 narratives out of 90 (23.3%), and in the third block it occurs in 7 narratives out of 82 (8.5%). Using the Chi-square test to compute the difference between the three blocks, we found that it was significant: χ^2 (2, N = 285) = 9.07 p = .011 Cramer's V = .18. In the third block, self-mastery is significantly lower than in the first or second block: χ^2 (1 195) = 8.51 p = .004 φ = .21, and χ^2 (1, 172) = 6.89 p = .009 φ = .20, respectively. This suggests that one reason for the decrease in agency overall might be the decrease in self-mastery. This means that the client expressed the mastering, controlling, perfecting, and expanding of the self to a lesser degree as psychotherapy progressed. This again contradicts our expectation of increasing agency as psychotherapy progresses. However, it is in line with our alternative hypothesis, that there might be fluctuations in agency, depending on the issues discussed at any given session. In the third phase of the observation period the analysand's issues discussed at the sessions may be related to the drop in self-mastery, as we mentioned above.

Looking at achievement, we can observe a steady reduction in the proportion of occurrence throughout the three phases of the observation period. In the first block we can find 32 occurrences out of the 113 narratives (28.3%); in the second block we can find it in 11 out of 90 narratives (12.2%); whereas in the third block we can find it in only 3 out of the 82 narratives (3.7%). There is a significant difference between the three blocks, χ^2 (2, N = 285) = 22.84 p < .001 Cramer's V = .28. Expression of achievement is significantly lower in the second block: χ^2 (1 203) = 7.78 p = .005 φ = .20. In the third block it is even lower than in the second block: χ^2 (1, 172) = 4.21 p = .040 φ = .16. So, we can conclude that the analysand expressed fewer and fewer successes and achievements regarding her tasks and instrumental objectives as psychoanalysis progressed. This result, again, is in contrast with our expectations of the increase of agency as psychotherapy progresses; however, it is in line with our alternative hypothesis suggesting that agency might fluctuate depending on the issues discussed at the sessions. So, the analysand's problems related to her lack of fulfilling her university requirements may have led to a decrease in the occurrence of the achievement theme.

It is also important to note here that differences in the proportions of the two categories of self-mastery and achievement should not be considered substantial, since if we use the Wilcoxon test to compare these categories by blocks, we find no significant differences between them: first block: p = .607, second block: p = .052, third block: p = 0.125.

Patiency

Expression of patiency occurred in 62.11% of the examined narratives during the observation period. This is more than double the proportion of agency, which suggests that using the category of patiency was useful in capturing an important aspect of the analysand's experience. Table 8.3 and Figures 8.4 and 8.5 contain the frequencies and proportions by subscale and total scores of patiency.

Differences in occurrence between patiency categories

Drawing together the overall data from all the sessions, using the Cochran Q-test, we found significant differences between the proportion of the patiency categories Q (df = 3; N = 285) = 303.624 p < .001. Using the Sign test as a post hoc test corrected by the Holm procedure, we can conclude that loss of self-control occurred in the highest proportion (average proportion 58.95%), and failure occurred at a significantly lower rate (p_H < ,001) (average proportion 28.07%). Loss of status occurred in significantly (p_H < ,001) lower proportion than failure. Finally the category of disempowerment was used at a significantly (p_H < ,001) lower rate than the rest of the categories (2.11%). Since the category of disempowerment has a very low occurrence (i.e. under 10%), we were not able to compute differences between the sessions.

Table 8.3 Patiency total score and subscales in narratives by blocks and sessions

		Total number of texts	Texts containing Patiency		Texts containing Loss of self-control		Texts containing Failure		Texts containing Loss o f status		Texts containing Disempowerment	
Block	Session	N	N	%	N	%	N	%	N	%	N	%
1	1	43	27	62.8	25	58.1	9	20.9	4	9.3	0	0.0
	2	38	24	63.2	24	63.2	18	47.4	7	18.4	0	0.0
	3	32	18	56.3	17	53.1	6	18.8	5	15.6	0	0.0
2	1	37	15	40.5	14	37.8	5	13.5	3	8.1	0	0.0
	2	21	13	61.9	13	61.9	0	0.0	0	0.0	0	0.0
	3	32	17	53.1	16	50.0	0	0.0	2	6.3	4	12.5
3	1	29	16	55.2	16	55.2	4	13.8	0	0.0	0	0.0
	2	28	25	89.3	23	82.1	21	75.0	8	28.6	0	0.0
	3	25	22	88.0	20	80.0	17	68.0	5	20.0	2	8.0

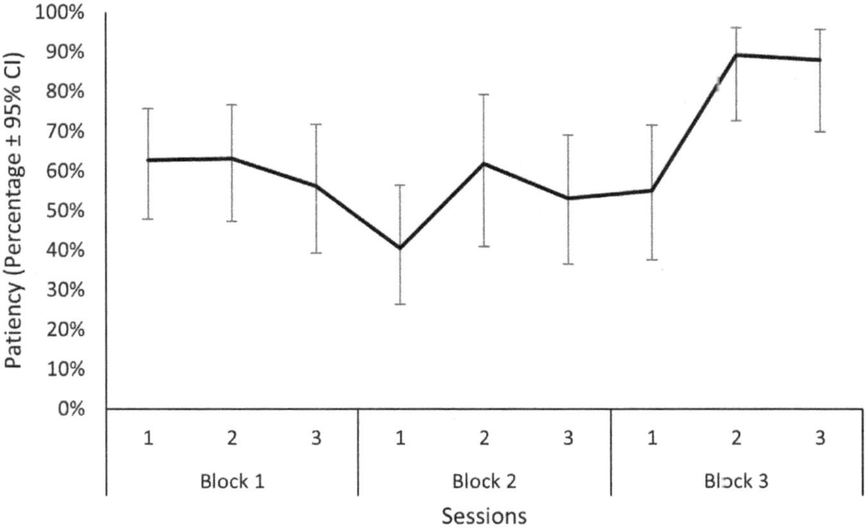

Figure 8.4 Changes of total scores and subscales of patiency in the course of the observation period

Note: On the graph we can see the percentage of the appearance of Patiency ± Wilson score confidence intervals for a binomial proportion

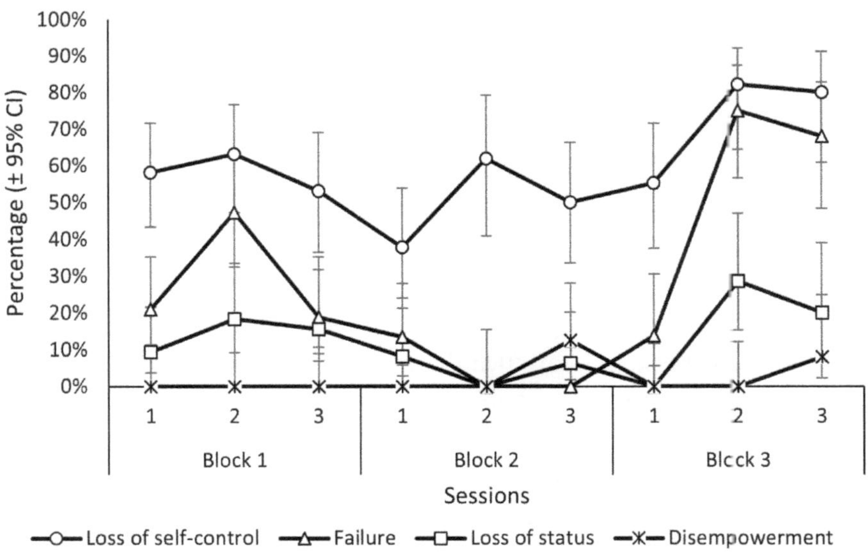

Figure 8.5 Changes of subscales of patiency in the course of the observation period

Note: On the graph we can see the percentage of the appearance of Patiency ± Wilson score confidence intervals for a binomial proportion

Differences between session blocks

The nine examined sessions were divided into three blocks, since there substantial time passed between these periods. Therefore, we have compared the sessions by blocks. The total amount of patiency expressed in the first block was 69 out of 113 narratives (61.1%), in the second block 45 out of 90 narratives (50%), and in the third block 63 out of 82 narratives (76.8%). The difference was significant between the three blocks, using the Chi-square test: $\chi^2(2, N = 285) = 13.21$ p < .001 Cramer's V = .22. There was no significant difference between the first two blocks: χ^2 (1 203) = 2.49 $p = .115$ $\varphi = .11$. In the third block patiency was significantly higher as either in the first block, χ^2 (1 195) = 5.40 $p = .020$ $\varphi = .17$, or in the second: χ^2 (1, 172) = 13.22 $p < .001$ $\varphi = .17$. So, as opposed to agency, which decreased significantly by the third phase of the observation period, patiency increased significantly by the third phase. These results are in harmony with each other, however. They both contradict our expectations, which predicted the opposite pattern to occur. So, from these results we can tell that the discussion of problems at the third phase sessions were possibly related to the decrease in agency. but they may also have been related to the increase in patiency at the same time, which might be explained by the analysand reporting more passivity, vulnerability, and failure in school assignments and home tasks (related to the mother's depression), as well as in intimate relationships.

Looking at the categories of patiency by blocks we found that narratives expressing the loss of self-control occurred 66 times out of 113 (58.4%) in the first block, 43 times out of 90 narratives (47.8%) in the second block, and in 59 out of 82 narratives (72%) in the third block. Using the chi-square test for showing the differences between the blocks we can say that there is a significant difference between them: $\chi^2(2, N = 285) = 10.38$ $p = .006$ Cramer's V = .19. There is no significant difference between the first two blocks, and between the first and the third block $\chi^2(1, N = 203) = 2.28$ $p = .131$ $\varphi = .11$; however, there is a significant difference between the second and the third blocks, since in the third block loss of self-control is higher $\chi^2(1, N = 172) = 10.39$ $p = .001$ $\varphi = .25$. An increase in the loss of self-control means that the analysand's narratives contained more themes of being a passive object/sufferer of other agent's actions, or environmental effects, which exercise control over them; as well as feeling weak and lost. So, by the third block, these topics became more dominant in the analysand's narratives, contrary to our expectations. However, these results are in harmony with our findings of a decrease in agency and an increase in patiency by the third phase of the observation period, possibly related to the problems discussed in the third phase therapy sessions.

Another theme, failure, occurs in the first block in 33 narrative out of 113 (29.2%), 5 out of 90 narratives in the second block (5.6%), and 42 out of 82 narratives (51.2%) in the third block. The difference between the blocks is significant using the Chi-squared test: $\chi^2(2, N = 285) = 44.431$ $p < .001$ Cramer's $V = .395$. Based on post hoc testing, failure is lower in the second block than in the first: $\chi^2(1, N = 203) = 18.414$ $p < .001$ $\varphi = .301$. However, by the third block failure increases, so it is higher than both in the first and in the second block: $\chi^2(1, N = 195) = 9.731$ $p = .002$ $\varphi = .223$ and $\chi^2(1, N = 172) = 45.053$ $p < .001$ $\varphi = .512$, respectively. An increase in failure means that in their narratives the analysand reports failure in tasks, requirements and in fulfilling responsibilities.

Loss of status occurs more rarely than the previous two variables in the psychoanalytic narratives. In the first block it occurs 16 times out of 113 (14.2%), in the second block in 5 out of 90 narratives (5.6%), in the third block in 13 out of 82 narratives (15.9%). As we can observe, the proportion of these patterns is identical to the previous variables; based on the Chi-square tests, these differences are not significant however $\chi^2(2, N = 285) = 5.22$ $p = .074$ Cramer's $V = .14$.

These results are in line with our earlier results of an increase in patiency and decrease in agency by the third phase of the observation period, and can be related to issues discussed during the third block session, especially at the last two sessions: relationship problems and failure in school assignments. It also supports our alternative hypothesis, which states that agency and patiency may fluctuate during treatment, depending on the topics and problems discussed at the given sessions. When the analysand experiences difficulties or faces new problems or a crisis situation, their sense of agency may temporarily decrease and patiency may increase accordingly.

Changes in agency and patiency in terms of narrative interaction at the session in the case of the female analysand

Looking at changes in agency, we found that the greatest drop in the total scores of agency occurred during the second session in the second phase of the observation period (5th session, L22). During this session the female analysand talks about her mother's depression, with whom she lives in the same household. Her mother fell ill from time to time, and such periods caused Clara a great deal of trouble because, as she explained to her analyst, she had to do all the housework alone and had no help from her mother. In addition, she had to actively help her mother's boyfriend with his car repair problems. According to the description she gave to her analyst at the session, these activities prevented her from completing her student assignments and studying for her university courses.

The NP patterns used by the analysand at the session point to her identification with her mother, taking on the mother's perspective by using pseudo-diegesis and, at the same time, using self-patiency, positioning herself in the role of a passive and vulnerable person (Berán & Unoka 2016). These perspectives show that the analysand was unable to consider the events from her own separate perspective. The boundaries of the self had grown unstable, and she was unable to act as an autonomous person independent of the people around her. The analysand also used internal focalization, the present tense, which suggests a deeper involvement of the self during the narrating process (Berán et al. 2017). We will analyse three excerpts from this session.

Antecedents to Excerpt 8.1

The analysand complains about her mother at the beginning of the session. The mother is going through a depressive episode; however, the analysand mentions that this is just hysteria on the mother's part. The mother is hysterical, according to the analysand, because her boyfriend, Feri, has been away, travelling for a while, and she needs to be at the centre of his attention. Meanwhile, Feri has returned, yet the mother is still in a depressive state. She asks the analysand to give Feri a lift to the car mechanics, because she (the mother) is unable to take him there. The analyst reacts to the situation in Excerpt 8.1. The following excerpts from this session have been previously analysed by Berán and Unoka (2016).

Excerpt 8.1 (session 5, L22)

345TER:	na de ha a Feri nincs ott,	well, but if Feri is not there,
346TER:	akkor nem tud rá figyelni.	then he cannot pay attention to her.
347PAT:	hát de most már itt van,	well, but he is here now,
348PAT:	aztán figyeljen.	then he should pay attention.
349PAT:	nem tudom+..	I don't know+...
comment:	pause 12 s	
350TER:	na de+..	well but+...
351TER:	amit én nem értek, hogy-	what I do not understand, is that-
352TER:	tulajdonképpen	in fact you join in as a third party.
		akkor maga beszáll harmadiknak.
353TER:	ebbe a # játékba, vagy játszmába.	in this # game, or match.
354PAT:	mer?	because?

In Excerpt 8. in line 345 the analyst uses hetero-diegesis—thus looking at the analysand's story from the outside—when she summarizes the reason for the family conflict, and the mother's growing need for attention, using internal focalization. Looking at her wording, it is important that she uses a demonstrative pronoun as a distal deixis ('there'), which, taken together with the hetero-diegetic perspective, emphasizes that she is outside the situation, and has a certain distance between herself and the events that happen to Clara. In lines 347–48 the analysand does not take on the distal perspective offered by the analyst in lines 345–46. Rather, she uses a close pointing pronoun as a proximal deixis (here), demonstrating that she is inside the story plane. She also uses pseudo-diegesis, talking in the mother's name, and taking on her perspective, this way identifying with her; she also uses internal focalization, as the analyst did. Hence, the analysand points out what she thinks is the reason for the mother's behaviour, namely that the boyfriend should be paying attention to her. In line 349 the analysand shifts perspective again. She shifts into homo-diegesis, first-person singular, internal focalization using self-agency while expressing uncertainty, maybe even helplessness about the situation. She also steps out of the story plane and shifts into the therapeutic here and now. This shift on the part of the analysand is a breaking away from the mother's perspective, signalling her readiness for some new ideas; at the same time, however, she is unable to give a different response to the situation, which is signalled by the long silence at this point (12 s).

After a while the analyst starts talking again using a rhetorical question and shifting perspective. She uses homo-diegesis this time, internal focalization and talking in the first-person singular in lines 350–51, suggesting that she is more involved in the conversation than before (when she used hetero-diegesis). In the analyst's utterance (lines 350–53) the analysand is put in the position of the agent, a person who 'joins' the 'game' (lines 352–53). Placing the analysand in the position of the agent also suggests that she is viewed by the analyst as an active, effective subject who has the opportunity of choosing a conscious, well-thought-out reaction to the situation. At the same time the analyst suggests that she thinks that the analysand consciously chooses to participate in the 'game'.

The analysand's portrayal as an agent consciously making a choice is in contrast with Clara's anger and frustration dominating in the situation (expressed in previous talk at the session), as well as with her uncertainty (expressed in line 349). In line 354 the analysand does not accept the analyst's interpretation of the situation; instead she challenges it. She expresses her doubt about the analyst's interpretation by asking for further explanation. This may also be considered a resistance in psychotherapy in analytic terms. What is clear, however, is that the analysand rejects the perspective taken by the analyst at this point.

The present analysis of the female analysand's narrative process during the session (Session 5, L22) can be enriched through the lens of contemporary psychoanalytic theories. These perspectives help us to understand the shifting dynamics of agency and patiency within the psychotherapeutic dialogue, and the evolving epistemic trust that structures the analytic relationship.

Relational psychoanalysis and intersubjectivity theory emphasize the co-construction of meaning within the analytic dyad (Atlas & Aron 2017) with the help of the process of mutual activation of multiple self-states of the analysand and analyst. In this case, the analysand's shifting between diegetic perspectives—oscillating between identification with her mother and a more distanced, self-reflective stance—is an illustration of her struggle with self-agency and relational entanglement. The analyst's focus of attention as it is expressed in NP, leads to new implicit relational knowing, by experiencing the mutual recognition and modifications of each other's perspectives (Lyons-Ruth et al. 1998). The narrative structure suggests a self-fragmentation that is characteristic of developmental disruptions in intersubjective experiences, as highlighted in Lyons-Ruth's work on disorganized attachment (Lyons-Ruth et al. 2006).

At the beginning of Excerpt 8.1, the analysand takes the pseudo-diegetic perspective, narrating from the perspective of the mother and thereby reinforcing her own self-patiency. This suggests a breakdown in self–other differentiation, a key aspect of intersubjective development. Tronick's mutual regulation model (Tronick 2003) posits that, when infants experience misattuned interactions without repair, their capacity to regulate distress through self-agency becomes compromised. In the analysed segment of the dialogue, this mechanism can manifest as difficulty in maintaining an autonomous perspective, as seen in the analysand's entrenchment in her mother's emotional reality. The shift observed in line 349—where the analysand moves into the first-person singular and expresses uncertainty—can be understood as an emergent 'moment of meeting' (BCPSG 2010). The analysand steps out of the rigid identification with her mother's perspective, momentarily engaging in a process of self-exploration. However, the 12-second pause signals an impasse, where the analysand encounters difficulty in fully internalizing her self-agency.

The analysand's challenge to the analyst's interpretation (line 354) can be examined in light of the tension between epistemic mistrust and the need for relational attunement. Resistance in therapy often signals a defensive stance and testing of the analytic relationship's reliability. Given the analysand's history of being enmeshed in care-giving roles within a family system characterized by dysregulated affect, it is plausible that she experiences the analyst's suggestion of agency as both liberating and threatening.

From a relational perspective, resistance can be reframed as a micro-regulation of trust within the analytic dyad. Tronick's (2003) work on interactive mismatch and repair provides a framework for understanding the necessity of these ruptures. Rather than a simple rejection of the analyst's interpretation, the analysand's 'because?' can be seen as an implicit bid for further attunement—an invitation for the analyst to refine the scaffolding of epistemic trust.

The analysand's shifting use of deixis, focalization, and narrative stance reflects her struggle to construct a coherent sense of self-agency. The intersubjective negotiation within the analytic dyad mirrors the broader developmental trajectory of narrative identity formation, where language mediates the transformation of lived experience into an articulated self-concept. Through the lens of relational psychoanalysis and intersubjectivity theory, we can appreciate how therapeutic change emerges not through unilateral insight but through the dynamic, co-constructed reworking of self-experience.

Excerpt 8.2 is a continuation of the Excerpt 8.1, where the analyst answers the analysand's question/challenge.

Excerpt 8.2 (session 5, L22)

355TER:	hát +..	well+...
356TER:	a mama azt mondja, hogy én nem tudok,	mother says that I cannot,
357TER:	akkor +..	and then+...
358TER:	itt van a lányom,	here is my daughter,
359TER:	támogassa ő a Ferit.	let her support Feri
360TER:	legyen +..	let her+...
361TER:	+, legyen ő az, aki a Feri mellett áll a bajban.	+, let her be the one, who stands by Feri, in his trouble.
362TER:	mondjuk.	so to say.
363PAT:	tényleg.	indeed.
364PAT:	én meg azt mondom, hogy nem,	and then I say no,
365PAT:	és utána meg iszonyú rosszul érzem magam.	and I feel terribly bad after that.

In line 356 the analyst shifts perspective again. She shifts into pseudo-diegesis talking in the first-person singular, taking on the perspective of the mother, continuing the narrative from her perspective, as was previously done by Clara.

She illustrates to the analysand the mother's thought process in lines 356–61, which makes it possible for her to see her mother from an outside point of view. So, this way the analysand has the chance to reflect to the situation demonstrated to her by the analyst. The use of this perspective on the part of the analyst helps the analysand to exercise her reflective functioning capacity (Katznelson 2014), which leads to an insight on the part of the analysand (lines 363–65).

At the same time we can see that the analyst changes her strategy in line 356, after she tried to look at the situation from hetero-diegetic (line 345) or homo-diegetic (lines 351–53) position. Instead, she reflects a pseudo-diegetic perspective used by the analysand earlier, which perspective, at the same time, consists of the rephrasing, and re-elaborating of the 'game' interpretation that she used before. This version of her interpretation was useful in inspiring the analysand to an insight (line 363). The analysand—as a response—uses homo-diegesis, first-person singular and self-agency in line 364, while expressing and describing her emotions: she explains how she reacts to the mother's 'line of thought' demonstrated by the analyst. Using internal focalization she recognizes that, since she rejects the pressure to help Feri, she experiences a great amount of guilt. She not merely recognizes her guilty emotions, but also the complex source of her bad feelings, and her guilt. However, she is still unable to defend herself from these emotions—and starts to talk about various other topics in the continuation of the session.

Excerpt 8.2 offers a nuanced view of the analyst's evolving intervention strategies and the analysand's emerging self-reflection. By examining it through the lens of relational psychoanalysis and intersubjectivity theory we can trace the analyst's attempt to facilitate a deeper understanding of agency and self–other differentiation in the analysand's experience.

In line 356, the analyst's use of a pseudo-diegetic perspective—speaking as the analysand's mother—is a non-interpretative intervention strategy, where the analyst mirrors the analysand's earlier mode of narration, rather than maintaining a distanced, interpretive stance. From an intersubjective perspective, this shift reflects an effort to provide a perspective for the analysand where she could reflect on her mother's words and, at the same time, give up the identification with her internalized mother's point of view, promoting a sense of mutual understanding and recognition (Atlas & Aron 2017).

The decision to momentarily 'inhabit' the mother's perspective allows the analysand to see her mother's expectations more clearly as an externalized construct rather than as an inescapable emotional reality. This technique aligns with the concept of scaffolding reflective functioning (Fonagy et al. 2002), wherein the analyst provides a structure through which the analysand can mentally step back and examine her own relational patterns. The analyst is reframing the mother's implicit demands in clear and structured terms (lines 356–61) and, by this intervention, the analyst offers a way for the analysand to engage in a reflective reappraisal rather than an automatic emotional response.

This moment represents an implicit 'moment of meeting' (BCPSG 2010), wherein the analyst's intervention allows for a micro shift in the analysand's self-perception. The mother's demand—previously experienced as an engulfing force—now appears as a constructed relational expectation that can be questioned.

A pivotal transition occurs in line 363 when the analysand responds with 'indeed', signalling a moment of recognition, followed by the analysand's self-reflective stance, which is accompanied by the emergence of self-agency and emotional distress. She states: 'and then I say no, and I feel terribly bad after that'. This utterance indicates a partial movement towards agency. On the one hand, she cognitively recognizes her reaction as a rejection of the mother's expectations, but on the other hand, she remains unable to disengage from the guilt attached to it emotionally. She can identify her feelings but has not yet regulated them effectively.

The analysand's guilt following her assertion of autonomy suggests a difficulty in affective self-regulation (Tronick 2003). The mutual regulation model posits that individuals who experience chronic misattunement in their early care-giving relationships develop maladaptive self-regulation strategies. The possible consequences of this are compliance, guilt, or distress when asserting their needs. The analysand's experience of feeling 'terribly bad' after refusing her mother's request exemplifies such a regulatory struggle.

From a relational psychoanalytic perspective, her difficulty in metabolizing her guilt may stem from an implicit belief that autonomy equals relational rupture. Clara's experience of guilt after attempting to assert her personal boundaries fits with Lyons-Ruth's (1999) research on disorganized attachment, where individuals struggle with both compliance and resistance. In this context, the analyst's role is to provide a containing function that allows her to tolerate the distress of differentiation from the mother, and co-regulate the analysand's emotional experience, and not merely to interpret it.

The analyst thus plays an important role in reconstructing the patient's agency. However, the analysand's persistent distress following her assertion of autonomy underscores the affective cost of self-differentiation, highlighting the need for continued therapeutic support in integrating these emerging insights. Her temporary withdrawal from the subject at the end of the excerpt suggests that self-regulatory processes have a stronger effect than interactive regulatory processes (Beebe & Lachman 2020), and moments of realization do not immediately translate into change—but, rather, they lay the groundwork for future transformation.

At a later point of the session (Excerpt 8.3) the analyst returns to this problem, and asks the analysand what happened, and whether she has found a solution to the problematic situation.

Excerpt 8.3 (session 5, L22)

544TER:	na és valahogy megoldódott ez a helyzet?	well, has this situation been resolved somehow?
545PAT:	bennem?	in me?
546PAT:	nem.	no.
547TER:	hogy a Feri konkrétan +..	with Feri, concretely+...
548PAT:	ja, eljött velem a Feri,	yes, Feri came with me,
549PAT:	és kiraktam a villamosnál.	and I have dropped him off at the tram.
comment:	the client laughs	
550PAT:	ennyi.	that's it.
551TER:	hát ez egy elég kézenfekvő megoldás.	well, this is a very obvious solution.
552TER:	mit kell ezen játszmázni?	why would one need to play games about it?
553PAT:	én az+/	that I/+
554PAT:	+, tehát én ezt nem tudom.	+, well, I don't know this.

In line 544 the analyst uses hetero-diegesis and the past tense again, but also the proximal deixis 'this' to point to the unresolved issue with the analysand's helping Feri to get to the car mechanics. By this perspective the analyst is again emotionally distancing herself from the events of the analysand's narrative, but at the same time redefining it as having clear boundaries and practically well-manageable details for herself and for the analysand. The analysand continues using the same perspective as the analyst in lines 545–46, except she logically uses homo-diegesis in her answer, discussing the problem. However, she interprets the analyst's question as if it were related to her inner world using homo-diegesis, at the same time distinguishing her inner world from the outside events in her answer when she asks: 'In me?'. She gives a negative answer to her own question in line 546, so showing that she still has doubts about her behaviour in the situation—whether it was the right solution or not.

It would be a reasonable assumption on the analysand's part to suppose that the analyst wants to talk about her inner response, her dilemma and feelings of guilt—as she acknowledged in lines 364–65. However, interestingly, that is not what the analyst wants to focus on in relation to this problem. She confirms in line 547 that what she means is whether Feri's concrete problem has been resolved. In lines 548–50 the analysand replies using the past tense, homo-diegesis, first-person singular to indicate her simple solution to the problem. In line 548 she puts Feri in the position of the agent, and in line 549 she puts herself in this position, thus showing her own capability to find a solution and to resolve the problem. Her laughter also confirms her relief and satisfaction about her solution. The feeling of relief and satisfaction is also expressed by the therapist in line 551. She uses the present tense and hetero-diegesis, the proximal deixis 'this' in pointing to the solution. These perspectives are similar to that used at the beginning of the discussion in line 345, with the difference of the deictic marker, which was distal in that utterance. This perspective again looks at the event from the outside, as something that has achieved closure at this point. Next, in line 552 the analyst again shifts perspective, uses the general subject and the present tense, which suggests that she is trying to draw a general conclusion or, rather, trying to help the analysand draw a general conclusion here by using a rhetorical question. In lines 553–54 the analysand answers the question, taking on the analyst's perspective (present tense), but using internal focalization and both proximal and distal deixis, which marks the statement as somewhat ambivalent, but still expressing agreement with the analyst. The ambivalence is also suggested by the analysand not using the general subject—as used by the analyst—but homo-diegesis, first-person singular—so, making her statement more subjective than the analyst's.

In this segment of this session (Excerpt 8.3) the analyst's shifting interventions and the analysand's responses highlight the ongoing struggle between cognitive resolution and emotional unrest.

At the beginning of Excerpt 8.3, the analyst asks, 'Well, has this situation been resolved somehow?' (544TER). By using hetero-diegesis and the past tense, the analyst frames the situation as an externalized, completed event. The use of proximal deixis ('this') subtly suggests that the issue, at least from the analyst's perspective, has clear boundaries and is now manageable. This linguistic choice fits with the analyst's earlier attempts (Excerpts 8.1 and 8.2) to guide the analysand towards a more objective, less emotionally entangled perspective on the events.

However, the analysand does not immediately adopt this perspective. Her response, 'In me?' (545PAT), signals a misalignment between the analyst's focus on practical resolution and the analysand's preoccupation with her internal emotional state. This moment exemplifies a rupture in epistemic trust (Fonagy &

Allison 2023), where the analysand initially assumes that the analyst is concerned with her inner turmoil rather than the pragmatic resolution of the external situation. Her subsequent response ('No', 546PAT) confirms that, while the practical issue may be resolved, her internal conflict remains unresolved.

This exchange is significant because it illustrates how affective experiences often persist beyond behavioural resolutions. From the perspective of mentalization theory (Fonagy et al. 2002), the analysand demonstrates partial mentalization—she recognizes her emotional response but has not yet fully processed or regulated it.

When the analyst reorients the conversation ('with Feri, concretely+…', 547TER), she implicitly shifts away from the analysand's unresolved feelings, directing attention towards a factual resolution of events. This move reflects a scaffolding strategy in which the analyst reinforces the analysand's ability to effect change in the external world. The analysand then narrates the resolution in a straightforward manner ('Yes, Feri came with me, and I dropped him off at the tram' 548–49PAT). Here, a significant linguistic shift occurs. Unlike earlier segments where she struggled with agency, the analysand now structures her narrative in a clear, agentic form: In 'Feri came with me' (line 548) Feri is the agent. In 'I dropped him off' (line 549), she assumes full agency. This shift regarding agency marks a moment of empowerment, reinforced by her laughter, which may suggest a sense of relief and mastery over the situation. The laughter may also indicate a release of tension, signalling that the weight of the dilemma has lifted.

The analyst's reaction ('Well, this is a very obvious solution', 551TER) acknowledges the analysand's newly found agency. The phrase 'very obvious' suggests a redefinition of the issue as one that did not actually require excessive emotional distress, reinforcing the idea that the analysand is capable of handling such conflicts more straightforwardly in the future. However, in line 552, the analyst asks, 'Why would one need to play games about it?' This intervention was aimed at generalizing the analysand's insight, potentially inviting her to recognize a broader pattern in her emotional responses. The analyst offers a shift into general subject and present tense, which is an attempt to transform the analysand's personal experience into a more universally applicable lesson.

Yet, the analysand's response ('That I/+ … well, I don't know this', 553–54PAT) reflects an ambivalence towards fully integrating this realization. Several linguistic markers reinforce this: The fragmented start ('That I/+') suggests hesitation. The return to homo-diegesis ('I' instead of a general subject) makes her response more personal and subjective. The phrase 'I don't know this' reflects lingering uncertainty, implying that, while she cognitively recognizes the analyst's point, she does not yet fully internalize it on an affective level.

This moment is crucial from an intersubjective and regulatory perspective. While the analysand demonstrates a capacity for behavioural agency, she remains emotionally unprepared to relinquish the habitual guilt and distress associated with asserting herself. Tronick calls incomplete dyadic repair the moments where an individual's emotional state is acknowledged but not fully metabolized within the relational context (2003). So, the analysand's response suggests a gap between intellectual insight and emotional transformation. This is a common phenomenon in psychoanalysis, where patients may gain cognitive clarity about their relational patterns but continue to struggle with deeply embedded affective responses (Beebe & Lachman 2020).

From a relational perspective, the analysand's laughter in line 549 can be seen as both a sign of relief and a subtle form of avoidance. While she acknowledges that the situation was, in fact, easy to solve, she does not fully resolve the emotional residue of the experience. Her concluding statement ('I don't know this', 554PAT) indicates that her guilt remains a structured part of her self-experience, despite behavioural changes.

So, this final segment of the session illustrates the delicate interplay between narrative restructuring, agency, and emotional ambivalence in psychoanalysis. The analysand's movement from distress to laughter, from uncertainty to pragmatic resolution, suggests progress in problem-solving and agency. However, her final hesitation reveals the ongoing challenge of affective self-regulation—a challenge that requires continued therapeutic engagement. As is often the case in relational psychoanalysis, such moments do not represent complete closure, but serve as groundwork for future therapeutic work—where cognitive insight can gradually be paired with affective integration, allowing for a more stable sense of agency and emotional clarity.

In summary, we can say that during the three excerpts analysed from session 5, L22, the analyst followed an unequivocal pattern of perspective shifts that show how she has tried in a series of shifts to help the analysand to shift her own perspective, and try to contemplate her situation from a different angle. At the beginning the analyst used hetero-diegesis, then homo-diegesis to approach the analysand's problem, but Clara did not respond by a coordination of perspectives. Then the analyst shifted into pseudo-diegesis, an identification with the mother, and this shift seemed to be helpful, by helping the analysand to an insight regarding her own emotional response to the situation. Finally, the analyst again distanced herself from the situation using hetero-diegesis, which helped the analysand to experience herself as an agent, who is able to resolve difficult situations. So, while at the session the analysand's sense of agency hits the lowest level, the analyst in her interventions helps the analysand to feel she still has self-agency, as expressed in her NP shifts.

Another interesting aspect of these three excerpts is that both the analysand and the analyst have frequently used internal focalization, hence manifesting the analysand's ability to reflect on her own as well as on other people's mental content. So, the main problem with this analysand regarding mentalization is not her lack of ability to use internal perspectives. Rather she has a problem with self-agency, which is also an important aspect of mentalization. This result contradicts previous conceptualizations of mentalization focusing solely on verbalizing mental content (Meins & Fernyhough 1999; Meins et al. 2001; Meins et al. 2002; Meins et al. 2003).

Looking at changes in the levels of patiency, we notice that it peaks at the second session of the third block, in other words, session 8, L32. We have discussed this session in Chapter 7 in connection to the 'understanding' reaction of others; so we will only summarize some aspects of that analysis here. During this session the analysand talks about her relationship anxiety, and her anxiety about her school assignments. A major source of her relationship distress is feeling misunderstood by her partner; she also often yields in conflicts because she cannot tolerate the emotional pressure of arguments. The perspectives used during this session, for example the first-person singular, internal focalization, the present tense, show that both the analyst and the analysand are highly involved in the discussion taking place at the session (Berán et al. 2017). The analyst also uses a series of perspective shifts during this session, perhaps with the intention to demonstrate to the analysand how she devalues her boyfriend (and others), and puts the analysand in the position of the agent, instead of letting her be the passive and vulnerable patient in her own narrative. The analysand herself is unable to thoroughly understand her contradictory inner states, and this situation seems to contribute to her relationship problems. The analyst in the course of this session helps the analysand to realize and accept this fact, and to experience 'being understood' first towards the self, and then towards the important other person (her boyfriend).

In the case of the female analysand–female analyst dyad our results show that agency and patiency does not change linearly during the course of psychoanalysis. Instead, the change of the frequency of these themes fluctuates from the beginning of the observation period to its end. The reason for this, according to our qualitative results, is the differences in ways various problems brought into a given session are processed. Thus in the case of the dominance of a given problem during a discussion of a session, agency might decrease or be stagnant, patiency may increase until the problem has been worked through, and an increase in agency may start again.

Shifts in perspective also may contribute to changes in agency and patiency, as we have illustrated in our qualitative analysis. The use of pseudo-diegesis, internal focalization, and the analysand's placing in the position of the agent in a series of shifts initiated by the analyst have major importance in the working-through process.

The findings from the analysis of the three excerpts from session 5, L22, and the broader trends in the case of the female analysand–female analyst dyad, provide valuable insights into the fluctuating nature of agency and patiency in psychoanalysis. By integrating perspectives from intersubjectivity theory, relational psychoanalysis, the Boston Change Process Study Group (BCPSG), Tronick's mutual regulation model, and the mentalization-based model, we can refine our understanding of how therapeutic change occurs through narrative restructuring, interactive regulation, and epistemic trust.

One of the key findings of this study is that agency and patiency do not follow a linear trajectory during the course of psychoanalysis. Instead, their fluctuation reflects the shifting nature of the analysand's engagement with different themes and relational patterns. This aligns with relational psychoanalysis, which posits that self-experience is not a fixed internal construct but rather co-created in the analytic dyad (Atlas & Aron 2017). The analysand's movement between agency and patiency mirrors the ongoing negotiation of self–other boundaries, a central focus in intersubjective developmental theory (Beebe & Lachmann 2020).

The analyst's perspective shifts throughout the session—from hetero-diegesis to homo-diegesis, to pseudo-diegesis, and back to hetero-diegesis—suggest that these fluctuations in agency and patiency are part of a dynamic mutual regulation process. In this context, Tronick's mutual regulation model (2003) provides a useful framework for understanding these shifts. Just as an infant's emerging sense of self is scaffolded by moment-to-moment interactions with a care-giver, the analysand's sense of agency is supported through the analyst's attuned responses and shifts in perspective.

From a relational psychoanalytic perspective (Atlas & Aron 2017), the analyst does not function as an objective observer but is instead an active participant in co-constructing the analysand's self-narrative. The use of pseudo-diegesis in Excerpt 8.2, where the analyst temporarily takes on the voice of the analysand's mother, illustrates an embodied relational intervention. By stepping into this perspective, the analyst helps the analysand momentarily externalize and re-encounter a familiar relational script in a more conscious, reflective manner.

This scaffolding of reflective functioning (Fonagy et al. 2002) is critical in helping the analysand reframe her experience. As relational theorists have suggested, therapeutic change is not achieved through intellectual insight alone but through experiencing new relational possibilities within the therapeutic interaction (Atlas & Aron 2017). The analyst's shifts into and out of the analysand's internalized relational roles provide an interactive demonstration of how perspectives can shift, creating the conditions for epistemic trust.

One of the most significant implications of this study is that the analysand's difficulty is not with taking an internal perspective—as she frequently uses internal focalization—but rather with self-agency within those perspectives. This distinction challenges traditional conceptions of mentalization, which have often focused on the ability to verbalize mental states (Meins et al. 1999, 2001, 2002). Instead, as Fonagy and Allison (2014) argue, epistemic trust—the ability to accept and integrate new perspectives from a trusted interlocutor—is crucial for therapeutic change.

In this case, the analysand's epistemic trust in the analyst fluctuates, as evidenced by her moments of resistance and ambivalence (e.g. Excerpt 8.3, lines 553–54). This suggests that, while she cognitively engages with the analyst's interventions, she does not yet fully trust the new relational narrative being offered to her. In moments where she expresses doubt or struggles with guilt (as in Excerpt 8.2, line 365), we see that her attachment history likely predisposes her to an unstable sense of self-agency—one that is easily undermined by interpersonal conflict or perceived criticism. From a mentalization-based therapy perspective, the analyst's role is to support the analysand in tolerating and regulating these uncertainties, rather than rushing to resolve them (Fonagy et al. 2015). This process takes time and, as the fluctuations in agency and patiency suggest, it does not happen in a linear fashion.

Regarding the analyst, her repeated shifts in perspective serve multiple therapeutic functions:

1. creating emotional distance (hetero-diegesis): When the analyst steps outside the analysand's emotional world (e.g. Excerpt 10.3, line 544);
2. helping to contain and regulate affect (Tronick 2003);
3. encouraging identification with the other's perspective (pseudo-diegesis): When the analyst speaks as the analysand's mother (Excerpt 10.2), she allows the analysand to engage in reflective reappraisal (BCPSG 2010);
4. restoring agency (homo-diegesis in the present tense): The analysand's gradual move towards speaking in the first-person singular with active agency reflects the reinternalization of a self-narrative in which she is not merely a passive victim but an active agent of change.

As relational theorists have argued (Atlas & Aron 2017), the ability to shift between positions in a relational narrative is a marker of increased psychological flexibility and a more developed self-structure. In contrast, rigidity in narrative stance (e.g. being stuck in victimization or omnipotence) is often indicative of developmental trauma or attachment disruption. From an intersubjective, relational, and mentalization-based perspective, the analyst's role is not to provide the 'correct' interpretation but to scaffold a process through which the analysand can develop a more flexible, agentic, and reflective sense of self. In this way, psychoanalysis functions not only as a method of uncovering unconscious material but as a relational practice of co-constructing new ways of being.

Results and discussion of the analysis of agency and patiency in the case of the male analysand–male analyst dyad

Occurrence of agency in self-narratives

In the case of the male analysand–male analyst dyad, agency occurred in 34% of the narratives. Table 8.4 and Figures 8.6 and 8.7 show the frequencies and percentages in total and for each category or subscale.

Differences in occurrence between agency categories

Drawing together data from all the sessions, using the Cochran Q-test we found a significant difference of the occurrences of categories of agency $Q(df = 3; N = 344) = 216.89$ $p < .001$.

While the occurrence of the theme of self-mastery is a relatively high proportion (average 29.36%) of the narratives, the rest of the categories are much lower (achievement: 5.52%; empowerment: 1.74%; status gain: 0.58%). Using the Sign test as a post hoc measure, and using the Holm procedure for correction for multiple testing, we can conclude that the proportion of self-mastery is significantly higher in the narratives than the rest of the categories $p_H < .001$; the occurrence of achievement is significantly higher than that of status gain $p_H = .002$, however, it does not differ significantly from the occurrence of empowerment, $p_H = .146$; and the occurrence of empowerment does not differ significantly from that of status gain $p > .999$. We must note, however, that since the occurrence of empowerment, status gain, and achievement is below 10%, the differences between sessions cannot be interpreted for these categories.

From these results we can conclude that among the agency categories, self-mastery was the category that occurred most frequently in the speech of the

Table 8.4 Frequencies and percentages of Agency and subscales of agency in the case of the male client

		Total number of texts	Texts containing Agency		Texts containing Self-mastery		Texts containing Achievement		Texts containing Status gain		Texts containing Empowerment	
Block	Session	N	N	%	N	%	N	%	N	%	N	%
1	1	45	**8**	**17,8**	3	6,7	4	8,9	1	2,2	2	4,4
	2	40	**15**	**37,5**	14	35,0	2	5,0	0	0,0	0	0,0
	3	30	**5**	**16,7**	5	16,7	0	0,0	0	0,0	0	0,0
2	1	35	**18**	**51,4**	13	37,1	5	14,3	0	0,0	4	11,4
	2	40	**6**	**15,0**	6	15,0	0	0,0	0	0,0	0	0,0
3	1	42	**10**	**23,8**	10	23,8	2	4,8	0	0,0	0	0,0
	2	61	**28**	**45,9**	27	44,3	1	1,6	0	0,0	0	0,0
	3	51	**26**	**51,0**	23	45,1	5	9,8	1	2,0	0	0,0

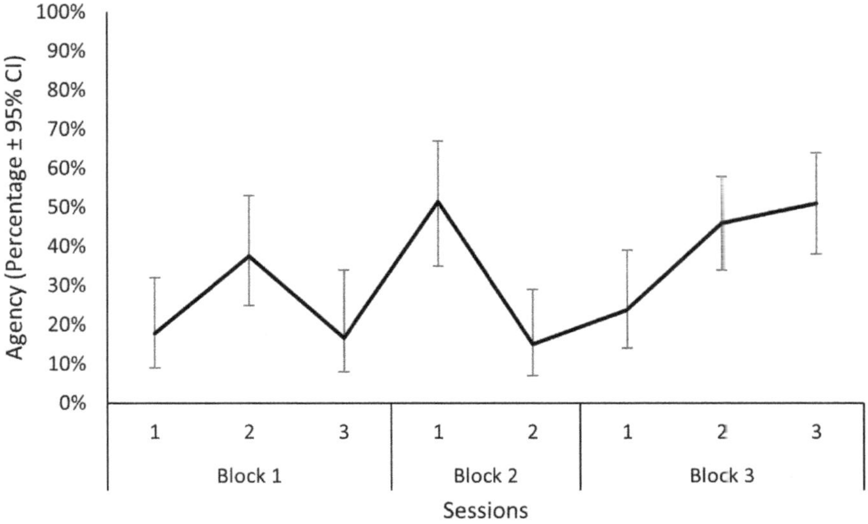

Figure 8.6 Changes in agency total scores by session and by block in the case of the male analysand

Note: In the figure, we can see the percentage of the appearance of agency ± Wilson score confidence intervals for a binomial proportion.

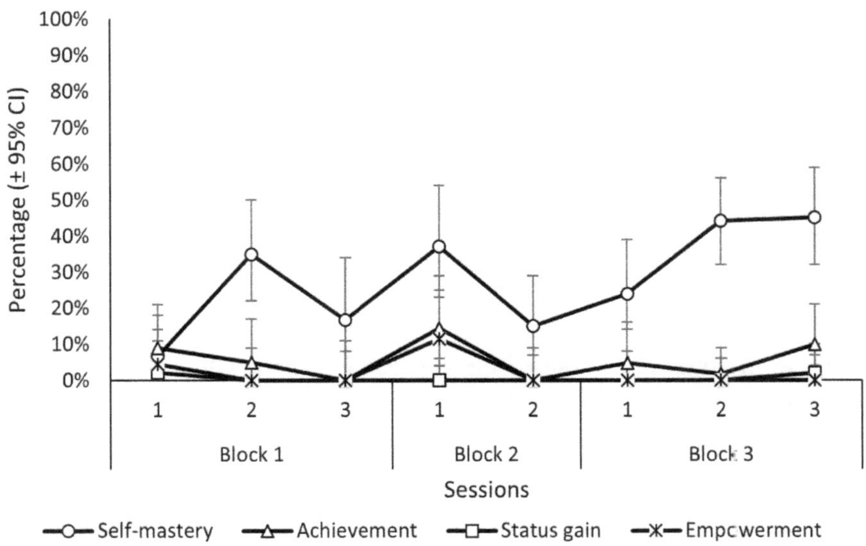

Figure 8.7 Changes in agency subscales by session and by block in the case of the male client

Note: In the figure, we can see the percentage of the appearance of agency ± Wilson score confidence intervals for a binomial proportion.

second analysand during the course of the observation period. Self-mastery includes activities of mastering, controlling, and perfecting the self, which activities are discussed in greatest proportion in the narratives told at the sessions. Since narrative agency was found to be positively related to purpose in life (Grossbaum & Bates 2002), we argue that the category of self-mastery should also be correlated with purpose in life, which would make its occurrence fruitful, and useful during the course of the psychoanalytic session.

Differences between session blocks

The eight examined sessions were divided into three blocks, since a substantial time passed between these periods. Therefore, we have compared the sessions by blocks. The comparison may be completed for total amount of agency, and for self-mastery.

In the first block, agency themes occurred in a total of 28 narratives out of 115 (24.3%), in the second clock it occurred in 24 narratives out of 75 (32.0%), and in the third block it occurred in 64 out of 155 narratives (41.3%). Using the Chi-squared test for testing differences between the blocks we found that there was a significant difference $\chi^2(2, N = 345) = 8.60$ p = .015 Cramer's V = .16, and frequency of agency has increased with time. This increase is apparent between the first and the third blocks, but it is so slight that it cannot be observed between either the first and second blocks or between the second and third blocks (for the first and third blocks χ^2 (1, 270) = 8.44 p=.004 φ = .18; for the first and second blocks χ^2 (1 190) = 1.34 p = .248 φ = .08; for the second and third blocks χ^2 (1, 230) = 1.85 p = .17 φ = .090).

The differences between the session blocks may be examined with respect to the category (subscale) of self-mastery—although the patterns are similar to those of agency, and therefore somewhat redundant. During the first block self-mastery can be found in 22 narratives out of 115 (19.1%), during the second block it is found in 19 out of 75 narratives (25.3%), and in the third block it can be found in 60 narratives out of 155 (38.7%). Using the Chi-squared test the difference between the three blocks is significant χ^2 (2, N = 345) = 12.94 p = .015 Cramer's V = .19, and the occurrence of self-mastery increases with time in the course of psychotherapy. The increase in self-mastery is manifest in the difference between the first and the third blocks, but it is so slight that it cannot be observed either between the first and the second blocks, nor between the second and third blocks (for the first and the third blocks χ^2 (1, 270) = 11.97 p = .001 φ = .21; for the first and the second blocks χ^2 (1 190) = 1.032 p = .37 φ = .07; for the second and the third blocks χ^2 (1, 230) = 4.01 p = .054 φ = .13).

These results regarding the differences between session blocks suggest that our hypothesis about the increase of agency in the course of therapeutic treatment was supported. However, nor do these results contradict our alternative hypothesis, according to which the fluctuation of agency may be due to the nature of the problems discussed in a given session. So, a decrease in agency may occur due to working through a difficult problem, or a crisis situation, and then an increase in agency occurs as a result of achieving closure or progress with a given problematic situation or relationship, for example.

Occurrence of patiency in self-narratives

Themes of patiency occurred in 54% of the narratives, which is again, in the case of this analysand, higher than that of agency. The frequencies by categories of patiency and its proportions by session are included in Table 8.5 and Figures 8.8 and 8.9.

Differences in occurrence between patiency categories

Drawing together data from all the sessions, using the Cochran Q-test we found a significant difference of the occurrences of categories of patiency Q (df = 3; N = 345) = 310.54 p < ,001. Whereas the occurrence of the category of loss of self-control is relatively high in proportion (average proportion 47.83%), the rest of the patiency categories are lower in occurrence (failure: 11.30%; disempowerment: 6.67%; loss of status: 3.48%). Using the Sign test as a post hoc test, and correcting for multiple testing with the Holms procedure, we can conclude that the occurrence of loss of self-control is significantly higher than the occurrence of the other three categories, p_H < ,001. The occurrence of failure is significantly higher than the occurrence of loss of status p_H = ,012, the occurrence of disempowerment is placed between failure and loss of status, not significantly differing from either of them, p_H < ,999.

Based on these results we can conclude that loss of self-control played a significant role in contributing to the total amount of patiency. Loss of self-control means that the analysand has attempted and failed in self-mastery, namely in his ability to master, control, or perfect the self. The mentioning of such failings at the session suggests that the analysand may feel inadequate and defeated regarding self-control. In addition, the category with the next greatest proportion for the male analysand is failure, which suggests that he did not succeed in achieving or accomplishing his instrumental goals, or was unsuccessfully taking on responsibilities, which in turn he was unable to fulfil.

Table 8.5 Frequencies and percentages of Patiency and subscales of patiency in the case of the male client

		Total number of texts	Texts containing Patiency		Texts containing Loss of self-control		Texts containing Failure		Texts containing Loss of status		Texts containing Disempowerment	
Block	Session	N	N	%	N	%	N	%	N	%	N	%
1	1	45	32	71,1	31	68,9	12	26,7	7	15,6	6	13,3
	2	40	20	50,0	15	37,5	8	20,0	0	0,0	2	5,0
	3	30	8	26,7	6	20,0	2	6,7	0	0,0	1	3,3
2	1	35	20	57,1	20	57,1	8	22,9	0	0,0	0	0,0
	2	40	33	82,5	33	82,5	4	10,0	3	7,5	3	7,5
3	1	43	18	41,9	17	39,5	0	0,0	1	2,3	4	9,3
	2	61	33	54,1	29	47,5	0	0,0	0	0,0	7	11,5
	3	51	16	31,4	14	27,5	5	9,8	1	2,0	0	0,0

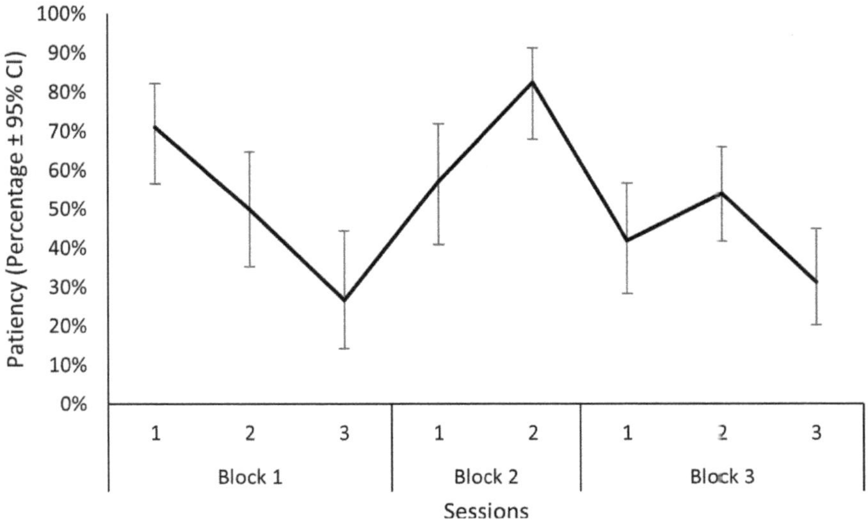

Figure 8.8 Changes in patiency total scores by session and by block in case of the male client

Note: On the figure, we can see the percentage of the appearance of patiency ± Wilson score confidence intervals for a binomial proportion.

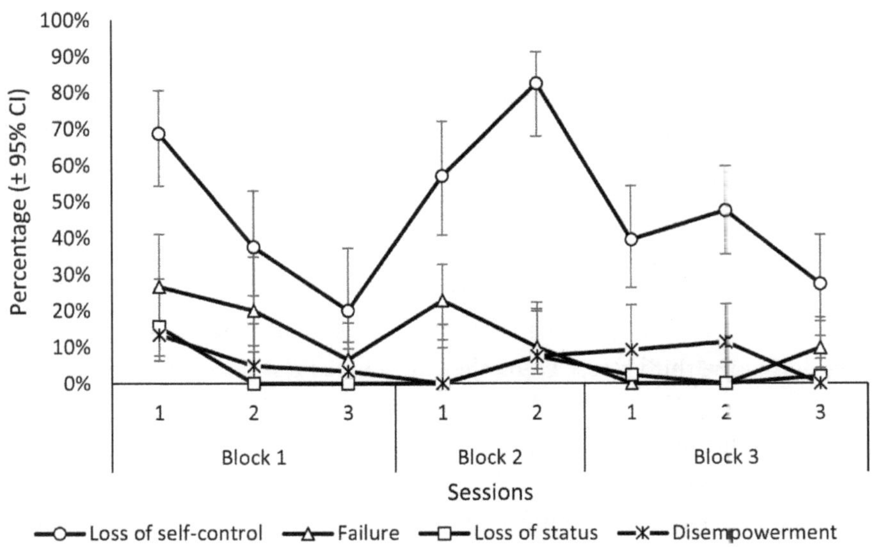

Figure 8.9 Changes in patiency subscales by session and by block in case of the male client

Note: On the figure, we can see the percentage of the appearance of patiency ± Wilson score confidence intervals for a binomial proportion.

The fact that he mentions these failures at the session suggests, again, feelings of inadequacy and defeat.

Since the occurrence of disempowerment and loss of status is below 10%, the differences between sessions cannot be calculated for these variables. The comparison among session blocks can be calculated for the total patiency score, as well as for the loss of self-control and failure variables.

Differences between session blocks

The eight examined sessions were divided into three blocks, since a substantial time passed between these periods (6–10 months). Therefore, we have compared the sessions by blocks. Patiency occurred in the first block in 60 out of the 115 narratives (52.2%), in the second block it occurred in 53 out of 75 narratives (70.7%), and in the third block in 67 out of 155 narratives (43.2%). Using a Chi-squared test for examining differences between the blocks we found that there was a significant difference, $\chi^2(2, N = 345) = 15.25$ $p < .001$ Cramer's V = .21 between the three blocks. The occurrence of patiency in narratives is fluctuating. During the second block there is a significant increase in comparison to the first block: χ^2 (1 190) = 6.41 $p = .011$ $\varphi = .18$. In the third block the occurrence of the patiency total score is significantly lower than during the second block: χ^2 (1, 230) = 15,25 $p <$,001 φ = ,26. There is no significant difference between the first and third blocks χ^2 (1, 270) = 2.12 $p = .145$ φ = ,09. These results confirm what we have discussed earlier with regard to the changes in agency of the female client; namely, our alternative hypothesis—changes in agency and patiency may fluctuate according to the nature of the problems discussed at a given session. In this case, patiency first increases, and then decreases again back to the level where it began.

Looking at the category of loss of self-control, narratives containing this theme occur in 52 out of 155 narratives during the first block (45.2%), in 53 out of 75 narratives (70.7%) during the second block, and in 60 out of 155 narratives during the third block. Using the Chi-squared test the difference between the blocks is significant: $\chi^2(2, N = 345) = 21.16$ $p < .001$ Cramer's V = .25. The pattern of differences here is similar to that of the total patiency score described above: occurrence of the loss of self-control fluctuates between the three blocks. During the second block it significantly increases in comparison to the first block: $\chi^2(1, N = 190) = 11.89$ $p = .001$ $\varphi = .25$. In the third block it is significantly lower than in the second block $\chi^2(1, N = 230)$ = 20,65 $p <$,001 φ = ,30, and there was no significant difference between the first and the third blocks $\chi^2(1, N = 270)$ = 1,15 p = ,283 φ = ,07. The explanation of the fluctuation of loss of self-control contradicts our hypothesis according to which patiency linearly decreases during the observation period. This result, however, again gives support to our alternative hypothesis.

The occurrence of failure is substantially lower than that of loss of self-control in narratives. During the first block it occurs in 22 narratives out of 115 (19.1%). During the second block it occurs in 12 narratives out of 75 (16%), and during the third block it occurs in 5 narratives out of 155 (3.2%). Using a Chi-squared test, the difference between the three blocks is significant: $\chi^2(2, N = 345) = 18.76$ $p < .001$ Cramer's V = ,23. However, there is no significant difference between the first and the second block: $\chi^2(1, N = 190) = 0.30$ $p = .582$ $\varphi = .04$. The third block has a lower occurrence of failure than the first and the second block, $\chi^2(1, N = 270) = 18.56$ $p < .001$ $\varphi = .26$ and $\chi^2(1, N = 230) = 12.05$ $p = .001$ $\varphi = .23$ respectively. So, in the case of failure, our data shows a decrease during the observation period, due to its decrease in the third phase. However, the decrease is not linear, because there is no difference between the first two phases. This, again, supports our alternative hypothesis, according to which failure could fluctuate depending on the issues discussed at the sessions.

Changes in agency and patiency in terms of narrative interaction at the session in the case of the male analysand–male analyst dyad

As can be seen from Figures 8.6 and 8.8, the total score of agency was lowest at session 5, F22 (the second session in the second phase of the observation period) and, at the same time, the total score of patiency was highest at the same session, which suggests that sense of agency and patiency, coded as separate variables independent from each other, may occur in a logically sound, asymmetrical way during a session. So, we decided to observe what happened during this salient session in terms of narrative interaction between analysand and analyst, in terms of the shifting of perspective. During the session the analysand and analyst discuss issues related to the analysand's health and mental health. The analysand was on anti-depressant medication during the time of the session; however, he is uncertain whether he should continue taking that medication or stop. The next topic of discussion is the analysand's story of his hospitalization due to his mental breakdown that happened years ago, before entering analysis. The analysand and the analyst discuss the reasons why the analysand thinks he has ended up in hospital care, what happened during the period he was hospitalized, and how he experienced his treatment in the hospital. The analysand has many complaints regarding his treatment and experiences in hospital, recollecting events that happened, as well as conversations with doctors and psychiatrists. The following four excerpts are chosen from session 5, F22. Some of these excerpts have been analysed previously from a different angle (Berán & Unoka 2016).

In Excerpt 8.4 the analysand discusses his hospital experiences with the analyst. During his stay at the hospital he caught a urinary infection, which was not recognized by the hospital staff until later. This may be considered a characteristic excerpt taken from this session, because it was typical during the session that the analysand recollected his hospital experiences one after the other, and complained about his hospital treatment to the analyst.

Excerpt 8.4 (session 5, F22)

410PAT:	és akkor az orvosomat megkerestem,	and then I have approached my doctor,
411PAT:	és mondtam,	and said,
412PAT:	hogy bocs baj van,	that sorry, there is something wrong,
413PAT:	de most állandóan így hirtelen rámjön,	but now I suddenly feel like,
414PAT:	hogy vécére kell járni állandóan,	that I need to go to the bathroom all the time,
415PAT:	és hogy véreset pisiltem.	and that I have blood in my pee.
416PAT:	**ugyan már, hogy ne képzelődjek, olyan nincs.**	**now, now, that I should not imagine things, there is no such a thing.**
417PAT:	**s akkor győzködhettem,**	**and then I had to persuade him,**
418PAT:	**hogy de van.**	**that there is.**
419PAT:	de olyan nincs.	but there isn't such a thing.
420PAT:	aztán végül aszonta,	then at the end he said,
421PAT:	na jó van,	well it is ok,
422PAT:	itt van egy kis izé,	here is a little thingy,
423PAT:	edény,	a bowl,
424PAT:	na jó, pisiljen bele,	well, its ok, pee in it,
425PAT:	és elküldöm a laborba.	and I send it to the lab.
426PAT:	adott egy kis edényt,	he gave me a little bowl,
427PAT:	belepisiltem,	I have peed in it,
428PAT:	elküldte a laborba,	he has sent it to the lab,
429PAT:	kiderült hogy tele van vérrel.	and it turned out that it was full of blood.

430PAT:	tehát hogy kimutatták a laborban is hogy az van.	thus they have shown that that's what I have in the lab as well.
431TER:	ühüm.	uhm.

In Excerpt 8.4 we can see that the analysand is recounting events in the hospital in a monological form, without interruption by the analyst. In lines 410–30 of the narrative he mainly uses external focalization, describing events, behaviours, and characters from the outside point of view, without discussing mental content (emotions, desires, goals, etc.). External focalization is a non-mentalizing perspective, where the speaker does not get involved either in their own emotional responses or thought processes regarding events, or in the emotional responses or thoughts of other characters of the narrative.

This perspective on the part of the analysand does not allow for the understanding and explaining of mental content, the working-through of emotions and desires, in contrast to internal focalization, which contains references to what is happening inside the narrator's and other characters' heads, and which perspective allows for mentalizing processes. During psychoanalysis, it is one of the main goals to discuss the mental contents of the analysand; therefore, psychoanalysts may try to shift the narrator's perspective—and hence the perspective of the analysand—from external to internal focalization.

Discussing hospital events, it would be useful for the analysand to better understand his own emotions, goals, motivations amid the interpersonal conflicts that he experiences in the hospital and to reflect upon them, especially while describing his conflicts with authority figures such as his doctor, or his painful emotions. However, using the NP of external focalization does not allow for such self-reflection and exploration of conscious and unconscious mental content and thought processes.

The exceptions to the use of external focalization in Excerpt 8.4 are lines 416–18 (printed in bold). Here the analysand shifts into internal focalizing mode spontaneously, without the help of the analyst. however soon he shifts back into external focalization (line 419), without elaborating on this perspective. In lines 416–18 the analysand describes what his doctor said (line 416) to him by quoting both directly and indirectly his words—so, mixing pseudo-diegetic and homo-diegetic perspectives. From line 419 the analysand continues quoting the conversation with the doctor using pseudo-diegesis again. These rapid shifts into internal and external focalization, and mixing of pseudo-diegetic and homo-diegetic perspectives, blur the line between the internal world of the analysand and the external world. In addition, the analysand describes a conflict situation, but in a way that he uses a NP in which he identifies with his doctor, as if he was re-experiencing the situation. This way of recounting the events creates emotional tension in the narration.

The analysis of agency and patiency in the narrative structure of Excerpt 8.4, situated within the broader context of the male analysand–male analyst dyad, reveals key psychoanalytic dynamics related to mentalization, epistemic trust, and intersubjective processes. In particular, the analysand's dominant use of external focalization, his ambivalent shifts into internal focalization, and his unresolved conflicts with authority reflect difficulties in integrating self-agency within his internal world. These elements can be interpreted through the lenses of relational psychoanalysis, intersubjectivity theory, mentalization-based therapy (MBT), and the mutual regulation model (Tronick 2003).

One of the most striking features of the analysand's narrative in Excerpt 8.4 is the predominance of external focalization, in which he recounts the events of his hospitalization as a detached sequence of behaviours and actions, devoid of emotional processing or self-reflection. The absence of internal focalization—where the narrator would engage with the emotional and psychological dimensions of the events—suggests a defence against the affective content of his experience. From the perspective of mentalization theory (Fonagy et al. 2003), this suggests that the analysand has difficulty reflecting upon his own mental states and those of others, particularly in situations of conflict and distress. Mentalization is crucial in psychoanalysis because it allows an individual to move beyond a rigid, action-driven engagement with the world to a reflective stance where emotions, desires, and interpersonal dynamics become accessible to conscious thought.

The lack of mentalization in the analysand's narrative suggests that his experiences in the hospital were not only distressing but remain psychologically unprocessed. The recounting of these events in a monological, emotionally distant manner may serve as a protective mechanism, shielding him from overwhelming affect. However, this mode of narration comes at the cost of emotional integration. As the Boston Change Process Study Group (BCPSG 2010) suggests, psychotherapeutic change is not just about cognitive insight but about the implicit reorganization of self-experience through relational processes. By maintaining an externalized, behaviourally focused narrative, the analysand unconsciously resists the intersubjective work of therapy that would allow him to explore his own feelings, conflicts, and agency in relation to the events.

While the analysand predominantly uses external focalization, there is a brief but significant shift into internal focalization in lines 416–18, where he quotes the doctor's dismissive response to his complaints. This moment of perspective shift is crucial, as it represents an implicit struggle between two modes of experiencing his own past: one in which he is emotionally detached, and one in which he momentarily re-experiences his frustration and helplessness. The analysand's switch between pseudo-diegetic and homo-diegetic perspectives in this moment also reflects a destabilization of narrative coherence, which may correspond to an underlying psychic conflict regarding his own agency in the situation. The quick reversion to external focalization in line 419 suggests that he cannot tolerate remaining in the mentalizing mode for long, instead retreating into a concrete, action-based account of events.

From the perspective of epistemic trust (Fonagy & Allison 2023), this hesitation in remaining in a reflective stance may indicate a fundamental mistrust in the analytic process as a space where his experience can be meaningfully processed. The dismissive attitude of the doctor, whom the analysand had to 'persuade' (417PAT) before his symptoms were taken seriously, mirrors a potential pattern of relational experiences where the analysand's distress was invalidated or minimized. The absence of an empathic and validating other in these past experiences could contribute to his difficulty in trusting the analyst—or the analytic process—as a space where his mental states are taken seriously.

Another notable feature of the analysand's narration is his implicit identification with the doctor's dismissive stance, particularly in the way he repeats the doctor's words without explicitly commenting on how they made him feel. Lines 416 and 419 ('There is no such thing') show an internalized authority voice, echoing the doctor's invalidation of his symptoms. This could indicate a learned pattern of emotional repression, where the analysand unconsciously aligns with the voices that have historically dismissed his distress, rather than asserting his own subjective experience.

Such a pattern is common in individuals who have experienced developmental trauma or attachment disruptions, where the child learns to suppress emotional needs in order to maintain a sense of relational stability with care-givers (Lyons-Ruth et al. 2006).

From a relational psychoanalytic standpoint (Mitchell 2022), this pattern could be seen as a defensive enactment of past relational dynamics, where the analysand unconsciously anticipates that his distress will not be validated by the analyst, just as it was dismissed by authority figures in his past. This can also be linked to Benjamin's (2004) concept of the 'doer and done-to' dynamic, where the analysand may vacillate between feeling like a powerless patient and identifying with those who dismiss him, in an attempt to exert some control over his own narrative.

The analyst's minimal verbal response ('ühüm', 431TER) is notable in Excerpt 8.4. While analytic silence is often used as a technique to allow the analysand to elaborate further, in this case it may inadvertently reinforce the analysand's resistance to engaging with his internal experience. Given the analysand's preference for external focalization and his avoidance of affective exploration, a more active relational intervention (e.g. a question that invites emotional reflection) might have encouraged him to pause and reflect on how he felt about the doctor's response.

From the mutual regulation model (Tronick 2003), emotional development occurs through dyadic interactive repair—that is, through moments when one individual (in this case the analyst) helps to regulate the emotional experience of another by providing an attuned, validating response. If the analysand is unable to mentalize his own emotions, a well-timed intervention from the analyst could serve as a scaffold for reflective processing, helping him transition from an action-oriented to a mentalizing stance.

Excerpt 8.5 is a continuation of Excerpt 8.4, still dealing with the problem of urinary infection during the analysand's hospital stay.

Excerpt 8.5 (session 5, F22)

435PAT:	ja meg meg kitenyésztették hogy izé+...	yeah, then then they developed it that whatever+...
436PAT:	+, ilyen baktérium fertőzés.	+, like a bacterial infection.
437PAT:	és hogy akkor és hogy akkor mm izét adtak végül rá,	and then so and then so mm they gave whatever for that,
438PAT:	antibiotikumot, hogy múljon el.	antibiotics, to get rid of it.
439PAT:	de mondom az első reakció mindenre ez volt,	but I'm telling you, the the first reaction to everything was this,
440PAT:	/olyan nincs.	/no such a thing.
441PAT:	ne beszéljen ilyen hhbutaságokat,	don't talk such hhnonsense,
442PAT:	/ilyen nincs.	/this is impossible.
443TER:	szóval végül nem volt elégedett a gondozással, ellátással?	so at the end weren't you satisfied with your treatment, care-giving?
444PAT:	nem tudom hát+...	I don't know, well+...
445PAT:	biztos jó az az osztály vagy valami,	it is probably a good department or something,
446PAT:	de mondom így emberileg a hozzáállással mindig ez volt.	but I am telling you like at the personal level it was always like this.

447TER:	hmm.	uhm.
448PAT:	tehát ez volt az alapattitüdjük.	so this was their basic attitude.
449%com:	pause 3 s	
450PAT:	de nem csak ilyenekben,	but not only in these kind of matters,
451PAT:	hanem+...	rather+...
452PAT:	+öö mikor bementem,	+erer when I went in,
453PAT:	rögtön# első nap vagy másnap,	immediately# on the first day or the next,

In lines 435–42 the analysand continues the story he began in Excerpt 8.4, about his urinary infection during his hospital stay. He, again, uses external focalization during his narration, and puts the hospital staff in the position of the agent. This perspective again does not allow him to reflect on his own emotions, desires, goals, and other mental content, and represents the narrator as a passive, vulnerable individual, who is, in a way, a victim of the hospital staff. Later the analyst's mentalizing question makes the analysand react with a shift of perspective, as far as he shifts into internal focalization, again, for a brief time-period.

The importance of focusing on external or internal events is conspicuous in Excerpt 8.5. The focus of the analysand's (lines 435–42) attention turns from external descriptions to mental events (lines 444–48). This is due to the analyst's shift of perspective in line 443. In his question the analyst directs the analysand's attention to his emotions, thought processes, opinions, the subjective experiences of the self, and the personal aspect of perceiving outside events. By this, the analyst demonstrates to the analysand that his thoughts and emotions are distinct from outside events, and they are present, and exist independently of those events. The external focalization mode is a non-mentalizing perspective, whereas the internal focalization mode is a mentalizing one. Introspective attention to mental events develops representations of the mind of the self and the other. It helps to develop behaviours like self-control, action planning and emotion-regulation (Fonagy et al. 2002). At the same time, in Excerpt 8.5 the analysand describes hospital staff as agents, and puts himself in the position of the patient. In line 443 the analyst shifts perspective by placing the analysand in the position of the agent. He is the one who can judge and evaluate the quality of the treatment in the hospital. The analysand responds to this by accepting the new perspective offered by the analyst. He uses self-agency in lines 444–46. So, using internal focalization and self-agency both contribute to a mentalizing perspective in the analysand's speech, and help him to take a position in which he is able to view others also as mentalizing agents in lines 446–48, when discussing the hospital staff. By considering them as mental agents, he is also able to better differentiate between their intentions and actions and his own reactions to the situation.

In addition, Excerpt 8.5 provides insights into the interactive processes underlying psychoanalytic change, particularly regarding mentalization, epistemic trust, and the relational co-construction of agency and patiency. The shifts in perspective between external and internal focalization and the analysand's vacillation between patiency and agency illustrate key intersubjective dynamics in the analytic dyad.

The analysand's reliance on external focalization is a hallmark of non-mentalizing discourse (Fonagy et al. 2002). By focusing on observable behaviours rather than internal mental states, the analysand avoids the affective dimension of his experience, which may be too overwhelming or threatening to fully process. From a relational psychoanalytic perspective (Mitchell 2022), this narrative stance may serve as a defensive strategy, helping him maintain a sense of control by organizing events into an objective, linear sequence rather than engaging with their subjective emotional impact. A pivotal moment occurs in line 443, when the analyst directly engages the analysand's subjective experience by asking: 'So at the end, weren't you satisfied with your treatment, care-giving?' This intervention represents a deliberate mentalizing shift, as the analyst:

- moves away from an externalized, action-driven recounting of events and instead invites the analysand to reflect on his own emotions and evaluative stance;
- positions the analysand as an agent, granting him the authority to assess and interpret his own experience;
- encourages self-reflective awareness, reinforcing the idea that his thoughts and emotions exist independently of external events.

From an epistemic trust perspective (Fonagy & Allison 2023), this shift plays a critical role in fostering the analysand's ability to engage with his own mental states. If past relational experiences have undermined his ability to trust his own perceptions and emotions, the analyst's question models a reflective stance, signalling that the analysand's subjective experience is valid and worth exploring.

The analysand's immediate reaction (line 444) is hesitant and uncertain: 'I don't know, well+…', which response suggests an initial resistance to the internal focalization shift. The pause and hesitation indicate that the analysand is not entirely comfortable engaging with his own emotions—a common reaction when epistemic trust was historically compromised.

However, a notable transition follows in lines 445–48, where the analysand begins to internalize the perspective shift:

- He acknowledges the legitimacy of the hospital department ('it is probably a good department'), suggesting an attempt to take a more balanced view.
- He moves from external descriptions to subjective evaluation ('but I am telling you, like at the personal level it was always like this'), marking a shift towards self-reflective awareness.
- He generalizes the hospital staff's behaviour ('so this was their basic attitude'), indicating a broader interpretation of interpersonal dynamics.

These shifts signal that the analysand is beginning to integrate his experience in a more complex way, where he can recognize both the objective aspects of his hospitalization and the subjective, interpersonal dimensions of his distress.

From a mutual regulation perspective (Tronick 2003), this exchange can be seen as a moment of co-regulated affective processing, where the analyst's intervention helps scaffold the analysand's movement from an action-based, externalized account to a more reflective, mentalized stance.

The analysand's shift into internal focalization and self-agency (lines 444–48) represents a crucial therapeutic moment, as he moves from:

- a passive, reactive stance (patiency) → towards a reflective, agentic stance (self-agency);
- viewing the hospital staff as monolithic figures → towards recognizing them as individuals with attitudes and mental states;
- a rigid, victimized self-narrative → towards a more nuanced understanding of the situation.

This progression is vital for mentalization because it allows the analysand to:

- differentiate between external reality and his subjective emotional experience;
- recognize the interplay between his own responses and the behaviours of others;
- begin to regulate his affect by assigning meaning to his distress.

In line 447, the analyst offers a minimal verbal response: 'Hmm'. This non-directive response can be interpreted in two ways: A facilitative stance, allowing the analysand to continue elaborating on his thoughts, or a missed opportunity for deeper engagement, where a more explicit mentalizing intervention might have further reinforced his shift towards self-agency.

Given the analysand's tendency to oscillate between external and internal focalization, a follow-up question aimed at deepening his self-reflection (e.g. 'How did that attitude affect you?') might have further encouraged a sustained mentalizing stance.

Excerpt 8.5 illustrates a pivotal shift in the analysand's capacity to mentalize his own experience, revealing several core dynamics essential to psychoanalytic transformation. First, it highlights the importance of mentalizing interventions in helping individuals move from an externalized, action-oriented, and emotionally detached stance to a more reflective and integrated sense of self. These interventions create space for the analysand to begin accessing inner states—his own and others'—thereby fostering emotional differentiation and psychological depth.

Equally significant is the role of self-agency within narrative discourse. As the analysand begins to engage with his experiences using first-person, internally focused language, he shifts from a position of patiency—of being acted upon—to one of agency. This shift is essential in the development of a coherent and resilient sense of self, particularly in the context of past relational injuries that may have undermined his autonomy and self-efficacy.

However, therapeutic change is not linear. Moments of hesitation, confusion, or resistance—such as the analysand's retreat from elaborating internal focalization—are not signs of failure, but indicators of epistemic transition. These are points at which the analysand is testing the safety and reliability of the analytic relationship, and gauging whether his own subjective experience will be received and validated. In these moments, epistemic trust is fragile, and must be carefully scaffolded by the analyst.

The analysand's brief engagement with internal focalization in the session signals real progress, yet it also underscores the tentative nature of reflective awareness in individuals whose early relational experiences may not have supported the development of stable mentalizing capacities. Continued analytic work is therefore necessary—not simply to deepen insight, but to reinforce the analysand's emerging sense of agency and trust in his own mental states.

This dynamic process can be further understood through Ed Tronick's mutual regulation model (2003), which posits that interactive regulation and self-organization are inextricably linked. Change in the analytic setting arises not solely from the dyadic interaction but from the reciprocal shaping of the analysand's internal rhythms and responses by the analyst's attunement, and vice versa. As

Tronick emphasizes, our self-rhythms—how we emotionally organize and regulate ourselves—are influenced by our partner's responses, making these processes partially dyadic, yet simultaneously governed by internal self-contingency.

Indeed, self-organizing processes may exert an even more powerful influence than interactive ones (Beebe & Lachman 2020). Within the analytic encounter, this means that, while the analyst plays a critical role in co-regulating affect and supporting reflective functioning, the analysand's own internal rhythms—his habitual modes of self-relating, his narrative habits, and the emotional logic of his psychic life—are actively shaping the therapeutic moment. The analytic process unfolds, therefore, in a mutual intertwining of self- and intersubjective regulation, with each influencing and transforming the other over time.

In sum, therapeutic change is not merely something that happens to the analysand through interpretation or insight—it is something that emerges through the complex, recursive interplay between self-regulation and relational experience. Recognizing this dialectic allows for a deeper understanding of why agency and patiency may fluctuate within treatment and why these fluctuations are not obstacles but integral parts of the psychoanalytic process of transformation.

Excerpt 8.6 is from a later point at the session. The analysand and the analyst are still discussing the hospital treatment, mainly the behaviour of the staff, which is criticized by the analysand.

Excerpt 8.6 (session 5, F22)

704PAT:	szal mindig megpróbáltak valamit belemagyarázni az emberbe ami ami nem igaz.	so they have always tried to construe something into one which which was not true.
705PAT:	én meg mondtam hogy-...	and I said that-...
706PAT:	hogy de nem úgy van!	that but it's not true!
707TER:	ühm.	uhm.
708PAT:	és és győzködtem őket,	and and I kept persuading them,
709PAT:	dehát asz asz őket nem érdekelte.	but they did not care about that.
710PAT:	mer hát ők jobban tudják.	because, well, they know better.
711TER:	ühüm.	uhm.
712TER:	tehát itt is az az élmény érte hogy hogy vádolják valami[vel-.]	so your experience here also has been that you were being blamed for some[thing.]
713PAT:	[velük] állandóan ilyenem volt–,	[with them] I permanently had this–,

714TER:	hogy [hibáztatják,]	that they were [blaming you,]
715PAT:	[velük velük] állandóan ilyenem [volt,]	[with them with them] I permanently had [this kind,]
716TER:	[nade nem csak] velük volt ilyenje.	[well, but you did not only] with them have this kind.
717PAT:	anyámmal is ilyen volt.	I had this kind with my mother also.
718PAT:	mindig.	always.
719PAT:	de de de ezekkel az orvoskkal ott ott ez ment állandóan.	but but but with these doctors there there this was on constantly.
720PAT:	nem tudom a többi beteggel mi+/	I don't know what with the other patients+/
721PAT:	mondjuk a többi beteggel is voltak ilyenek.	I guess such things happened with the other patients too.

In Excerpt 8.6 the analyst draws the analysand's attention to a new aspect of his complaints about the hospital staff. The analysand's hospital experiences reminded the analyst of the analysand's childhood experiences or his way of relating to his mother. In terms of shifts in perspective, the analyst offers a radically new point of view to the analysand, from which he could compare his previous experiences in two different stories—or memories—about himself; in other words, he could compare his two previous (narrative) selves: the childhood one, and the one in the hospital.

In lines 704–10 the analysand continues his complaints about the hospital staff, because, as he claims, they repeatedly tried to construe something about him that he did not feel fitting or true. The analyst answers only with listening cues (uhm), but in line 712 he shifts into internal focalization when talking about the analysand, putting him in the patient's position: 'your experience here also has been that you were being blamed for something'. By adding 'also' the analyst gives a hint to the analysand that his experience with the hospital staff was a repetition of earlier experiences, or similar to earlier ones. In his reply, interrupting the analyst, the analysand emphasizes that he is not recounting other experiences but the ones with the hospital staff. In line 716 the analyst uses the narrator level, as the analysand has done before, and repeats the analysand's use of wording in the expression 'I had this kind'—which expression refers to the quality of the analysand's experiences using language in an unconventional way: 'well, but you did not only with them have this kind'. In his interpretation the therapist reminds the client for the second time that his experiences with the hospital staff are a repetition of previous, similar experiences. By using the narrator level he offers a perspective to the analysand in which he can see, and compare, two similar experiences. The analysand accepts the position offered by the analyst and reacts in line 717 by admitting that he had this kind of (experience) with his mother. In line 718 he adds emphasis to his statement by confirming: 'always'. At this point it would be possible for the analysand to talk about his childhood experiences with his mother, or to explicitly compare the experiences with the hospital staff to his earlier experiences at the narrator level. The insight that he repeats the interaction patterns he used to have with his mother is made possible for the analysand by directly comparing the two experiences, and elaborating on this perspective. Elaboration would also explicate the reasons why such experiences with the mother were so fundamental for the analysand. Instead of elaborating this perspective, however, the analysand returns to the discussion of the behaviour of the hospital staff, and the analyst does not interrupt this turn of the narrative.

In Excerpt 8.7 the analysand continues to try to convince the analyst about his experiences in the hospital, about how the hospital staff treated him badly. In the excerpt the analysand and analyst succeed in clarifying a misunderstanding between them regarding a trust issue: the analysand's thinking that the analyst does not believe what he says about his hospital experiences.

Excerpt 8.7 (session 5, F22)

828PAT:	hát mondom, konkrét példákat el tudok mondani.	well I am telling you I can give concrete examples.
829TER:	ühmm.	uhm.
830PAT:	hogy hogy zajlottak, amikor ilyenek voltak.	how how these happened, when there were this kind of things.
831TER:	ühm.	uhm.
832%com:	pause 19 s	
833TER:	hmm most mire gondol?	what are you thinking about now?
834PAT:	hát most erre,	well about this,
835PAT:	hogy ezt még hogy mondjam el, hogy ez ilyen volt.	how else I could tell you, what this was like.
836PAT:	meg hát+...	and well+...
837TER:	[föl fölmerül magában+.]	[does it occur occur to you+...]
838PAT:	[most ez attól] hogy ez hasonlít attól+//	[now just] because this is similar to it it does not+//

839TER:	+, hogy én nem hi hiszem el amit mondott?	+, that I do not be believe what you have said?
840PAT:	hát igen,	well yes,
841PAT:	minthogyha azo az+,	as if that that+,
842PAT:	az merül fel bennem,	that occurs to me,
843PAT:	hogy ez maga most itt,	that this you now here,
844PAT:	tehát ahogy itt maga utalgatni próbál,	well that you are trying to imply,
845TER:	aha.	uhm.
846PAT:	hogy ez nekem arra,	that this for me to that,
847PAT:	minthogyha arra akarna rávezetni,	as if you were trying to lead me to that,
848PAT:	hogy tulajdon képen ez nem is így történt meg,	that as a matter of fact this did not happen like this,
849PAT:	csak én az anyám analógiája kapcsán ezt ezt úgymond+...	only as related to the analogy of my mother this this so to speak+...
850PAT:	rájuk is rájuk húztam,	I pull on them them also,
851PAT:	ezt a ruhát.	this dress.
852TER:	ühm.	uhm.
853TER:	értem.	I see.
854TER:	nem, énbennem kiváncsiság van, hogy akkor mi lehet ez.	No, there is curiosity in me about what this could be.

In lines 828 and 830 the analysand continues recounting his hospital experiences using external focalization, and the analyst reacts in using minimal responses (ühm). In line 832 there is a long silence, after which the analyst starts talking by shifting into internal focalization, and the here and now of the therapeutic session: 'What are you thinking about now?' The analysand replies, discussing his mental content dilemma, shifting also into internal focalization mode. The analyst asks a question in lines 837–39, which has to do with an important issue: the trust between him and his patient: 'Does it occur to you that I do not believe what you have said?'

The analysand's reply indicates that this is indeed the case. In lines 841–51 the analysand explains what he thinks of the analyst's intentions, why he brought up the analogy of his childhood experiences with his mother. He uses the level of the therapeutic here and now, and present tense, internal focalization, which perspective is suitable to discuss current interpersonal experiences with the analyst. From lines 846–51 the analysand describes his worries regarding the analyst's intensions, namely that the analyst is trying to suggest that the hospital experiences described by the analysand are not his true experiences, but merely his projections, based on his previous experiences with his mother. It is worth mentioning that there seems to be a concurrence here: the analysand is recounting his hospital experiences where he was misunderstood and misconstrued by the hospital staff and, at the same time, when he is telling this narrative to the analyst, he experiences that the analyst misconstrues or misunderstands him. There is a parallel here when emotions represented by the analysand's narrative infiltrate into the therapeutic relationship, resulting in a crisis of trust between analysand and analyst.

We also must note that this belief on the part of the analysand may also contribute to his inability or lack of willingness to elaborate on childhood experiences in Excerpt 8.6. In other words, the analysand resists working with the problem of being misconstrued in his childhood by his mother, while the same experience surfaces at the therapeutic session towards the analyst.

The analyst's first reaction to the situation is an expression of understanding in line 853. He uses the same perspective as the analysand: the therapeutic here and now, present tense, and homo diegesis to express his own involvement in this situation. His expression of understanding contradicts the analysand's story of being misconstrued; however, in addition, in line 854 the analyst also explicitly denies the analysand's hypothesis of what he is trying to imply. Instead he clearly states what he feels in connection to the analysand's hospital story. Not much later in the session (not quoted here) the analyst explains to the analysand what he meant and why he brought up the parallel between the hospital experiences and his childhood experiences with his mother. He repeatedly states that he does not doubt the validity of the hospital experiences that the analysand has been discussing. The analysand's reaction to the analyst's explanation is an expression of acceptance of the analyst's idea of a possible influence of childhood experience on his emotional reaction in the hospital but, following this acceptance, he returns to the discussion of the hospital staff again. Therefore, in conclusion, we can say that he overall puts up a resistance in the analysis, by thwarting the analyst's attempts to talk about his childhood experiences with his mother.

Based on our analysis of session F22, we can say that the topics discussed at the session, such as the hospital treatment and related events regarding therapeutic alliance, may have both contributed to the analysand's lower levels of expressed agency, and higher levels of patiency. Our detailed qualitative analysis of one of the main threads of discussion at the session can reveal why and how this might have occurred. Namely, in the analysand's experiences at the hospital he felt ineffective in communicating with the staff, and therefore felt vulnerable and helpless, despite trying to stand up for himself. It is important to note, however, that during the session the analyst's goal of increasing the analysand's agency by placing him in the agent's position, and developing his mentalization skills by fostering internal focalization, was conspicuous.

Excerpt 8.7 represents a turning point in the therapeutic process, as the analysand's persistent complaints about the hospital staff begin to reveal deeper relational patterns from his past. What starts as an externally directed complaint about mistreatment transforms into an instance of transference, where the analysand begins to feel that the analyst—just like the hospital staff and, more broadly, his mother—fails to understand him.

These excerpts highlight fundamental psychoanalytic dynamics, including the interplay between agency and passivity in personal narratives; the role of mentalization in distinguishing past from present experiences; the development of transference and the emergence of epistemic mistrust; as well as the significance of narrative breakdown and repair in the analytic process.

In lines 837–51, the analysand expresses a deep concern: He misinterprets the analyst's intervention as an attempt to discredit his hospital experience ('as if you were trying to lead me to that this did not actually happen like this'.). His language suggests a projection of past relational traumas, particularly his experiences of being misunderstood by authority figures (hospital staff, his mother). The metaphor 'I pull this dress onto them also' (line 850) is a powerful expression of his fear that he unconsciously distorts reality based on past experiences—a realization that is itself unsettling. At this moment, the analysand perceives the analyst not as a neutral observer but as yet another figure who dismisses and misconstrues his reality, reinforcing the transference dynamic. The analyst's clarification in line 854 ('No, there is curiosity in me about what this could be') serves as an attempt to repair the rupture, signalling that his intent is to understand, not to discredit.

These excerpts illustrate the analysand's struggle with integrating past and present relational experiences. He initially resists connecting his hospital experiences to earlier relational patterns but briefly acknowledges the connection. However, when this connection is made too explicit, he perceives it as a challenge to the legitimacy of his personal narrative.

They also underscore the role of transference in shaping the analytic relationship. The analysand projects past experiences of mistrust onto the analyst, experiencing him as invalidating or manipulative. This dynamic highlights the importance of epistemic trust: The analysand oscillates between moments of self-reflection and defensive reassertion of his original narrative, revealing a fragile capacity for mentalization (Fonagy & Allison 2023).

Finally, these moments emphasize the necessity of narrative repair in psychoanalytic work. The analysand's misinterpretation of the analyst's intervention threatens the therapeutic alliance. The analyst's response in line 854 aims to rebuild trust and encourage continued reflection.

These excerpts mark a critical juncture in the analysis, where unresolved relational wounds resurface in the analytic space. The analysand's pattern of feeling misunderstood and misconstrued by authority figures is re-enacted in the therapeutic relationship, creating a moment of transference crisis. While he briefly acknowledges the connection between his past and present experiences, this insight remains fragile and emotionally charged. Moving forward, the analyst's task will be to reinforce epistemic trust while helping the analysand differentiate between genuine external mistreatment and unconscious projections shaping his perceptions. Ultimately, greater narrative coherence and self-agency will emerge when the analysand can hold both perspectives simultaneously—recognizing his past wounds without feeling that his present experiences are being invalidated.

Conclusion: agency and patiency changes during long-term psychoanalytic treatment

In summary, we may say that, contrary to our expectation, using a quantitative analysis of agency and patiency revealed that in the case of both our analysands there has not been a significant linear increase in agency and decrease in patiency during the observation period of psychoanalytic treatment. These results contradict previous studies, but they are coherent in themselves. Instead of a linear increase in agency and decrease in patiency, there was a fluctuation in the level of agency and patiency as a function of time—as we stated in our alternative hypothesis—and in some time periods agency decreased while patiency increased during the course of the observation period. Our qualitative analysis of the topics discussed at crucial sessions has shown that the nature of the problems discussed at the sessions, as well as changes affecting therapeutic alliance, may have influenced expression of agency and patiency at the sessions.

The findings of our study demonstrate that agency and patiency fluctuate over time rather than following a predictable trajectory of increasing agency and decreasing patiency. This pattern aligns with contemporary theories of relational psychoanalysis (Mitchell 2022), intersubjectivity theory (Stolorow et al. 2002), epistemic trust and mentalization theory (Fonagy & Allison 2023), Ed Tronick's mutual regulation model (2003), and the Boston Change Process Study Group's (BCPSG 2005, 2010) conceptualization of therapeutic change as an emergent, dynamic process.

Rather than viewing psychoanalytic progress as a linear increase in agency and decrease in patiency, the observed fluctuations suggest that shifts in agency and patiency are co-regulated within the therapeutic dyad. Tronick's mutual regulation model emphasizes that affect and self-states are not developed in isolation but are continuously shaped and reorganized through relational interactions. These interactions include mismatches and repair processes, where temporary disruptions in agency (e.g. feelings of subjugation) may actually serve as moments of deep therapeutic engagement, provided that these disruptions are recognized and worked through within the analytic relationship.

For instance, the analysands' recurrent experiences of patiency during certain phases of treatment may indicate not a regression but a necessary moment of relational and affective reworking. Rather than reflecting a failure to develop agency, these moments could represent a phase in which the analysand re-experiences a past relational dynamic within the analytic space, allowing for the possibility of its mentalization and transformation. Our analyses of mutual regulation of perspective shifts during the analyst–analysand interaction consider the subtle, discursive, micro-regulatory, and social-emotional processes that unfold in analysand–analyst interactions. Our aim with this is to show how the analysand's self-organizing capacities are scaffolded in the analysand–analyst's dyadic regulatory system and, by their co-creativity, lead to a more complex agency experience in the interpersonal space, and agentic mentalization (Fonagy 2015).

From a relational psychoanalytic perspective (Mitchell 2022), agency is not merely an individual trait but an intersubjectively negotiated experience in the process of 'at-one-ment', that is the interaction between the activated multiple self-states of the analyst and analysand (Atlas & Aron 2017). The absence of a linear increase in agency suggests that psychoanalytic change does not occur through an isolated, internal reorganization of self-experience but rather through repeated intersubjective engagements in which the analyst's perspective helps shape and scaffold the analysand's evolving self-narrative. This process aligns with the Boston Change Process Study Group's (BCPSG 2005, 2010) model of therapeutic change, which argues that implicit relational knowing—the way individuals unconsciously organize relationships—undergoes transformation not through explicit insight alone but through ongoing relational experiences that are 'felt' before they can be fully articulated. This learning from interpersonal experience gives a new meaning to Freud's concept of after-education (Nacherziehung), as discussed by Fonagy and Allison (2023).

In some sessions, the analysand's experience of patiency might be heightened, not as a sign of failure but as a necessary step in the working-through process, where previously unconscious patterns of helplessness or submission in relationships become activated in the analytic space. These moments may then be followed by an increase in agency, as the analysand internalizes a new relational pattern—one in which agency is recognized and validated rather than dismissed or overwhelmed by past relational scripts. This cyclical pattern of activation and integration helps explain the fluctuation of agency and patiency rather than a steady, linear change.

A key finding in our study was the importance of perspective shifts, both in the analysands' own narratives and in the analyst's interventions. In many of the key sections analysed, analysands initially adopted an external focalization mode, recounting their experiences in a detached, factual manner without engaging with their own emotions. These non-mentalizing moments often coincided with increased patiency, where the analysand positioned himself as a passive victim of external circumstances (e.g. hospital staff, parental figures, authority figures), whereras the analyst's interventions were often aimed at shifting perspective:

- encouraging internal focalization (e.g. moving from an externalized narrative to an exploration of how the experience felt);
- using relational interpretations (e.g. linking present difficulties with past relational patterns);
- reframing patiency into agency (e.g. helping the analysand recognize choices, interpretations, and reactions as part of an active process rather than a predetermined script).

These shifts in narrative stance often coincided with subsequent increases in agency, suggesting that the ability to change one's self-narrative in response to new relational input is central to psychoanalytic change. The findings in this study support a nonlinear, dialectical model of change, rather than a simple accumulation of agency over time. Change occurs through:

- moments of increased patiency: when past relational patterns become reactivated in the analytic space;
- therapeutic interventions and relational repairs: where these past patterns are recognized, validated, and restructured within the analytic relationship;
- subsequent increases in agency: as the analysand internalizes a new relational script, where self-expression and autonomy feel safe and supported rather than threatening or invalidated.

This oscillation between agency and patiency is not a sign of resistance or stagnation but a necessary part of the therapeutic process, reflecting the way individuals integrate new relational experiences. The findings in this study align with Ed Tronick's mutual regulation model, relational psychoanalysis, intersubjectivity theory, mentalization-based therapy, and the Boston Change Process Study Group's research on implicit relational knowing. We can conclude that, rather than being an isolated cognitive shift, the development of agency in psychoanalysis is a relationally co-constructed process, emerging not in a linear process but through moments of rupture, repair, and reorganization.

9 Working in the here and now of the therapeutic session

In this chapter we will focus on the use of one specific perspective, namely the here and now of the therapeutic session. This perspective—as we have discussed in detail in Chapter 3—is associated with the discourse-level aspect of our NP model. The discourse level—which is also close to what is referred to as speaker roles (Koven 2012)—focuses on the identifications enacted in narrative discourse, and its associations with different modes of remembering. The three levels of discourse we distinguished are 1) the narrator level, 2) the character level and 3) the level of the here and now of the therapeutic session. The here-and-now level of the therapeutic session is defined as interchanges between analysand and analyst that are focusing on events, emotions, affective states, etc. that occur in the actual reality and real time of the therapeutic session. Although much of analytic work focuses on past events, looking for causes of current problems in earlier—typically childhood—traumas, working with current events and emotions may also be the choice of the analyst or the analysand. Such work in psychoanalytic psychotherapy may focus on emotional or affective states, anxieties, transference or countertransference issues, and so on, in the here and now of the session. In this chapter, first we will discuss briefly some psychoanalytic views on the here and now, and then relate this to our own narrative model of the discourse-level aspect of narrative perspective (NP). Following this, in the bulk of this chapter we will discuss here-and-now work based on examples of excerpts from the Budapest Psychotherapy Database, and show how the use of this perspective contributes to the psychotherapy process.

Psychoanalytic view of the here and now

There has been much debate during the past century in psychoanalytic literature on the function, importance, or even the definition of the therapeutic work in the here and now of the session (Blass 2011; Busch 2011; Joseph 2013). Blass (2011) distinguishes four approaches to the here and now within the psychoanalytic literature: 1) cathartic, 2) interpersonal, 3) experiential, 4) Kleinian (mainly represented by Betty Joseph).

Cathartic. The earliest proponents of the concept of the here and now according to Blass (2011) were Ferenczi and Rank, who, in their early writings in *The Development of Psychoanalysis* (1925, quoted by Blass 2011) used the expression 'immediacy' to refer to therapeutic work that was focused on reproduction of early (traumatic) events at the session, rather than interpreting them as the 'there-and-then' events.

Interpersonal. Focuses on the interpersonal relationship between analysand and analyst, what the analysand experiences and understands of the transference now—as it is manifested at the session. Blass criticizes this approach, because it lacks depth: 'unconscious determinants' and the analysand's history as a causal factor play a less important role in such interpretations. The proponents of the interpersonal view, according to Blass are Gill (1983, quoted by Blass 2011), and ego-psychologists such as Kernberg (1968, quoted by Blass 2011).

Experiential. What is crucial in this approach is the focus on the immediately available subjective experience of the analysand, and the way they feel at a given moment of the session. Interpretations, therefore, should not go beyond this level (Blass 2011). Moreover, the interpretation of transference—according to this view of the here and now—is not prioritized over other, perhaps more urgent problems of the analysand.

Klenian. According to Joseph, using the here and now expression means:

> 'here' refers primarily to what is going on between the two participants in the room, but in addition, it conveys the immediate, often concrete, reality of the individual's experience ... The *now*, when we speak of *here and now*, implies a sense of time, not just past and future, but an awareness of the patient's situation at the moment, one that is dynamic, never static, and that changes from moment to moment. The analyst is in a position to witness the movement and thus to gauge the forces operating in the patient. (Joseph 2013: 2)

From this quotation it becomes clear that Joseph—and the other psychoanalytic authors referred to—defined here and now based on the analyst's view of how the analysand might feel, and how the analyst understands their patient through transference and countertransference. In contrast, the here-and-now perspective we use in our discourse analysis is based on objective verbal information that appears in the 'text'—transcript—of the session. We are not dealing here with the psychoanalytic conceptual arsenal to interpret what is going on at the session. Rather, we use our discourse-based definition of NP to define units in the text that are identified as references to the here and now. The 'text' that we analyse from a linguistic point of view may still be structured and organized by unconscious motivations, desires, and intentions; however, we analyse the point of view of the analyst and the analysand as individuals considered as participating in an interaction. Our starting points are the system of two persons being watched over by a third person, in contrast to the analyst's position, who is participating in the system of two individuals and at the same time observing and interpreting the system itself, as well as the analysand, as an individual. We can also claim, at the same time, that there is some interconnection of the use of here and now in the way we use it in our discourse analysis, with the psychoanalytic notion, namely its reference. In other words, the reference to what is actually happening at the session, in terms of the emotions and thoughts of the participants (also regarding alliance) that is voiced by them in the present; and hence it is observable by a third party, or in the psychoanalytic case by the analyst.

The concept of the here and now in relational psychoanalysis, as well as in the frameworks of the Boston Change Process Study Group (BCPSG 2010), Ed Tronick's mutual regulation model (2003), mentalization-based therapy, and epistemic trust theory (Fonagy et al. 2015; Fonagy & Allison 2023) emphasizes the therapeutic encounter as a dynamic, co-constructed process. Rather than focusing solely on past events, these models view the present relational moment between analyst and analysand as the primary site of change. In this intersubjective space, affective states are co-regulated (Tronick 2003), implicit relational knowing is reshaped (BCPSG 2010), and reflective functioning is scaffolded (mentalization theory). Epistemic trust is fostered when the analysand feels recognized and emotionally understood in the here and now, enabling the integration of new relational experiences and supporting lasting therapeutic transformation.

The significance of working in the here and now of the session was shown to be important by psychoanalysts describing their own work, as well as by analysts of other therapeutic orientations (Kivlighan 2014, Yalom & Leszcz 2005). According to Kivlighan, for example, here-and-now work in individual and group psychotherapies helps working with relationships within the therapy, as opposed to relationships outside the therapeutic setting; such work enhances the therapeutic relationship and fosters the analysand's problem-solving.

Examples of working in the here and now from the Budapest Psychotherapy Database

In this chapter we will discuss excerpts with the male analysand–male analyst dyad as well as with the female analysand–female analyst dyad, both of them from the third phase of the observation period, during the working phase of therapy. We chose these excerpts using a theoretical sampling method, which means choosing sessions and excerpts where discussions in the here and now take an important or central role. Using these examples, we would also like to illustrate how shifting among the three levels of the discourse-level aspect of NP can have various functions, and be fruitful during psychoanalytic work.

Excerpt 9.1 is from the psychotherapy of the male analysand–male analyst dyad. It is the continuation of a situation discussed in Chapter 6 (Excerpt 6.8), when the analysand has brought chairs to her mother as a present on Mother's Day. The mother's reaction was a positive one; she liked the chairs, and was grateful to her son. However, in the further discussion of the mother's reaction, the analysand argues that his mother acted much more kindly to him in an otherwise conflictual relationship, because others were present. In fact, when he visited her mother on Mother's Day, his sister, and his nephew (T.) were also present. Therefore—he argues—the occasion should not be interpreted as an improvement in their communication.

Excerpt 9.1 (F32)

1103PAT:	éppen amikor vittem ott voltak,	exactly when I brought them they were there,
1104PAT:	és letettem a cuccot,	and I put the stuff down,
1105PAT:	és akkor már a T-val jöttünk el, hogy+…	and we were leaving already with T., so+…
1106TER:	aha.	uhm.
1107PAT:	+, mer ők éppen indulóban voltak.	+, because they were about to leave.
1108%com:	pause	
1109TER:	**értem.**	**I see.**
1110TER:	**tehát akkor ne örüljek neki,**	**so I should not be glad,**
1111TER:	**hogy pozitív kommunikáció történt.**	**that it was a positive communication.**
1112PAT:	**nem, mer erre mondom,**	**no, because I say to this,**
1113PAT:	hogy ilyen máskor is volt,	that similar thing has happened already before,
1114TER:	**hogyha+//**	**if+//**
1115PAT:	**ha érti mire gondolok?**	**if you know what I mean?**
1116PAT:	**remélem hogy miről beszélek?**	**I hope, what I am talking about?**
1117TER:	**persze.**	**sure.**

1118PAT:	hogyha mások is ott vannak,	if other people are also there,
1119PAT:	meg máskor is amit mondtam magának,	in other occasions as I have told you,
1120PAT:	meg van hogy úgy másoknak előadja,	there are situations when she performs to others,
1121PAT:	hogy jaj hogy ő hogy kitenné a lelkét a fiáért,	that oh my god, how she would give her soul for her son,
1122PAT:	jaj, nem is tudja hogy hogy segíthesssen,	oh, she does not even know how she could help,
1123PAT:	meg mi,	and so on,
1124PAT:	érti?	**do you understand?**

In lines 1103–07 the analysand describes the circumstances of his visit to his mother on Mother's Day. He just arrived, gave his present to her mother, and left swiftly with his nephew and sister. He uses the character level, first person, homo-diegesis to describe this episode. In lines 1109–11 the analyst intervenes and shifts his perspective to the here-and-now level. He summarizes the situation based on his own feelings, in the first-person singular: 'I should not be glad'. The first person is a relatively rarely used perspective on the part of the analyst (in the actual session his use of the first person is about 17% in comparison to the second and third person). The analyst also sparsely expresses his own emotions so openly, giving a strong feedback to the analysand. In this case, he is asking for confirmation from the analysand about how the situation should be interpreted according to him. In line 1112 the analysand also shifts to the discourse level of the here and now, followed by the narrator level, and then again in 1115–16 back to the here and now, the use of which level is also repeated in line 1117 by the analyst.

The use of the here-and-now level here first by the analyst, then by the analysand, signals an important turning point in the analysand's story, and a clarification of the evaluation of what exactly has happened, what emotions the analyst should experience while listening to the recounted events. This is followed by the analysand's asking for confirmation that the analyst has understood him correctly, since, based on his question, the analysand has doubts.

In the excerpt we witness a key example of how here-and-now interventions, understood within the frameworks of relational psychoanalysis (Atlas & Aron 2017), intersubjectivity theory, and the Boston Change Process Study Group (2010), can create opportunities for therapeutic clarification and meaning-making. By entering the discourse from a subjective, emotionally present position, the analyst positions himself not only as a listener but as a relational participant in the dialogue. His comment, 'so I should not be glad', is not a neutral interpretation but an implicit emotional inquiry, inviting the analysand to co-construct the emotional meaning of the event.

This shift marks a transition into the here-and-now level of discourse, emphasizing the immediacy of shared experience in the therapeutic space. Drawing on Tronick's mutual regulation model (2003), this moment can be seen as part of a dyadic regulation process, where the analyst's emotional self-disclosure opens the door for affective attunement and repair. The analysand responds by echoing this shift—moving from recounting past events to addressing the analyst directly and requesting understanding (lines 1115–16, 1124). This reflects an emergent need for epistemic trust: the analysand offers a narrative and tests whether the analyst truly grasps its emotional significance. From a mentalization-based perspective, this exchange supports the analysand's reflective functioning, as it enables him to consider not only his mother's behaviour but how it is received, interpreted, and understood in the analytic relationship (Fonagy 2015). These perspective shifts—from the narrative level to the here and now—illustrate how affective meaning and relational clarity are co-constructed moment by moment, aligning with the BCPSG's emphasis on implicit relational knowing and the transformative potential of intersubjective moments.

The discussion is then continued by the analysand using the narrator level in lines 1118–23. He describes his mother's behaviour very vividly, at times using pseudo-diegesis—lines 1121–23—and then again asking for the analyst's confirmation using the level of the here and now in line 1124. Shifting to the level of the here and now in this excerpt was employed in the function of clarifying meanings, expressing emotions on the part of the analyst, and asking for the analyst's confirmation on the part of the analysand.

Excerpt 9.2 is a continuation of the discussion in Excerpt 9.1 with the same dyad. The analysand continues to complain about his mother, because she treats him badly if other people are not present.

Excerpt 9.2 (F32)

1125PAT:	miközben meg ha velem beszéli ugyanezt akkor meg+...	whereas if she talks about the same thing with me+...
1126PAT:	micsoda?	what?
1127PAT:	méghogy én neked?	should I, for you?
1128PAT:	ér+/	you k+/
1129PAT:	emlékszik ilyenekre,	you remember things like that,

1130PAT:	nem?	don't you?
1131PAT:	hogy beszéltük.	that we discussed.
1132TER:	igen.	yes.

In lines 1125–27 the analysand states that, when his mother discusses the same issue with him in private, she behaves unkindly, in fact in lines 1126–27 he shifts from his previous homo-diegesis, narrator level (line 1125) into pseudo-diegesis, character level, identifying with the mother's voice, and expressing her humiliating and aggressive tone. In lines 1129–31 the analysand shifts into the level of the here and now, in order to relate to the analyst in the present. Once again, he is asking for his confirmation, that he remembers such situations, because they have already discussed them in previous occasions. In line 1132 the analyst confirms that he recalls such previous mentions of the issue. So, in this case the shifting into the level of the here and now on the part of the analysand serves the function of asking for confirmation from the analyst, and on the part of the analyst it serves the function of complying with the request.

In the excerpt the analysand's shift into pseudo-diegesis is emotionally charged and suggests a deep internalization of her invalidating stance. Drawing on relational psychoanalysis and intersubjectivity theory (Atlas & Aron 2017), this moment can be seen as an enactment of a traumatic interpersonal pattern—where the self is not only diminished by the other but also adopts the other's voice in a self-directed, critical mode. That enactment of the mother's voice is consistent with what the Boston Change Process Study Group refers to as 'implicit relational knowing'—the procedural, non-verbalized knowledge of self-in-relation that emerges spontaneously in the therapeutic dialogue.

What is particularly striking here is the analysand's immediate return to the here-and-now level (lines 1129–31), asking the analyst to confirm that this experience was previously discussed. This move reveals a need for epistemic validation—a hallmark of the process of restoring epistemic trust. From the perspective of mentalization-based theory, the analysand is seeking reassurance that his subjective reality is being recognized and remembered. The analyst's brief but attuned affirmation (lines 1132) supports this process, functioning as a moment of co-regulation (Fonagy 2015; Tronick 2003). This exchange underscores how the here-and-now function of discourse can become an emotionally significant vehicle for repairing relational ruptures, supporting reflective functioning, and enabling the analysand to safely mentalize difficult interpersonal content. In this way, the analytic process moves beyond interpretation, working instead through the fine-grained affective calibration of presence, recognition, and memory—what the BCPSG describes as the 'micro-processes' of therapeutic change.

These two examples demonstrate that shifting into the here and now serves both analysand and analyst by 1) securing confirmation of understanding and 2) enabling the listening to and discussion of emotions. However, looking at more complex situations and longer processes during a given session, we can see how shifting in and out of the three levels of the discourse-level aspect of NP can be fruitful in terms of the psychoanalytic work during the session. We would like to illustrate this by a series of excerpts from the psychotherapy of the female analysand–female analyst dyad. In this example, the whole session is dedicated to discussing the problem of thesis-writing, which is a major issue for the analysand at the time of the session. More specifically, they discuss various sub-questions related to this greater issue. The topic of the analysand's thesis is the sociological analysis of the life history of Holocaust survivors, based on interview data. The analysand is confused about how to start analysing the interviews and, in general, she feels stuck about getting started with her project.

Excerpt 9.3 (L31)

105 %com:	pause 3s	
106PAT:	hát hogy azon gondolkodom,	well, what I am thinking about now,
107PAT:	hogy +...	is that +...
108PAT:	hogy most minden történetet,	that now all the stories,
109PAT:	tehát minden interjúalany történetét összefoglaljam-e egy pár sorba.	well that whether I should summarize the biography of each interviewee in a few lines.
110PAT:	tehát ilyen maximum ilyen öt hat sorba.	well, like five-six lines maximum.
111TER:	hányan vannak?	how many are they?
112PAT:	tizenöten.	fifteen.
113PAT:	khmm khmm.	khm khm.
114%com:	pause 4s	
115PAT:	ne nem tudom.	I don don't know.
116PAT:	most van aki azt mondta hogy kell,	now there are people who said that it was necessary,
117PAT:	van aki azt mondta hogy nem kell,	and there were those who said it was not,
118TER:	maga szerint?	what do you think?
119PAT:	őszintén?	honestly?
120PAT:	fogalmam sincs.	I have no idea.

121PAT:	de én már olyan döntéseket se tudok meghozni hogy éhes vagyok e vagy se?	but I cannot even decide whether I am hungry or not?
122PAT:	tehát így+...	well, it's like+...
123PAT:	nem tudom.	I do not know.
124TER:	hát ö+...	well ö+...
125TER:	lehet belőle baj,	can it become a problem,
126TER:	ha leírja,	if you write about it,
127TER:	vagy ha nem írja le?	or if you do not write about it?

In Excerpt 9.3, we can observe the use of the different levels of the discourse-level aspect of NP. In lines 106–10 the analysand uses the here-and-now level and present tense to discuss her problems with thesis-writing, whether she should summarize the life stories of each interviewee. The analyst in line 111 also uses the present tense, but asks a question about a piece of general information ('How many are they?'), at the narrator level, to which the analysand replies at the same level in line 112. Following this exchange, the analysand hems and keeps a longer silence suggesting her undecidedness, which she expresses also verbally in lines 115–17. She describes the opinion of others, placing them in the agent position, in the past tense, narrator level. The analyst shifts perspective in line 118, putting the analysand into the position of the agent, using the level of the here and now: 'What do you think?'. With this shift the analyst offers the opportunity for the analysand to express her own opinion instead of the opinion of others, and opens the space for the analysand to air her feelings about her situation in the here and now. So, we may observe that the analyst is trying to help Clara in dealing with her difficulties in the present, discussing the practical aspects of her problems, as opposed to asking for her associations, dreams or looking for the root of the problem in her childhood traumas. The analysand in lines 119–23 expresses her feelings in the here and now, present tense, self-agency, thus repeating or mirroring the analyst's previously used perspective. Although she expresses her feelings, and opinion (or the lack of it) as an agent, regarding the content of her utterance she expresses her indecision and hesitation. In lines 124–27 the analyst shifts perspective again, to the character level, future tense (line 125), and once again her intervention focuses on the practical aspect of the analysand's problem.

The analyst's use of different levels of the here and now in this excerpt suggests that she alternates the narrator, character and the here-and-now levels, while using each level in different functions. By offering the here-and-now position to the analysand Clara is able to focus on her current emotions regarding the problematic situation. By the analyst focusing on the character level, she is able to offer the analysand a point of view, where she is able to anticipate as well as consider the outcomes, and the consequences of her choices. Furthermore, by using the narrator level, the analyst and the analysand are able to consider the situation from a more distant point of view.

Excerpt 9.4 (Berán & Unoka 2018) is another discussion of the same topic, initiated by the analyst a few minutes later in the session.

Excerpt 9.4 (L31)

148TER:	mondja,	tell me,
149TER:	szeretné leírni?	would you like to write about it?
150TER:	azt úgy érzi hogy öö informatív?	do you feel that it is erer informative?
151TER:	vagy maga magának fontos?	or is it important for yo you?
152TER:	hogy szerepeljenek ezek a személyek a rövid élettörténetükkel együtt?	that these people should be included together with their short biographies?
153PAT:	nem.	no.
154PAT:	nem.	no.
155PAT:	nem fontos.	it's not important.
156TER:	akkor hogyan merült föl hogy leírná?	then how did it come to your mind to write about it?
157PAT:	papa mondta.	papa has told me.
158TER:	aha.	I see.
159TER:	de maga nem ért egyet?	but do you disagree?
160TER:	de bizonytalan.	but you are uncertain.
161TER:	hogy vajon a+//	that whether the+//
162PAT:	akár egyet is érthetek.	I could even agree.
163PAT:	dehát hogy így+...	but it's like, well+...
164PAT:	ne nem tudom.	I don don't know.
165PAT:	hogy ez most+...	that this is now+...
166PAT:	kell,	necessary,
167PAT:	vagy nem kell,	or unnecessary,

The analyst in lines 148–49 again uses the here-and-now level, present tense, to address the analysand, and to ask her feelings about including the short biographies of participants. In lines 150–52 she shifts into the narrator level, and asks the analysand about her feelings in general, in a straightforward manner. The analysand replies in lines 153–55, using the same perspective (narrator level), indicating in a very succinct way that it is not important for her to include the short biographies. The analyst continues to ask the analysand while trying to understand why including the biographies became such a dilemma for her (line 156), while shifting to the past tense, character level. In the analysand's answer in line 157, the analysand is again uses the perspective (past tense, character level) offered by the analyst. However, the analysand's giving here very brief answers while the analyst continues asking her questions suggests that there is something more going on here, untold by the analysand. The analyst continues from lines 159–61 asking questions about the analysand's general attitude, shifting again into the narrator level, present tense. The analysand, although she interrupts the analyst, answers this question, using the same perspective the analyst used before: the narrator level, present tense (lines 162–67).

In Excerpt 9.4 we saw that the analysand was unable to verbalize her feelings and attitudes towards the problem of thesis-writing, more specifically whether or not she should include short biographies of the participants. The analyst's strategy to deal with this situation was focusing on the present problem: asking questions from various perspectives, and shifting into various levels of the discourse-level aspect of NP. This latter strategy proves to be useful here. For example, using the character-level perspective the analyst is able to focus on the concrete reasons of why the analysand wanted to include short biographies in the first place. This turned out to be the idea of the analysand's father. The analysand, as we may understand from other intertextual contexts of this conversation (i.e. transcripts of other sessions), has an ambivalent relationship with her father. Her parents are divorced, and she is living with her mother and her mother's partner at the time of the psychoanalysis. The use of the narrator level allows the analysand and analyst to clarify the analysand's position form a more general perspective.

Excerpt 9.5 (Berán & Unoka 2018) is a continuation of this conversation:

Excerpt 9.5 (L31)

168TER:	de,	but,
169TER:	hát álljunk meg!	well, let's stop (here)
170TER:	ezek szerint a papa azt ajánlotta, papa hogy ez legyen benne.	then according to this has suggested that this should be included.
171TER:	származhat e bármi baj abból ha benne van?	can it cause any problem if it is included?
172PAT:	nem.	no.
173TER:	nem.	no.
174TER:	legfeljebb az olvasó azt mondja,	perhaps the reader says,

175TER:	hogy na én ezt most nem olvasom tovább.	that well, I am not going to continue reading this.
176TER:	de bajnak nem baj.	but it is not a problem.
177TER:	nem?	isn't it?
178PAT:	de.	yes.
179TER:	jobb jobb ha valami benne van.	it is better better if something is included.
180TER:	mintha hiányozna.	than if it would be missing.
181TER:	persze nem kell bő lére ereszteni,	of course it does not need to be spinned out,
182TER:	meg nem kell hogy minden benne legyen.	it does not need to include everything.

In lines 168–69 the analyst shifts her perspective to the discourse level of the here and now, using the homo-diegetic perspective, first person, plural subject. With her utterance, she interrupts the analysand's story. Despite this, however, the fact that she uses a homo-diegetic perspective signals that she includes herself as an agentic participant of events, and thus emphasizes her presence, and attention towards what the analysand is saying at the moment, and also towards its significance. This becomes even more clear in line 170, when the analyst returns to the analysands story in hetero-diegesis, character level, repeating the analysand's earlier statement in a modified form: 'papa has suggested that this should be included'. By repeating the analysand's statement, she emphasizes the importance of the father's role in the analysand's dilemma. However, in line 171 the analyst, shifting into the narrator level, third-person subject, continues her argument about including the short biographies of participants in the form of a question, as opposed to drawing the analysand's attention to her problematic relationship with her father, and taking up that line of discussion. The analyst's choice suggests she repeatedly and persistently steers the conversation towards solving the problem at the session, instead of free-associating, expanding the discussion, and approaching the analysand's problem from a more traditional psychoanalytical point of view.

In line 172 the analysand answers the analyst's question by stating that there would not be a problem if she included the short biographies and, by this, she takes on the analyst's point of view. In line 173 the analyst repeats the analysand's answer, emphasizing the point made by her. The analyst shifts perspective in lines 174–75, approaching the question from the point of view of the future reader, and expressing their potential response by using pseudo-diegesis, character level, identifying with the future reader's position, but also demonstrating their potential reaction to the analysand. In line 176 the analyst shifts to the narrator level and, in this position, she repeatedly states that it would not cause any problems if the analysand included the short biographies. In line 177 she turns to the analysand for confirmation, which she gives in line 178, by accepting the analyst's point of view. In lines 179–82 the analyst continues to argue why it would be better to include the short biographies, and advises the analysand how to include them while shifting into the narrator level.

In summary, we can say that in Excerpt 11.5 the analyst is trying to help the analysand to arrive at a decision on the question of including short biographies in her thesis. She focuses her frequent interventions on dealing with problems in the present. As for the use of NPs, she shifts between various levels of the discourse-level aspect, using the here and now in the function of helping the analysand to focus on her problems, and the narrator's position to approach the problem practically. In order to succeed, the analyst must help the analysand to shift perspective several times. She achieves this in a step-by-step manner, asking for the analysand's opinion or agreement at each turning point of her argument. The analyst's strategy can be explained by her underlying goal to help the analysand to focus on the practical aspect of her problem, as opposed to being overwhelmed by her anxious feelings underlying her writing process.

The series of excerpts from the female analysand–female analyst dyad illustrate how therapeutic progress may occur through a sustained, step-by-step engagement with current life difficulties, rather than a return to childhood or unconscious fantasy. The analysand's paralysis around the question of whether to include biographical summaries in her thesis serves as the central dilemma across Excerpts 11.3–11.5. Rather than interpreting this indecision as simple resistance, the analyst works within the here and now to explore the practical and emotional dimensions of the problem, using strategic shifts across the narrator level, character level, and the present moment to support the analysand's reflective process. As Ed Tronick's mutual regulation model (Tronick 2003) suggests, self-organization and interactive regulation co-determine therapeutic outcomes. The analyst alternates between guiding, containing, and prompting Clara's agency, creating a rhythm of inquiry and confirmation that enables Clara to mentalize her impasse.

In Excerpt 9.5, the analyst explicitly brings herself into the interaction ('Let's stop!') using first-person, homo-diegetic discourse, signalling heightened presence and commitment. She then recontextualizes Clara's narrative by revoicing the father's suggestion, highlighting an unconscious transference element without interpreting it directly. Importantly, the analyst avoids expanding into associations or psychogenetic explanations. Instead, she foregrounds decision-making and consequently helps Clara to see her dilemma through multiple lenses: from her own ambivalence, her father's influence, and potential reader reception. These shifts in narrative position—from concrete detail to reflective evaluation—are not random but relationally and affectively timed interventions aimed at building Clara's sense of agency and reducing her overwhelming uncertainty. From a mentalization-based perspective (Fonagy 2015), the analyst scaffolds Clara's ability to hold multiple perspectives in mind simultaneously—a capacity that had temporarily collapsed under stress.

Excerpt 9.6 is from a later point of the same session (Berán & Unoka 2018). The analyst continues the discussion of short biographies of interviewees, this time bringing up the problem related to summarizing the participants' lives in a short paragraph.

Excerpt 9.6

373%com:	pause 2s	
374TER:	most hirtelen az jutott eszembe,	now it suddenly occurred to me,
375TER:	hogy ö+…	that er+…
376TER:	ebből a sorsból khm mit lehet összefoglalni öt mondatban?	how can you summarize this fate in five sentences?
377PAT:	hát ez egy jó kérdés!	well that is a good question!
378TER:	mit írna?	what would you write?
379PAT:	nem tudom.	I don't know.
380TER:	mit írna ezekben az öt mondatokban?	what would you write in these five sentences?
381PAT:	fogalmam sincsen.	I have no idea.
382PAT:	nem tudom!	I don't know!
383PAT:	nem igazán+/	not really+/
384PAT:	nem tudom megírni az öt mondatokat,	I cannot write those five sentences,
385PAT:	hogy úgy nem tudom.	that like I don't know.
386TER:	akkor ez a baj?	then is this the problem?
387TER:	hogy öt mondatba nem tudja összefoglalni?	that you cannot summarize it in five sentences?
388TER:	úgy érzi?	is this how you feel?
389%com:	pause 2s	
390PAT:	hát ez is.	well, this also.
391PAT:	mer nem+/	because I don+/

392PAT:	én nem hiszem,	I don't believe,
393PAT:	hogy valakinek az életét össze lehet foglalni öt mondatba.	that someone's life could be summed up in five sentences.

In Excerpt 9.6 from lines 374–76 the analyst returns to the question of the biographies, using the here-and-now level perspective, first-person subject, and past and present tenses. The analysand responds in line 377 using the same perspective (i.e. the level of the here and now). By both interlocutors using the here-and-now perspective they express feelings and thoughts that occur to them spontaneously at the session, focusing still on the practical aspect of the analysand's problem. In line 378 the analyst shifts into the character-level perspective, placing the analysand in the position of the agent, using the second-person subject, and the future tense, while asking a question. The use of the character level and agency here is an invitation for the analysand to imagine what she could write in a hypothetical situation. In line 379 the analysand answers while shifting again to the here-and-now level, thus not engaging in the perspective offered to her by the analyst in line 378. Shifting into the character level would have meant that she was able to anticipate or to imagine what she would write. Despite this, however, she places herself in the position of the agent in this utterance, thus emphasizing her own ability to act, be effective and responsible—although denying it at the content level ('I do not know'). This point is perhaps more conspicuous if we compare it with the analysand's previously relying on opinions of others in Excerpt 9.3, or on her father's opinion in Excerpt 9.4. Here she takes on the responsibility of summarizing the biographies in five sentences.

In line 380 the analyst repeats the same question, using the same perspective she used before. The analysand also repeats her answer using identical perspective in lines 381–82. These repetitions suggest that the interlocutors are firmly committed to their own points of view. The analyst tries to encourage the analysand to think about her problem in a hypothetical situation, while the analysand resists this by refusing to imagine what she would write. Clara continues in lines 383–85 in the present tense, first person, homo-diegesis, at the level of the here and now—suggesting that she would be unable to summarize the short biographies. The analyst accepts her feelings, and interprets the situation in lines 386–88 in the form of questions, shifting into the present tense, therapeutic here and now perspective in line 389, a perspective that the analysand used before. So, here the analyst accommodates the analysand's perspective, while putting the analysand in the position of the agent, and using internal focalization in line 388: 'Is this how you feel?' In line 390 the analysand answers the analyst's previous question ('Is this the problem?'), shifting into the narrator level, and explains her problem from the position of the agent, first-person subject, present tense in lines 391–93 in more detail.

Summarizing our analysis of Excerpt 9.6, we can say that we observed a gradual shifting of perspectives, both in the case of the analysand and the analyst, which lead to a deeper understanding of the analysand's problem with the thesis-writing, and helping to arrive at a turning point of the session in one of its major themes. The analyst returns to this problem several times during the session; she seems to be committed to help the analysand to solve the writer's block she has regarding her thesis in the here and now of the session. The analysand resists the analyst's attempts, but finally shifts into the perspective the analyst offers her, and explains her main difficulty more precisely and exactly (perhaps even realizing this for the first time)—which is a step forward in solving her problem. This is a turning point at the session because, following the analysand's verbalization of her problem, they discuss the various characteristics of life stories in the interviewees, and suggest different ways of summarizing them. These suggestions come from both the analysand and the analyst. This discussion takes up much of the time of the session.

In Excerpt 9.6, we observe a pivotal moment in the analytic work with the female analysand, where the therapeutic conversation, grounded in the here and now, deepens the analysand's understanding of her writer's block. Drawing on Ed Tronick's mutual regulation model (2003), the analyst and analysand engage in a fine-tuned interactional process, in which shifting among discourse levels—particularly between the character level and the here and now—is employed to navigate Clara's difficulty articulating and acting on her academic task. The analyst introduces a problem in the present tense, first-person perspective (line 374), inviting Clara into the immediacy of the session and prompting a shared space of reflection. Clara's adoption of first-person agency marks a subtle yet significant shift: unlike earlier excerpts where she deferred to others' views, here she takes ownership of her difficulty, signalling growing epistemic trust and the analyst's successful scaffolding of a more agentic self-position (Fonagy & Allison 2023).

This interaction reflects the dynamic interplay between interactive and self-organizing processes, a hallmark of relational psychoanalytic theory and the Boston Change Process Study Group's emphasis on implicit relational knowing (2010). The analyst gradually accommodates Clara's resistance, matching her perspective and emotional tone (lines 386–88), which facilitates a safe environment for reflective mentalization. Clara eventually moves from a diffuse and affectively loaded 'I can't write' position to a more nuanced and integrated stance:

she recognizes that the act of compressing an entire life into five sentences feels ethically and emotionally constraining (lines 391–93). This realization marks a turning point in the session. It is not merely an intellectual insight but a felt shift in how Clara relates to the task. Through recursive perspective-taking, the analyst helps Clara to verbalize the unspoken moral conflict underlying her writer's block, bridging her felt experience and the narrative demand of her thesis work. This exchange reflects a successful instance of therapeutic movement from emotional dysregulation towards reflective functioning, enabled by the analytic dyad's shared navigation of narrative perspectives and emotional meaning.

Excerpt 9.7 is an example of a discussion of how to summarize life stories. The analyst suggests that the analysand should summarize the life stories of Holocaust survivals and their descendants based on some common theme of their Holocaust-related trauma. The analysand immediately comes up with an example of transgenerational trauma that repeatedly occurred in one survival family.

Excerpt 9.7

443TER:	hát, akkor talán azt kellene kiemelni,	well then, perhaps what you should stress,
444TER:	hogy a szülők milyen traumát szenvedtek el?	that what kind of trauma the parents suffered from?
445TER:	melyik szülő hogyan,	which parent how,
446TER:	milyen módon,	in what way,
447TER:	khm.	uhm.
448PAT:	hát igen.	well, yes.
449TER:	aztán +…	then+…
450TER:	hogy egy ff+…	that a ss+…
451TER:	a gyereküк+//	their child+//
452PAT:	egy van.	there is one.
453PAT:	egy nagyon érdekes van például.	one very interesting. for example.
454PAT:	most így,	now like,
455PAT:	amit így fel+/	which like re+/
456PAT:	amit most így kapásból fel	which I can like relate here off the bat. tudok fűzni ennek a mentén.
457PAT:	hogy ö+…	that er+…
458PAT:	hogy van egy+…	that there is one+…
459PAT:	tehát én,	well I,

460PAT:	én a legfiatalabbik generációval	I have talked to the youngest generation, beszéltem,
461PAT:	tehát az ő szempotjából.	well, from their point of view.
462TER:	az az melyik korosztály?	that that which generation is that?
463PAT:	az én korosztályom.	my generation.
464TER:	aha khm khm.	yeah hm hm.
465PAT:	olyan 27 éves.	about the age of 27.
466TER:	ühm.	uhm.
467PAT:	és az ő ##,	and his ##,
468PAT:	az ő anyukája,	his mother,
469PAT:	már a háború után született,	she was born after the war,
470PAT:	és ö +...	and she+...
471PAT:	és két éves koráig nem is ismerte az anyukáját.	and until the age of two she did not even know her mother.
472PAT:	tehát a nagymamát.	well, the grandmother.
473PAT:	és a+...	and the+...
474PAT:	na jó ezt most így bonyolult	well, now this is difficult to explain elmagyarázni,
475PAT:	tehát a+...	well, the+...
476PAT:	ő tan a dédnagymamam nevelte.	she was taken care of by the great- grandmother
477PAT:	és aztán+/	and then+/
478PAT:	két éves koráig,	until the age of two,
479PAT:	és aztán két éves korába előkerült a nagymama,	and then when she was two years old the grandmother turned up
480PAT:	tehát az anyuka,	well the mother,
481PAT:	és ö+...	and she+...
482PAT:	ő végül is ő nevelte fel,	at the end she brought her up

In lines 443–51 the analyst begins to advise the analysand on how she should summarize the life stories of interviewees. She uses an impersonal general subject, narrator level, and hetero-diegesis, starting in the present tense then shifting into the past tense from line 444. The analysand agrees with the analyst's idea in line 448, and then interrupts her in line 452, because she starts recounting a concrete example that came into her mind. She uses the present tense in lines 452–56, and she shifts into the here-and-now perspective to indicate her thinking process. In lines 457–61 the analysand begins to describe her work with one particular survivor family using the narrator level, past tense. The analyst takes the floor in line 462, asking a question related to the analysand's story, also using the narrator level. The analysand then continues in lines 467–82 to describe the traumatized family, uninterrupted by the analyst, using the narrator level, past tense, hetero-diegesis. The story continues even after Excerpt 9.7 ends, and it describes how the trauma of the disappearance of the grandmother was repeated in the succeeding (third) generation of the survivor family.

It is important to note here that, in contrast to previous excerpts from this session, the analysand becomes very active while discussing the survivor family in detail and at length, while staying in the same perspective for an extended time period. In contrast, the analyst, who was very active previously, is now silently listening to the analysand, and only encourages her to talk by giving minimal responses and listening cues. So, it seems that, at this part of the session, the analysand is less anxious, and able to focus more on her problem, while her perspective—the narrator level, past tense, hetero diegesis—suggests she is able to keep a distant view on her subject matter, allowing for reflecting on her problem.

After the analysand has finished her narrative about the survivor family, she draws a conclusion about how to organize the biographies in Excerpt 9.8.

Excerpt 9.8

529PAT:	tehát hogy ezt+…	well that this+…
530PAT:	ezt így fel tudom fűzni ennek a mentén.	I can relate this along these lines.
531PAT:	jó nyilván sok más szempontból is fel lehet fűzni ez a történeteket,	well obviously these stories could be related from several different aspects,
532TER:	ühm.	uhm.
533TER:	tehát hogy a+…	well that the+…
534TER:	az az látszik ebből a történetből,	that that is clear from this story,
535TER:	hogy a trauma megismétlődött.	that the trauma was repeated.
536PAT:	igen.	yes.
537TER:	generációkon keresztül.	across generations.
538PAT:	igen.	yes.
539TER:	és ez úgy tűnik hogy jellegzetes az összes többi történetben is?	and does this seem typical in all the other stories as well?
540PAT:	hát az eltűnés mint motívum az igen.	well the disappearance motif does.
541TER:	ühm.	uhm.

In Excerpt 9.8 from lines 529–30 the analysand uses the here-and-now level, first-person subject, present tense to summarize her thought process regarding the story of the Holocaust survivor family, and relate herself to their story. In line 531 she shifts perspective, and talks in general terms—using the narrator level, hetero-diegesis, present tense—about the possibility of different approaches to summarizing the biographies. In lines 532–37 the analyst takes the floor and also draws her own conclusions from the analysand's Holocaust survival story, using the narrator level, present and past tenses, hetero-diegesis, third person—so keeping her distance from the survivor narrative. The analysand expresses her agreement with the analyst's conclusion in lines 536 and 538. Then in line 539 the analyst again tries to further the analysand's thinking about the problem of summarizing the narratives, asking a question about whether cross-generational trauma is typical in all the survivor stories—using the same perspective as before. The analysand replies, using the perspective offered by the analyst. This excerpt illustrates how both the analyst and the analysand contribute to solving the analysand's problem of summarizing the biographies of survivors. So, after going into the details of one survival family's story, mainly told by the analysand, the analyst becomes active again in this excerpt, and both interlocutors contribute to drawing conclusions from the given story, and generalizing that conclusion to other survival stories. The here-and-now level of the session is being used by the analysand to indicate her thought process, whereas the narrator level is used in the function of reasoning about survivor stories in general, looking at events from a distance.

In the final excerpt from this session, Excerpt 9.9, the analyst suggests another method for summarizing survivor stories:

Excerpt 9.9

551TER:	de lehet szerintem másképp is megközelíteni.	it is possible to approach this in a different manner in my opinion.
552TER:	hogy mindegyik történetből a +/	that from all the stories the+/
553TER:	vagy minden történetet egyedileg szemlél,	or to look at each story individually,
554TER:	és annak a lényegét írja le,	and to summarize its essence,
555TER:	vagy a különlegességét,	or its specificity,
556TER:	vagy a legfőbb sajátosságát.	or its major characteristics.
557PAT:	ühm.	uhm.
558TER:	és akkor+…	and then+…

559TER:	hmm akkor talán nem annyira koncepciózus,	hm then perhaps it is not as conceptual,
560TER:	vagy van+/	or there is+/
561TER:	pontosabban nem annyira tendenciózus a leírás,	to be more precise, the description is not as tendentious,
562TER:	viszont+...	however+...
563TER:	viszont lehet az.	however, it could be that.
564TER:	mert lehet hogy minden történet ugyanolyan lesz,	because it is possible that all stories come out the same,
565TER:	ennek ellenére.	despite this.
566PAT:	hú ez jó ötlet.	wow, this is a great idea.
567TER:	nem tudom.	I don't know.
568PAT:	ez jó ötlet.	this is a great idea.
569PAT:	erre még nem gondoltam,	I haven't thought about that,
570PAT:	hogy külön külön kezeljem őket.	to treat them each individually.
571PAT:	csak annyira össze akartam csoportosítani az egészet.	I just really wanted to group them together.
572TER:	igen.	yes.
573PAT:	mer mindegyik más.	because they are all different.
574PAT:	egyébként meg.	otherwise.
575TER:	hát persze.	well, of course.
576%com:	pause 5s	

In line 551 the analyst shifts into a new perspective: the narrator level, general subject, homo-diegesis, present tense, internal focalization. The use of these perspectives suggests that the analyst speaks in general terms; however, she uses a mentalizing expression ('in my opinion') describing her thinking about the analysand's problem. In lines 552–56 she suggests a new approach to the analysand for summarizing the biographies, addressing the analysand in the second person, but staying at the narrator level. Using this perspective, she directly talks to the analysand, to which the analysand reacts in line 557, with a listening clue, which may signal the analysand's agreement with what the analyst is saying. The analyst stays at the narrator level, present tense, but at the same time shifts into the third person in lines 558–65, discussing the new way of summarizing biographies. In line 566 the analysand speaks for the first time since the analyst started discussing the new way of summarizing biographies, shifting into the here-and-now level of the therapeutic session, but staying in the present tense, third person, internal focalization, mirroring the analyst's previous perspective. She expresses her opinion, using an interjection, which signals her enthusiasm for the analyst's idea, and places 'idea' in the agent's position. In line 567 the analyst expresses uncertainty about her own idea, shifting into the first-person subject, homodiegesis, internal focalization, and also shifting into the here and now of the session, as the analysand did before. Despite the uncertainty of the analyst, the analysand repeats her previous statement in line 568, using the same perspective as before, while stating that the analyst's idea is a good one. In lines 569–71 the analysand shifts into the past tense, first-person subject, narrator level, placing herself in the position of the agent, describing her now previous attitude towards summarizing the biographies, and the difference between her previous way of thinking, and the new method suggested by the analyst. So, the analyst's idea helps the analysand towards a new insight and, hence, towards a turning point in dealing with her problem of summarizing biographies, and of thesis-writing. In line 572 the analyst expresses her agreement with the analysand, and the analysand continues in lines 573–74, shifting into the third person, present tense, and staying at the narrator level, and placing the biographies in the position of the agent. In line 575 the analyst expresses her agreement repeatedly. The analyst's contribution is followed by a longer pause, which suggests the discussion of this topic came to a conclusion. During the rest of the session, neither interlocutor brings up the question of biographies again. We might assume that closing the discussion on summarizing biographies may have reduced the analysand's anxiety regarding her thesis-writing, at least temporarily. Since the analyst did not bring up the problem again at the session, we may assume that she found the solution suggested by her and accepted by the analysand for summarizing biographies satisfactory.

As the session unfolds in Excerpts 9.7–9.9, we observe Clara moving from a paralyzed stance to an increasingly coherent narrative engagement with her subject matter. After voicing the ethical unease of summarizing Holocaust survivors' life stories in Excerpt 9.6, she becomes able, in Excerpt 9.7, to generate a detailed narrative from one interview. This shift demonstrates a movement from fragmented emotional responses to organized autobiographical reasoning, paralleling what the BCPSG (2010) describes as the transformation of procedural to narrative knowing. Clara's extended and uninterrupted storytelling, grounded in narrator-level, hetero-diegetic, past-tense discourse, shows her capacity to take a reflective, composed stance on the interview content. Notably, the analyst becomes more silent here, using only minimal responses—demonstrating trust in Clara's narrative competence. This marks a key moment of analytic containment, where the analyst's earlier scaffolding gives way to the analysand's independent elaboration. From a mentalization-based perspective, Clara is now capable of holding multiple generational perspectives in mind, reflecting on intergenerational trauma without becoming overwhelmed.

In Excerpt 9.8, Clara takes a further step by summarizing her insight in the here and now, indicating that the story can be 'related along these lines' (line 530). This moment of conceptual consolidation is a powerful demonstration of epistemic mastery—Clara is now not only narrating but interpreting her material. The analyst joins this integrative moment in Excerpt 9.9, proposing another structuring principle for the biographical summaries. Her intervention—offered at the narrator level, with internal focalization and addressed in a general but personally attuned way—invites Clara to evaluate a new narrative framework. Clara's enthusiastic reaction ('this is a great idea') marks an affective shift, one of excitement and mastery replacing confusion and anxiety. The oscillation between narrator-level generalization and here-and-now affective engagement in these final excerpts reflects the therapeutic function of co-constructed meaning-making, whereby both analysand and analyst collaboratively arrive at new narrative forms that integrate affect, ethics, and structure.

Together, these excerpts offer a vivid demonstration of how perspective shifting, relational attunement, and narrative co-construction function as core mechanisms of change in psychoanalysis. Through recursive exchanges grounded in the here and now and balanced with narrative distance, the analytic dyad transforms confusion and emotional obstruction into insight and generative action—an outcome made possible by the continuous interplay of mutual regulation, mentalization, and epistemic trust.

This sequence of excerpts from the session illustrate how focusing work on the here and now of the session may be carried out in the case of a very specific problem causing anxiety in the analysand. Instead of using free association, or analysing the early childhood roots of the analysand's anxiety, the analyst helps the analysand to focus on one important aspect of her problem—the summarizing of biographies being one aspect of the problem of writer's block. So, by helping the analysand to think about the specific problem, and suggesting various solutions, engaging the analysand to do the same, and start her own thinking process about the given question, the analyst helps to reduce the analysand's anxiety by focusing on her problem.

The analyst's solution here is rather unusual in psychoanalytic psychotherapy. Looking at the practical consequences of the analyst's choice, we can see that she is very active at the session—perhaps unusually so. She brings up the problem repeatedly, asks questions related to it, finds potential solutions and brings up ideas and arguments in support of certain solutions. Finally, the analysand also becomes active, and decides on one of the solutions suggested by the analyst. For this, it was necessary for the analyst actively and frequently to use different perspectives of the discourse-level aspect of NP. The level of the here and now made it possible for the analysand to express her emotions, feelings, and actual thought processes. the character level—although rarely used here—allowed her to engage in concrete episodic details. and the narrator level made it possible to think about events in a more distant and general way. Another important perspective change was shifts in agency. The analyst's placing the analysand into the agent's position, and the analysand's shift into self-agency emphasized the analysand's role as an active shaper of events, her efficacy, and taking responsibility for outcomes.

It is also important to note that by these series of shifts in the speakers' perspective the problem could be seen in a different light at the end of the given part of in-session dialogue. At the beginning, the analysand had trouble deciding whether or not she should write about the biographies of the interviewees at all; at the end she has arrived at the question of how to summarize them, and found a solution to that question. The analyst, who offered various perspectives to the analysand, fostered the gradual changes in the analysand's perspective. So, the change in the analysand's perspective took place through the process of coordination of perspectives between her and the analyst.

The analysis of the female analysand–female analyst dyad highlights how working within the here and now can become a powerful therapeutic tool, particularly in cases where anxiety is connected to a specific, present-day problem rather than to unconscious material from early development. Drawing from the frameworks of relational psychoanalysis (Atlas & Aron 2017), mentalization-based therapy (Fonagy et al. 2015; Fonagy & Allison 2023) and Tronick's mutual regulation model (2003), our analysis has shown how shifting among narrator, character, and here-and-now levels of NP enables a flexible and finely attuned response to the analysand's evolving needs. The analyst's active engagement, including repeated returns to the problem, offering practical solutions, and coordinating discourse levels with the analysand, created a space of co-regulated exploration where anxiety could be reduced not by interpretation alone, but by collaborative meaning-making and emotional clarification. In this shared narrative field, the analyst supported the analysand's growing epistemic trust and self-agency, not only by inviting her to articulate her current emotional state but also by guiding her to experiment with new cognitive and emotional perspectives.

Most importantly, the case illustrates how perspective coordination between the analyst and analysand can lead to significant therapeutic shifts. As shown through the progressive elaboration across the excerpts, the analysand moved from being overwhelmed by indecision to adopting an active, agentic stance, ultimately arriving at a workable and emotionally satisfying solution. This transformation was not driven by insight into early relational trauma, but by the analyst's strategic and sustained use of discourse-level positioning, enabling the analysand to differentiate her own thoughts and feelings from those of others, reflect on them in real time, and reorganize her relation to the present problem. The movement between the levels of narrative stance—particularly the grounded use of here-and-now utterances for clarifying affect, seeking confirmation, and formulating decisions—demonstrates how psychoanalytic progress can occur through co-constructed relational and cognitive operations. In this way, the analyst does not interpret from above but collaborates from within, helping the analysand to become the author of her own experience through a process that is dialogic, emotionally attuned, and structured by narrative positioning.

Conclusion

The nine excerpts in this chapter have illustrated the use of various levels of the discourse-level aspect of NP, in other words of shifting in and out of the narrator, character, and here-and-now level. Table 9.1 summarizes the functions of shifting into these levels on the part of the analysand and the analyst separately.

Table 9.1 shows that some functions of using the discourse-level aspect of NP can be generalized over the analysands' and the analysts' use of discourse levels, whereas other functions are specific for the analysts or the analysands as speakers. The functions described in Table 9.1 are not exhaustive, however; rather, they merely exemplify the kinds of functions the various levels of the discourse-level variable may be used for. More specifically, we can observe in the third column of Table 9.1 what functions the here and now of the session can be used for according to our data. These show, one might argue, how essential this level is for reflecting on the analysands' current feelings and emotions, as well as clarifying their problems. In the course of the analysis of the narrative construction process in case of both dyads we showed how both sets of participants, and especially the analysts, took advantage of the use of this level in order to accomplish therapeutic goals, and advance analysis in the desired direction. In terms of the psychoanalytic functions of the here and now described at the beginning of this discussion based on Blass (2011) we can say that the functions revealed by our analysis do not contradict psychoanalytic interpretations of this level of discussion at the session; in fact, we have seen examples of the interpersonal and experiential aspects as defined above. So, in case of both dyads we have demonstrated that shifting between narrative levels (here and now,

Table 9.1 Functions of shifting into levels of the Discourse-level aspect of NP

Speaker	Narrator-level	Character-level	Here-and-now level
Analysand	• expressing general ideas • describing general aspects of events • distancing the narrator from described events and/or characters	• describing concrete events	• asking for confirmation from the analyst • expressing emotions • expressing thought process • describing current problems occurring at the session
Analyst	• expressing general ideas • describing general aspects of events • approaching the problem in a practical way • drawing conclusions • distancing the narrator from described events and/or characters	• focusing on concrete aspect of the problem • creating future model of solution • describing concrete events • asking for concrete reasons of actions	• clarifying meanings • expressing emotions • complying with analysand's confirmation request • asking about analysand's emotions • helping the analysand to focus on her problem

character, and narrator) can function as a powerful clinical tool, helping to regulate affect, restore epistemic trust, and foster reflective functioning. Whether in the emotionally charged context of the male dyad's family re-enactments or in the female dyad's structured work on academic paralysis, the analytic conversation becomes a field of co-created meaning, where relational patterns are not only revealed but reshaped in real time.

Conclusion

In this conclusion, we revisit the original aims of this book and summarize some of the theoretical, empirical, and technical contributions developed across the previous chapters. Drawing from the integration of discourse-based narrative analysis and autobiographical memory theory we propose that joint narrative construction taking place at the psychoanalytic session contributes to therapeutic transformation and change. At the core of our approach lies the notion of the shifting of narrative perspective (NP) and the linguistic construction of agency. Together, these concepts form the basis for understanding how narratives evolve within the psychoanalytic setting, and how therapeutic change can be systematically observed and facilitated. Finally, we argue that our understanding of NP shifting behaviour at the psychoanalytic session may be further developed and potentially used as a tool by psychoanalysts, thus serving as a contribution to psychoanalytic technique.

Revisiting the major goals of the studies included in our book

The major aim of our book was the observation and description of narrative interaction processes taking place at the psychoanalytic session in order to trace changes in the narrative self during psychoanalysis. We have accomplished this goal by describing and analysing shifts in NP of speakers at the psychoanalytic sessions of the Budapest Psychotherapy Database, and related these narrative processes to the psychotherapy process taking place at the same time. We have analysed, throughout Part 3 of the book, joined narrative construction processes while studying various aspects of the psychotherapy process, such as regulation of affective involvement, mentalization, empathy—expressed on the part of the analyst—alliance, working in the here and now of the session, long-term changes in interpersonal relating, and expressing sense of agency. Our findings provide evidence for the claim that narrative interaction taking place at the session contributes to the psychotherapy process through the transformation of the analysand's self-narratives, and hence contributes to structural changes in the narrative self taking place during psychoanalysis. Moreover, we suggest that, based on the evidence discussed in this book, the transformation of narratives is rooted in processes of shifting of NP on the part of both speakers during the interaction. Analysing two aspects of NP shifting behaviour, self-regulation and interactive regulation, we have traced these transformations in the analysand's self-narratives.

Related to our first aim, our more specific goal in the studies included in the book was to describe and analyse the process of interactive regulation of NP shifting behaviour, in other words the coordination of NP between speakers during the joint construction of narratives, and to show how interactive regulation of NP relates to the psychotherapy process. We have accomplished this goal through studying the analyst's active role in influencing the analysand's NP shifting behaviour, and by showing how the analysand shifted their perspective following a similar shift in the analyst's intonation unit. In addition, we have also shown how the analyst shifted perspective following the analysand's shifts—hence providing evidence that NP shifting behaviour is influenced mutually by both speakers throughout the studies included in Part 3.

Shifting of NP as a basis for psychoanalytic transformation of the narrative self

Narrative development begins in early life, shaped by affectively attuned care-giver–child interactions. Following Tronick's theory of mutual regulation, we frame early dyadic coordination as the prototype for narrative co-construction. As language emerges, children begin to structure self-experience into narratives, often scaffolded by the care-giver's elaborative support. These narrative practices evolve into autobiographical memory systems, which in adulthood are revisited and reshaped within the analytic encounter. Psychoanalysis, in this light, becomes a site for relationally mediated narrative reconstruction.

Our discursive framework for analysing the speakers' NP shifting behaviour introduces several key innovations related to narrative interaction observable at the psychoanalytic session. First, we treat NP shifts as functional cues for memory retrieval and emotional regulation. By helping how the analysands vary grammatical person, temporal stance, and focalization through the coordination of NP, analysts support flexible memory access, particularly episodic memories embedded within over-general schemas. This iterative practice facilitates the enrichment of abstract concepts with emotional detail, and the reframing of concrete episodes within broader meaning systems. The dynamic oscillation between conceptual and episodic elements fosters integration and coherence in the analysand's self-narrative.

Crucially, the shifting and coordinating of NP also promotes mutual memory transformation. As narratives are co-authored, both participants experience shifts in internal representations. Analysts may reconfigure their understanding of the analysand, while analysands encounter new ways of remembering, feeling, and symbolizing their experience. These changes align with procedural and declarative memory integration, offering a bridge between implicit relational knowledge and explicit autobiographical meaning.

Second, we introduce a method for tracking shifts in agency that are embedded in language. These shifts signal how analysands relate to responsibility, choice, and self-representation. By identifying moments where analysands shift from active to passive constructions, or attribute agency to dissociated parts of the self, analysts can intervene to clarify ownership and promote psychological integration. Our method of analysis based on our model of NP thus focuses on micro-level linguistic interventions—instead of traditional interpretive techniques—that reflect, challenge, or scaffold the analysand's evolving sense of self.

Third, a cornerstone of our model of NP is the concept of pseudo-diegesis—an NP shift wherein the speaker adopts the voice of another, real or imagined. These shifts often mark the emergence of dissociated self-states or internalized object voices. By recognizing and joining these perspectives, analysts can engage in coordinated regulation of NP shifting during narrative reconstruction. This technique echoes Ferenczi's play analysis, but emerges organically through narrative attunement rather than premeditated role play. Pseudo-diegetic shifts provide a rich terrain for exploring affect-laden experiences and for facilitating corrective emotional moments within the analytic dyad.

Fourth, we propose a redefinition of the psychoanalytic 'here and now' grounded in narrative analysis. Traditionally understood as the immediate transference–countertransference field or shared affective moment, we argue that the here and now is also a linguistic and structural event. It is recognizable through shifts to the present tense, and first-person constructions, focusing on emotions, ideas that emerge during the session. These linguistic markers signal moments of heightened subjectivity and intersubjective negotiation. By attending to these cues, analysts can intervene with greater precision, distinguishing reflective engagement from regressive enactment or affective flooding.

Our redefinition of the here and now introduces a precise, observable structure to what was a mostly intuitive or affectively felt phenomenon. This clarity offers a new level of control and sensitivity in clinical practice, enhancing the analyst's capacity to intervene with both attunement and narrative precision. It bridges the gap between language and emotion, experience and structure, allowing psychoanalysis to address the fundamental question: not only what is felt in the here and now, but how it is told, and by whom.

A potential contribution to psychoanalytic technique

Finally, we suggest that an understanding of NP shifting behaviour may help the analyst in their practice of psychoanalysis at the session. The analyst's own narrative choices—whether to mirror, challenge, or shift perspective—serve as micro-interventions that shape the evolving story. In adopting or stepping out of shared narrative frames, analysts signal containment, empathy, or invitation for reappraisal. This practice of linguistic attunement enhances the analyst's capacity to regulate affect, and guide reflective function through the shifting of NP. In practical terms, the analyst is equipped with a toolbox of linguistic interventions: mirroring emerging agency, reframing passive voice, initiating or responding to perspective shifts, and modulating the affective tone of a session through grammatical stance. These tools extend traditional psychoanalytic technique into a new domain of narrative-based relational work, providing both interpretive depth and structural clarity.

Our understanding of joint narrative construction in psychoanalysis is compatible with diverse psychoanalytic traditions—Freudian, intersubjective, relational, and MBT—but adds a unique language-based lens. It offers a codifiable grammar of therapeutic transformation and change. By tracking how narratives are told, who speaks, and how agency is distributed, we offer clinicians a precise and flexible method for engaging with the moving edge of subjectivity.

In closing, we believe that the future of psychoanalytic work lies not only in the exploration of affect or the decoding of unconscious content, but in the shared authorship of narrative. Through the analytic dialogue, analysands do not simply recall what has happened to them; they learn new ways of narrating it. This narrative transformation fosters a sense of agency, coherence, and emotional vitality. As we have shown throughout this book, these techniques observed in our sample of the Budapest Psychotherapy Database offer psychoanalysts a powerful new path to therapeutic transformation and change—one that begins not merely with what is said, but how it is told.

This book is grounded in the detailed linguistic and narrative analysis of audio-recorded psychoanalytic sessions. By systematically examining naturally occurring dialogue between analysts and analysands, we have brought into focus aspects of psychoanalytic work that have traditionally remained in the domain of clinical intuition. Through this empirical lens, we make explicit a subtle yet pervasive layer of the therapeutic process—how meaning is co-constructed through shifts in NP and agency. Our findings aim to transform what was once only vaguely felt by practising analysts into a conscious, observable structure of intervention. In doing so, we offer a new grammar for understanding and participating in the psychoanalytic dialogue.

References and Bibliography

Abargil, M. & Tishby, O. (2021). Countertransference as a reflection of the patient's inner relationship conflict. *Psychoanalytic Psychology*, *38*(1): 68–78. https://doi.org/10.1037/pap0000312

Abargil, M. & Tishby, O. (2024). Changes in countertransference and changes in patient working alliance and outcome: an empirical study. *Journal of Counseling Psychology*, *71*(5): 447–58. doi: 10.1037/cou0000743. Epub 2024 Jul 8. PMID: 38976443.

Abargil, M., Wiseman, H., Yonatan-Leus, R. & Tishby, O. (2023). Changes in clients' relational patterns with parents and therapist during psychodynamic psychotherapy: their association and relation to treatment outcome. *Journal of Clinical Psychology*, *79*(10): 2422–38. doi: 10.1002/jclp.23559. Epub 2023 Jun 21. PMID: 37341459.

Adler, J.M. (2012). Living into the story: agency and coherence in a longitudinal study of narrative identity development and mental health over the course of psychotherapy. *Journal of Personality and Social Psychology*, *102*(2): 367–89. doi: 10.1037/a0025289. Epub 2011 Sep 12. PMID: 21910554.

Adler, J.M. & McAdams, D.P. (2007). The narrative reconstruction of psychotherapy. *Narrative Inquiry*, *17*(2): 179–202. https://doi.org/10.1075/ni.17.2.03adl

Adler, J.M, Turner, A.F., Brookshier, K.M., Monahan, C., Walder-Biesanz, I., Harmeling, L.H., Albaugh, M., McAdams, D.P. & Oltmanns, T.F. (2015). Variation in narrative identity is associated with trajectories of mental health over several years. *Journal of Personality and Social Psychology*, *108*(3): 476–96. doi: 10.1037/a0038601. PMID: 25751718; PMCID: PMC4395856.

Agnew-Davies, R., Stiles, W.B., Hardy, G.E., Barkham, M. & Shapiro, D.A. (1998). Alliance structure assessed by the Agnew Relationship Measure (ARM). *British Journal of Clinical Psychology*, *37*(2): 155–72. doi: 10.1111/j.2044-8260.1998.tb01291.x. PMID: 9631204.

Arnold, K. (2005). Intersubjectivity, multiplicity, and the dynamic unconscious. *Contemporary Psychoanalysis*, *41*(3): 519–33. DOI: 10.1080/00107530.2005.10747262

Aron, L. (2003). The paradoxical place of enactment in psychoanalysis: introduction. *Psychoanalytic Dialogues*, *13*: 623–31. https://doi.org/10.1080/10481881309348760

Aron, L. & Atlas, G. (2019). Dramatic dialogue: dreaming & drama in contemporary clinical practice. *Psychoanalytic Perspectives*, *16*(3): 249–71. https://doi.org/10.1080/1551806X.2019.1653660

Atkinson, J.W. (1958). *Motives in fantasy, action, and society: a method of assessment and study*. Van Nostrand.

Atlas, G. & Aron, L. (2017). *Dramatic dialogue: contemporary clinical practice*. Routledge.

Avdi, E. (2008). Analysing talk in the talking cure: conversation, discourse, and narrative analysis of psychoanalytic psychotherapy. *European Psychotherapy*, *8*(1): 69–87. https://doi.org/10.1111/bjp.12444

Avdi, E. & Georgaca, E. (2007). Discourse analysis and psychotherapy: a critical review. *European Journal of Psychotherapy and Counselling*, *9*(2), 157–76. https://doi.org/10.1080/13642530701363445

Bakan, D. (1966). *The duality of human existence: an essay on psychology and religion*. Chicago, IL : Rand McNally.

Baker, R. (2020). The patient's discovery of the psychoanalyst as a new object 1. In: *The Contemporary Freudian Tradition* (pp. 251–68). Routledge.

Bal, M. (2004). Narration and focalization. *Narrative theory: critical concepts in literary and cultural studies*, *1*: 263–96.

Bal, M. & Lewin, J.E. (1983). *The narrating and the focalizing: a theory of the agents in narrative*. Style.

Baldwin, D.A., Baird, J.A., Saylor, M.M. & Clark, M.A. (2001). Infants parse dynamic action. *Child Development, 72*(3): 708–17. https://doi.org/10.1111/1467-8624.00310

Bamberg, M., Demuth, C. & Watzlawik, M. (eds) (2021). *Cambridge handbook of identity* (pp. 193–214). Cambridge University Press.

Bandura, A. (2006). Toward a psychology of human agency. *Perspectives on Psychological Science, 1*(2): 164–80. https://doi.org/10.1111/j.1745-6916.2006.00011.x

Barber, J., Crits-Christoph, P. & Luborsky, L. (1990). A guide to the CCRT standard categories and their classification. In: L. Luborsky & P. Crits-Christoph (eds), *Understanding transference* (pp. 37–51). Basic Books.

Barber, J.P., Crits-Christoph, P. & Luborsky, L. (1996). Effects of therapist adherence and competence on patient outcome in dynamic therapy. *Journal of Consulting and Clinical Psychology*, *64*(3): 619–22. https://doi.org/10.1037//0022-006x.64.3.619.

Barry, T.J., Lenaert, B., Hermans, D., Raes, F. & Griffith, J.W. (2018). Meta-analysis of the association between autobiographical memory specificity and exposure to trauma. *Journal of Traumatic Stress*, *31*(1): 35–46. doi: 10.1002/jts.22263. PMID: 29513912.

Barsness, R.E. (2021). Therapeutic practices in relational psychoanalysis: a qualitative study. *Psychoanalytic Psychology, 38*(1): 22–30. https://doi.org/10.1037/pap0000319

Barthes, R. & Duisit, L. (1975). An introduction to the structural analysis of narrative. *New Literary History*, *6*(2): 237–72. https://doi.org/10.2307/468419

Bateman, A. & Fonagy, P. (2016). *Mentalization-based treatment for personality disorders: a practical guide*. Oxford University Press.

Bauer, P.J. & Burch, M.M. (2004). Developments in early memory: multiple mediators of foundational processes. In: J.M. Lucariello, J.A. Hudson, R. Fivush & P.J. Bauer (eds), *The development of the mediated mind: sociocultural context and cognitive development* (pp. 101–25). Lawrence Erlbaum Associates Publishers.

Becker, T. & Quasthoff, U.M. (2005). Different dimensions in the field of narrative interaction. In: U.M. Qusthoff & T. Becker (eds), *Narrative interaction* (pp. 1–12). John Benjamins Publishing Company.

Beebe, B. & Lachmann, F. (2020). Infant research and adult treatment revisited: cocreating self- and interactive regulation. *Psychoanalytic Psychology, 37*(4): 313–23. https://doi.org/10.1037/pap0000305

Benjamin, J. (1995). *Like subjects, love objects: essays on recognition and sexual difference*. Yale University Press.

Benjamin, J. (2004). Beyond doer and done to: an intersubjective view of thirdness. *The Psychoanalytic Quarterly*, 73(1): 5–46. https://doi.org/10.1002/j.2167-4086.2004.tb00151.x

Benjamin, J. (2010). Where's the gap and what's the difference? The relational view of intersubjectivity, multiple selves, and enactments. *Contemporary Psychoanalysis, 46*(1): 112–19. https://doi.org/10.1080/00107530.2010.10746042

Benjamin, J. (2013). *The bonds of love: psychoanalysis, feminism, and the problem of domination.* Pantheon.

Benveniste, E. (1971). Subjectivity in language. In: M.E. Meek (ed.), *Problems in general linguistics*, 1 (pp. 223–30). University of Miami.

Berán, E. (2009). A narratív perspektíva szabályozó szerepe a terápiás diskurzusban [The regulative role of narrative perspective in psychotherapeutic discourse] (Doctoral dissertation, ELTE, PPK).

Berán, E. (2013). Páciencia kódolása önéletrajzi narratívumokban. Kézirat [The coding of patiency in self-narratives] (Unpublished Manuscript).

Berán, E., Czobor, P. & Unoka, Z. (2017). Regulating affective involvement in in-session verbal interaction by shifting perspective: a longitudinal study of one client-therapist dyad in psychodynamic psychotherapy. *Language and Psychoanalysis, 6*(2): 76–98.

Berán, E., Richman, M.J. & Unoka, Z. (2019). Autobiographical memory impairment in borderline personality disorder: a quantitative meta-analysis interpreted in terms of the CaR-FA-X model. *Journal of Personality Disorders, 33*(6): 818–31. https://doi.org/10.1521/pedi_2018_32_368

Berán, E. & Unoka, Z. (2005). Construction of self-narrative in psychotherapeutic setting: an analysis of a mutual determination of narrative perspective taken by patient and therapist. In: U.M. Quasthoff & T. Becker (eds), *Narrative interaction* (pp. 151–69). John Benjamins Publishing Company.

Berán, E. & Unoka, Z. (2015). Önéletrajzi emlékezet és narratív perspektíva váltás Ferenczinél és a mai terápiás gyakorlatban [Autobiographical memory and the shifting of perspective in Ferenczi and in current psychotherapy practice]. *Lélekelemzés, 10*(2): 249–69.

Berán, E. & Unoka, Z. (2016). Élettörténetek a pszichoterápiában [Life-stories in psychotherapy]. Oriold és Társai.

Berán, E., Unoka, Z. & Czobor, P. (2011). A szelf affektív bevonódása a pszichoterápiás folyamatba: érzelmi intenzitás kifejezése narratív perspektívahasználattal a terápia kezdeti szakaszában. *Pszichológia, 31*(3), 237–57.

Berman, R.A. & Slobin, D.I. (2013). Narrative structure 1. In: *Relating events in narrative* (pp. 39–84). Psychology Press.

Bion, W.R. (1962a). The psycho-analytic study of thinking. *International Journal of Psychoanalysis, 43*(4–5): 306–10.

Bion, W.R. (1962b). *Learning from experience.* Heinemann/Basic Books.

Bion, W.R. (1963). *Elements of psycho-analysis.* Heinemann.

Bird, A. & Reese, E. (2006). Emotional reminiscing and the development of an autobiographical self. *Developmental Psychology, 42*(4): 613–26. https://doi.org/10.1037/0012-1649.42.4.613

Bird, A., Reese, E. & Tripp, G. (2006). Parent–child talk about past emotional events: associations with child temperament and goodness-of-fit. *Journal of Cognition and Development, 7*(2): 189–210. https://doi.org/10.1207/s15327647jcd0702_3

Blass, R.B. (2011). On the immediacy of unconscious truth: understanding Betty Joseph's 'here and now' through comparison with alternative views of it outside of and within Kleinian thinking. *International Journal of Psychoanalysis, 92*: 1137–57. doi: 10.1111/j.1745-8315.2010.00361.x

Bluck, S. & Habermas, T. (2000). The life story schema. *Motivation and Emotion, 24*(2): 121–47. https://doi.org/10.1023/A:1005615331901

Bluck, S. & Habermas, T. (2001). Extending the study of autobiographical memory: thinking back about life across the life span. *Review of General Psychology, 5*(2): 135–47. https://doi.org/10.1037/1089-2680.5.2.135

Bohanek, J.G., Marin, K.A., Fivush, R. & Duke, M.P. (2006). Family narrative interaction and children's sense of self. *Family Process, 45*(1): 39–54. https://doi.org/10.1111/j.1545-5300.2006.00079.x

Bohleber, W. (2013). The concept of intersubjectivity in psychoanalysis: taking critical stock. *International Journal of Psychoanalysis, 94*(4): 799–823. https://doi.org/10.1111/1745-8315.12021

Bohleber, W., Fonagy, P., Jiménez, J.P., Scarfone, D., Varvin, S. & Zysman, S. (2013) Towards a better use of psychoanalytic concepts: a model illustrated using the concept of enactment. *International Journal of Psychoanalysis, 94*: 501–30. https://doi.org/10.1111/1745-8315.12075

Bortolussi, M. & Dixon, P. (2003) *Psychonarratology: foundations for the empirical study of literary response*. Cambridge University Press.

Boston Change Process Study Group. (2005). The 'something more' than interpretation revisited: sloppiness and co-creativity in the psychoanalytic encounter. *Journal of the American Psychoanalytic Association, 53*(3): 693–729. https://doi.org/10.1177/00030651050530030401

Boston Change Process Study Group (2008). Forms of relational meaning: issues in the relations between the implicit and reflective-verbal domains. *Psychoanalytic Dialogues, 18*: 125–48. DOI: 10.1080/10481880802473357

Boston Change Process Study Group (2010). *Change in psychotherapy: a unifying paradigm*. W.W. Norton & Company.

Boyd, R.L., Blackburn, K.G. & Pennebaker, J.W. (2020). The narrative arc: revealing core narrative structures through text analysis. *Science Advances*, 7.6(32): eaba2196. doi: 10.1126/sciadv.aba2196. PMID: 32821822; PMCID: PMC7413736.

Brand Bartlett, A. (2002). Current perspectives on the goals of psychoanalysis. *Journal of the American Psychoanalytic Association, 50*(2): 629–38. https://doi.org/10.1177/00030651020500020401

Branje, S., de Moor, E.L., Spitzer, J. & Becht, A.I. Dynamics of identity development in adolescence: a decade in review. *Journal of Research on Adolescence, 31*(4): 908–27. doi: 10.1111/jora.12678. PMID: 34820948; PMCID: PMC9298910.

Bremond, C. (1973). *Logique du récit*. Seul.

Bromberg, P.M. (1996). Standing in the spaces: the multiplicity of self and the psychoanalytic relationship. *Contemporary Psychoanalysis, 32*(4), 509–35. https://doi.org/10.1080/00107530.1996.10746334

Bromberg, P.M. (2014). *Standing in the spaces: essays on clinical process trauma and dissociation*. Routledge.

Brooks, C. & Warren, R.P. (1959). *Understanding fiction*. Appleton-Century–Crofts. Inc.

Brown, L.J. (2013). *Intersubjective processes and the unconscious: an integration of Freudian, Kleinian and Bionian perspectives*. Routledge.

Bruner, J. (1985). Narrative and paradigmatic modes of thought. In: E. Eisner & E.W. Eisner (eds), *Learning and teaching the ways of knowing*, vol. 84(2) (pp. 97–115). University of Chicago Press.

Bruner, J. (2004). Life as narrative. *Social Research: an International Quarterly, 71*(3): 691–710. DOI: 10.1353/sor.2004.0045.

Brunyé, T.T., Ditman, T., Mahoney, C.R. & Taylor, H.A. (2011). Better you than I: perspectives and emotion simulation during narrative comprehension. *Journal of Cognitive Psychology, 23*(5): 659–66. https://doi.org/10.1080/20445911.2011.559160

Brunyé, T.T., Ditman, T., Mahoney, C.R., Augustyn, J.S. & Taylor, H.A. (2009). When you and I share perspectives: pronouns modulate perspective taking during narrative comprehension. *Psychological Science, 20*(1): 27–32. https://doi.org/10.1111/j.1467-9280.2008.02249.x

Bruschweiler-Stern, N., Lyons-Ruth, K., Morgan, A.C., Nahum, J.P., Sander, L.W. & Stern, D.N. (2007). The foundational level of psychodynamic meaning: implicit process in relation to conflict, defense and the dynamic unconscious. *International Journal of Psychoanalysis., 88*(4): 843–60. doi: 10.1516/t2t4–0x02–6h21–5475. PMID: 17681896

Bucci, W. (1995). The power of the narrative: a multiple code account. In: J.W. Pennebaker (ed.), *Emotion, disclosure, and health* (pp. 71–92). American Psychological Association.

Bucci, W. (2001). Pathways of emotional communication. *Psychoanalytic Inquiry, 21*(1): 40–70. https://doi.org/10.1080/07351692109348923

Bucci, W. (2002). The referential process, consciousness, and the sense of self. *Psychoanalytic Inquiry, 22*(5): 766–93. https://doi.org/10.1080/07351692209349017

Bucci, W.S. (2018). The uncertainty principle in the psychoanalytic process. In: *Knowing, not-knowing and sort-of-knowing* (pp. 203–14). Routledge.

Buchheim, A. & Mergenthaler, E. (2000). The relationship among attachment representation, emotion-abstraction patterns, and narrative style: a computer-based text analysis of the adult attachment interview. *Psychotherapy Research, 10*(4), 390–407. https://doi.org/10.1093/ptr/10.4.390

Bunia, R. (2010). Diegesis and representation: beyond the fictional world, on the margins of story and narrative. *Poetics Today*, 31(4): 679–720. DOI: 10.2307/25835336

Burt, R.S. (1987). A note on strangers, friends, and happiness. *Social Networks, 9*(4): 311–31. DOI:10.1016/0378-8733(87)90002-5

Busch, F. (2011). The workable here and now and the why of there and then. *International Journal of Psychoanalysis, 92*: 1159–81. doi: 10.1111/j.1745-8315.2010.00375.x

Carson-Wong, A.C. (2016). The effect of therapist use of validation strategies on change in client emotion in an individual DBT treatment session. (Doctoral Dissertation, Graduate School-New Brunswick, Rutgers, State University of New Jersey).

Cash, T.F. & Hrabosky, J.I. The effects of psychoeducation and self-monitoring in a cognitive-behavioral program for body-image improvement. *Eating Disorders: The Journal of Treatment & Prevention, 11*(4): 255–70. doi: 10.1080/10640260390218657. PMID: 16864292

Castonguay, L.G., Constantino, M.J. & Holtforth, M.G. (2006). The working alliance: where are we and where should we go? *Psychotherapy: Theory, Research, Practice, Training, 43*(3): 271–79. https://doi.org/10.1037/0033-3204.43.3.271

Chafe, W. (1988). Linking intonation units in spoken English. In: J. Haiman & S.A. Thompson (eds), *Clause combining in grammar and discourse* (pp. 1–27). John Benjamins Publishers.

Chafe, W. (1994). *Discourse, consciousness, and time: the flow and displacement of conscious experience in speaking and writing.* University of Chicago Press.

Chatman, S. (1986). Characters and narrators: filter, center, slant, and interest-focus. *Poetics Today*, 7(2): 189–204. https://doi.org/10.2307/1772758

Chen, L., Xu, X. & Lv, H. (2023). How literary text reading is influenced by narrative voice and focalization: evidence from eye movements. *Discourse Processes, 60*(10): 675–94. https://doi.org/10.1080/0163853X.2023.2260247

Clark, H.H. (1996). *Using language.* Cambridge University Press.

Coates, J. (1998). Gossip revisited: language in all female groups. In: C. Jennifer (ed.), *Language and gender: a reader* (pp. 226–54). Blackwell Publishers.

Cogan, R. (2007). Therapeutic aims and outcomes of psychoanalysis. *Psychoanalytic Psychology, 24*(2): 193–207. https://doi.org/10.1037/0736-9735.24.2.193

Coleman, R. A., & Neimeyer, R. A. (2015). Assessment of subjective client agency in psychotherapy: A review. *Journal of Constructivist Psychology, 28*(1), 1-23.

Conway, M.A. (1992). A structural model of autobiographical memory. In: *Theoretical perspectives on autobiographical memory* (pp. 167–93). Springer.

Conway, M.A. (2001) Sensory-perceptual episodic memory and its context: autobiographical memory. *Philosophical Transactions of the Royal Society of London. Series B, Biological Sciences. 356*(1413): 1375–84. doi: 10.1098/rstb.2001.0940. PMID: 11571029; PMCID: PMC1088521.

Conway, M.A. (2005). Memory and the self. *Journal of Memory and Language, 53*(4): 594–628. https://doi.org/10.1016/j.jml.2005.08.005

Conway, M.A. (2009). Episodic memories. *Neuropsychologia, 47*(11): 2305–13. doi: 10.1016/j.neuropsychologia.2009.02.003. Epub 2009 Feb 11. PMID: 19524094.

Conway, M.A., Justice, L.V. & D'Argembeau, A. (2019). The self-memory system revisited: past, present, and future. In: J.H. Mace (ed.), *The organization and structure of autobiographical memory* (pp. 28–51). Oxford University Press. https://doi.org/10.1093/oso/9780198784845.003.0003

Conway, M. A., Loveday, C., & Cole, S. N. (2016). The remembering–imagining system. *Memory Studies, 9*(3), 256-265.

Conway, M.A. & Pleydell-Pearce, C.W. (2000). The construction of autobiographical memories in the self-memory system. *Psychological Review, 107*(2): 261–88. https://doi.org/10 1037/0033-295X.107.2.261

Conway, M.A., Singer, J.A. & Tagini, A. (2004). The self and autobiographical memory: correspondence and coherence. *Social Cognition, 22*(5): 491–529. https://doi.org/10.1521/soco.22.5.491.50768

De Jong, P., Bavelas, J.B. & Korman, H. (2013). An introduction to using microanalysis to observe co-construction in psychotherapy. *Journal of Systemic Therapies, 32*(3): 17–30. https://doi.org/10.1521/jsyt.2013.32.3.17

Deppermann, A. (2020) Unpacking parental violence in narratives: agency, guilt, and pedagogy in narratives about traumatic interpersonal experiences, *Applied Linguistics, 41*(3): 428–51. https://doi.org/10.1093/applin/amz068

Deppermann, A., Scheidt, C.E. & Stukenbrock, A. (2020). Positioning shifts from told self to performative self in psychotherapy. *Frontiers in Psychology*, 11: 572436. https://doi.org/10.3389/fpsyg.2020.572436

Dimaggio, G., Salvatore, G., Azzara, C. & Catania, D. (2003). Rewriting self narratives: the therapeutic process. *Journal of Constructivist Psychology, 16*(2): 155–81. https://doi.org/10.1080/10720530390117920

Ditman, T., Brunyé, T.T., Mahoney, C.R. & Taylor, H.A. (2010). Simulating an enactment effect: pronouns guide action simulation during narrative comprehension. *Cognition, 115*(1): 172–78. https://doi.org/10.1016/j.cognition.2009.10.014

Duchan, J.F., Bruder, G.A. & Hewitt, L.E. (2012). *Deixis in narrative: a cognitive science perspective.* Psychology Press.

Dylgjeri, A. & Kazazi, L. (2013). Deixis in modern linguistics and outside. *Academic Journal of Interdisciplinary Studies, 2*(4): 87–96. DOI: 10.5901/ajis.2012.v2n4p87

Eder, R.A. (1989). The emergent personologist: the structure and content of 3½-, 5½-, and 7½-year-olds' concepts of themselves and other persons. *Child Development*, *60*(5): 1218–28.

Eder, R.A. (1990). Uncovering young children's psychological selves: individual and developmental differences. *Child Development*, *61*(3): 849–63. https://doi.org/10.2307/1130969

Eichenberg, C., Aranyi, G., Rach, P. & Winter, L. (2022). Therapeutic alliance in psychotherapy across online and face-to-face settings: a quantitative analysis. *Internet Interventions*, 29: 100556. doi: 10.1016/j.invent.2022.100556. Epub 2022 Jul 10. PMID: 35942217; PMCID: PMC9350857.

Eisenberger, N.I. & Cole, S.W. (2012). Social neuroscience and health: neurophysiological mechanisms linking social ties with physical health. *Nature Neuroscience*, *15*(5): 669–74. doi: 10.1038/nn.3086. PMID: 22504347.

Ericsson, K.A. & Kintsch, W. (1995). Long-term working memory. *Psychological Review*, *102*(2): 211–45. https://doi.org/10.1037/0033-295X.102.2.211

Erikson, E. (1959). *Identity and the life cycle*. International Universities Press.

Ezriel, H. (1956). Experimentation within the psycho-analytic session. *British Journal for the Philosophy of Science*, 7(25): 29–48.

Farrant, K. & Reese, E. (2000). Maternal style and children's participation in reminiscing: stepping stones in children's autobiographical memory development. *Journal of Cognition and Development*, *1*(2): 193–225. https://doi.org/10.1207/S15327647JCD010203

Ferenczi, S. (1931). Child-analysis in the analysis of adults. *International Journal of Psycho-Analysis*, *12*: 468–82.

Fivush, R. (1991). The social construction of personal narratives. *Merrill-Palmer Quarterly*, *37*(1): 59–81. http://www.jstor.org/stable/23087339

Fivush, R. (2004). Voice and silence: a feminist model of autobiographical memory. In: J.M. Lucariello, J.A. Hudson, R. Fivush & P.J. Bauer (eds), *The development of the mediated mind: sociocultural context and cognitive development* (pp. 79–99). Lawrence Erlbaum Associates Publishers.

Fivush, R. (2011) The development of autobiographical memory. *Annual Review of Psychology*, *62*: 559–82. doi: 10.1146/annurev.psych.121208.131702. PMID: 20636128.

Fivush, R., Haden, C.A. & Reese, E. (2006). Elaborating on elaborations: role of maternal reminiscing style in cognitive and socioemotional development. *Child Development*, *77*(6): 1568–88. doi: 10.1111/j.1467-8624.2006.00960.x. PMID: 17107447.

Fivush, R. & Salmon, K. (2023). Maternal reminiscing as critical to emotion socialization. *Mental Health & Prevention*, *30*: 200281. doi: 10.1016/j.mhp.2023.200281. Epub 2023 May 6. PMID: 37193550; PMCID: PMC10163791.

Fivush, R. & Vasudeva, A. (2002). Remembering to relate: socioemotional correlates of mother–child reminiscing. *Journal of Cognition and Development, 3*(1): 73–90. https://doi.org/10.1207/S15327647JCD0301_5

Flückiger, C. & Grosse Holtforth, M. (2008). Focusing the therapist's attention on the patient's strengths: a preliminary study to foster a mechanism of change in outpatient psychotherapy. *Journal of Clinical Psychology*, *64*(7): 876–90. doi: 10.1002/jclp.20493. PMID: 18484601.

Flückiger, C., Del Re, A.C., Wampold, B.E. & Horvath, A.O. (2018). The alliance in adult psychotherapy: a meta-analytic synthesis. *Psychotherapy*, *55*(4): 316–40. https://doi.org/10.1037/pst0000172

Fludernik, M. (2002). *Towards a 'natural' narratology*. Routledge.

Fonagy, P. (2015). Mutual regulation, mentalization, and therapeutic action: a reflection on the contributions of Ed Tronick to developmental and psychotherapeutic thinking. *Psychoanalytic Inquiry, 35*(4): 355–69. https://doi.org/10.1080/07351690.2015.1022481

Fonagy, P. & Allison, E. (2013). What is mentalization?: the concept and its foundations in developmental research. In: N. Midgley & I. Vrouva (eds). *Minding the child mentalization-based interventions with children, young people and their families.* (pp. 11–34). Routledge.

Fonagy, P. & Allison, E. (2023). Beyond mentalizing: epistemic trust and the transmission of culture. *Psychoanalytic Quarterly, 92*(4): 599–640. https://doi.org/10.1080/00332828.2023.2290023

Fonagy, P., Gergely, G., Jurist, E. & Target, M. (2002). *Affect regulation, mentalization, and the development of the self.* Other Press.

Fonagy, P., Luyten, P. & Allison, E. (2015). Epistemic petrification and the restoration of epistemic trust: a new conceptualization of borderline personality disorder and its psychosocial treatment. *Journal of Personality Disorders*, 29(5): 575–609. doi: 10.1521/pedi.2015.29.5.575.

Freud, S. (1912). *The dynamics of transference. Classics in psychoanalytic techniques.* Hogarth Press and Institute of Psycho-Analysis.

Freud, S. (1915/1957). Repression. In: J. Strachey et al. (eds), *The standard edition of the complete psychological works of Sigmund Freud*, vol. XIV (pp. 141–58). Trans. C.M. Baines & J. Strachey. Hogarth Press.

Freud, S. (1957). Instincts and their vicissitudes. In: J. Strachey et al. (eds), *The standard edition of the complete psychological works of Sigmund Freud*, vol. XIV (pp. 109–40). Trans. C.M. Baines & J. Strachey. Hogarth Press.

Fried, D., Crits Christoph, P. & Luborsky, L. (1990). The parallel of narratives about the therapist with the CCRT for the people. In: *Understanding transference: the CCRT method* (pp. 147–58). Basic Books.

Fusaroli, R., Gangopadhyay, N. & Tylén, K. (2014a). The dialogically extended mind: language as skilful intersubjective engagement. *Cognitive Systems Research, 29*: 31–39. https://doi.org/10.1016/j.cogsys.2013.06.002.

Fusaroli, R., Rączaszek-Leonardi, J. & Tylén, K. (2014b). Dialog as interpersonal synergy. *New Ideas in Psychology, 32:* 147–57. https://doi.org/10.1016/j.newideapsych.2013.03.005

Fusaroli, R. & Tylén, K. (2012). Carving language for social coordination: a dynamical approach. *Interaction Studies: Social Behaviour and Communication in Biological and Artificial Systems, 13*(1): 103–24. https://doi.org/10.1075/is.13.1.07fus

Gallagher, I.I. (2000). Philosophical conceptions of the self: implications for cognitive science. *Trends in Cognitive Sciences, 4*(1): 14–21. doi: 10.1016/s1364-6613(99)01417-5. PMID: 10637618.

Garrod, S. & Anderson, A. (1987). Saying what you mean in dialogue: a study in conceptual and semantic co-ordination. *Cognition, 27*(2): 181–218. https://doi.org/10.1016/0010-0277(87)90018-7

Garrod, S. & Pickering, M.J. (2004). Why is conversation so easy? *Trends in Cognitive Sciences, 8*(1): 8–11. https://doi.org/10.1016/j.tics.2003.10.016

Garrod, S. & Pickering, M.J. (2009). Joint action, interactive alignment, and dialog. *Topics in Cognitive Science, 1*(2): 292–304. https://doi.org/10.1111/j.1756-8765.2009.01020.x

Gelso, C.J. & Hayes, J.A. (1998). *The psychotherapy relationship: theory, research, and practice.* John Wiley & Sons Inc.

Genette, G. (1972). *Figures I–III.* Editions du Seuil.

Genette, G. (1980). *Narrative discourse. an essay in method.* Cornell University Press.

Genette, G. (1983). *Narrative discourse: an essay in method*, vol. 3. Cornell University Press.

Gergely, G. & Watson, J.S. (1996). The social biofeedback theory of parental affect-mirroring: the development of emotional self-awareness and self-control in infancy, *International Journal of Psycho-Analysis*, *77*: 1181–212.

Gergely, G. & Watson, J.S. (1999). Early socio-emotional development: contingency perception and the social-biofeedback model. In: Philippe Rochat (ed.), *Early social cognition: understanding others in the first months of life* (pp. 60, 101–36). Psychology Press.

Gergen, K.J. (1999). *An invitation to social construction*. Sage.

Gorlin, E.I. & Békés, V. (2021). Agency via awareness: a unifying meta-process in psychotherapy. *Frontiers in Psychology*, *12*: 698655. doi: 10.3389/fpsyg.2021.698655. PMID: 34335416; PMCID: PMC8316855.

Grecucci, A., Frederickson, J. & Job, R. (2017). Editorial: advances in emotion regulation: from neuroscience to psychotherapy. *Frontiers in Psychology*, *8*: 985. doi: 10.3389/fpsyg.2017.00985. PMID: 28680409; PMCID: PMC5479113.

Green, K. (2022). *New essays in deixis: discourse, narrative, literature*, vol. 103. Brill.

Grenyer, B.F.S. & Marceau, E.M. (2022). Helping patients master core conflictual relationship themes in psychotherapy. *Journal of Clinical Psychology*, *78*(3): 386–95. doi: 10.1002/jclp.23314. Epub 2022 Jan 19. PMID: 35043390; PMCID: PMC9306742

Grossbaum, M.F. & Bates, G.W. (2002). Correlates of psychological well-being at midlife: the role of generativity, agency and communion, and narrative themes. *International Journal of Behavioral Development*, *26*(2): 120–27. https://doi.org/10.1080/01650250042000654.

Gülich, E. & Quasthoff, U.M. (1985). Narrative analysis. In: T.A. van Dijk (ed.), *Dimensions of discourse. Handbook of discourse analysis*, vol 2 (pp. 169–97). Academic Press.

Habermas, T. (2006). Who speaks? Who looks? Who feels? Point of view in autobiographical narratives. *International Journal of Psychoanalysis*, 87(2): 497–518. https://doi.org/10.1516/AXWM-QRNF-H69K-9K3C

Habermas, T. (2011) Autobiographical reasoning: arguing and narrating from a biographical perspective. *New Directions for Child and Adolescent Development*, *131*: 1–17. doi: 10.1002/cd.285. PMID: 21387528.

Habermas, T. (2019). *Emotion and narrative: perspectives in autobiographical storytelling*. Cambridge University Press.

Habermas, T. & Bluck, S. (2000). Getting a life: the emergence of the life story in adolescence. *Psychological Bulletin*, *126*(5): 748–69. https://doi.org/10.1037/0033-2909.126.5.748

Habermas, T. & Kemper, N. (2021). Psychoanalytic perspectives on identity: from ego to life narrative. In: M. Bamberg, C. Demuth & M. Watzlawik (eds), *The Cambridge handbook of identity* (pp. 193–214). Cambridge University Press

Habermas, T. & Paha, C. (2001). The development of coherence in adolescent's life narratives. *Narrative Inquiry*, *11*(1): 35–54. https://doi.org/10.1075/ni.11.1.02hab

Habermas, T. & de Silveira, C. (2008). The development of global coherence in life narratives across adolescence: temporal, causal, and thematic aspects. *Developmental Psychology*, *44*(3): 707–21. doi: 10.1037/0012-1649.44.3.707. PMID: 18473638.

Haden, C.A., Haine, R.A. & Fivush, R. (1997). Developing narrative structure in parent–child reminiscing across the preschool years. *Developmental Psychology*, *33*(2): 295–307. https://doi.org/10.1037/0012-1649.33.2.295

Hayes, A.F. & Krippendorff, K. (2007). Answering the call for a standard reliability measure for coding data. *Communication Methods and Measures, 1*(1): 77–89. https://doi.org/10.1080/19312450709336664

Haynal, A. (2011). On psychoanalysis in Budapest. In: P. Loewenberg & N. Thompson (eds), *100 years of the IPA. The centenary history of the International Psychoanalytical Association 1910–2010. Evolution and change* (pp. 95–106). Karnac.

Helgeson, V.S. & Palladino, D.K. (2012). Agentic and communal traits and health adolescents with and without diabetes. *Personality and Social Psychology Bulletin, 38*(4): 415–28. https://doi.org/10.1177/0146167211427149

Housby, H., Thackeray, L. & Midgley, N. (2021). What contributes to good outcomes? The perspective of young people on short-term psychoanalytic psychotherapy for depressed adolescents. *PLoS ONE, 16*(9): e0257334. doi.org/10.1371/journal.pone.0257334

Hymes, D. (1992). The concept of communicative competence revisited. In: R. Dirven (ed.), *Thirty years of linguistic evolution: studies in honour of René Dirven on the occasion of his sixtieth birthday*, vol. 61 (pp. 31–57). John Benjamins Publishing.

Ikeo, R. (2022). Contemporary present-tense fiction: crossing boundaries in narrative. *Language and Literature, 32*(1): 98–128. https://doi.org/10.1177/09639470221117674 (Original work published 2023).

Inbar, M., Genzer, S., Perry, A., Grossman, E. & Landau, A.N. (2023). Intonation units in spontaneous speech evoke a neural response. *Journal of Neuroscience, 43*(48): 8189–200. https://doi.org/10.1523/JNEUROSCI.0235-23.2023

Jackendoff, R.S. (1992). *Languages of the mind*, vol. 10. MIT Press.

Jacobson, E. (1964). *The self and the object world.* International Universities Press.

Jin, J. & Liu, S. (2023). Shifts in narrative perspectives consume attentional resources and facilitate reading engagement. *Scientific Studies of Reading, 27*(5), 393–407. https://doi.org/10.1080/10888438.2023.2179922

Joseph, B. (2013). Here and now: my perspective. *International Journal of Psychoanalysis, 94*: 1–5. doi: 10.1111/j.1745-8315.2012.00558.x.

Joyce, A.S., McCallum, M., Piper, W.E. & Ogrodniczuk, J.S. (2000). Role behavior expectancies and alliance change in short-term individual psychotherapy. *Journal of Psychotherapy Practice and Research, 9*(4): 213.

Katznelson, H. (2014). Reflective functioning: a review. *Clinical Psychology Review, 34*(2): 107–17. doi: 10.1016/j.cpr.2013.12.003. Epub 2013 Dec 29. PMID: 24486522.

Kernberg, O. (1975). *Borderline conditions and pathological narcissism.* Jason Aronson.

Kernberg, O. (2004). *Contemporary controversies in psychoanalytic theory, techniques, and their applications.* Yale University Press.

Kernberg, O.F. (2011). Divergent contemporary trends in psychoanalytic theory. *Psychoanalytic Review, 98*(5): 633–64. https://doi.org/10.1521/prev.2011.98.6.633

Kernberg, O.F. (2016). New developments in transference focused psychotherapy. *International Journal of Psychoanalysis, 97*(2), 385–407. https://doi.org/10.1111/1745-8315.12289.

Kivlighan, D.M., Jr. (2014). Three important clinical processes in individual and group interpersonal psychotherapy sessions. *Psychotherapy, 51*(1): 20–24. https://doi.org/10.1037/a0032162

Kohut, H. (1971). *The Analysis of the Self.* International Universities Press.

Koven, M. (2012). Speaker roles in personal narratives. In: J.A. Holstein & J.F. Gubrium (eds), *Varieties of Narrative Analysis* (pp. 151–80). Sage Publications.

Kukkonen, K., Hühn, P., Meister, J.C., Pier, J. & Schmid, W. (2014). *The living handbook of narratology.* University of Hamburg Press.

Labov, W. (1972). *Language in the inner city: studies in the Black English vernacular (no. 3).* University of Pennsylvania Press.

Labov, W. (2006). Narrative pre-construction. *Narrative Inquiry, 16*(1): 37–45. https://doi.org/10.1075/ni.16.1.07lab

Labov, W. & Fanshell, D. (1977). *Therapeutic discourse: psychotherapy as conversation.* Academic Press.

Labov, W. & Waletzky, J. (1967). Narrative analysis: oral versions of personal experience. In: J. Helm (ed.), *Essays on the verbal and visual arts* (pp. 12–44). University of Washington Press.

Lacan, J. (1988). *Freud's papers on technique 1953–1954.* W.W. Norton & Company.

Lakoff, G. & Turner, M. (1989). *More than cool reason: a field guide to poetic metaphor.* University of Chicago Press.

Lambert, M.J. & Barley, D.E. (2001). Research summary on the therapeutic relationship and psychotherapy outcome. *Psychotherapy: Theory, Research, Practice, Training, 38*(4): 357–61. https://doi.org/10.1037/0033-3204.38.4.357

Lane, R.D., Ryan, L., Nadel, L. & Greenberg, L. (2015). Memory reconsolidation, emotion arousal, and the process of change in psychotherapy: new insights from brain science. *Behavioral and Brain Sciences, 38.* doi.org/10.1017/S0140525X14000041

Laplanche, J. & Pontalis, J.B. (1973). *The language of psycho-analysis.* Trans. D. Nicholson-Smith. W.W. Norton.

Leonardi, J., Gazzillo, F. & Dazzi, N. (2022). The adaptive unconscious in psychoanalysis. *International Forum of Psychoanalysis, 31*(4): 201–17.

Levenkron, H. (2009). Engaging the implicit: meeting points between the Boston Change Process Study Group and relational psychoanalysis. *Contemporary Psychoanalysis, 45*(2): 179–217. https://doi.org/10.1080/00107530.2009.10745995

Lilgendahl, J.P. & McAdams, D.P. (2011) Constructing stories of self-growth: how individual differences in patterns of autobiographical reasoning relate to well-being in midlife. *Journal of Personality, 79*(2): 391–428. doi: 10.1111/j.1467-6494.2010.00688.x. PMID: 21395593; PMCID: PMC3386782.

Longo, D.A., Lent, R.W. & Brown, S.D. (1992). Social cognitive variables in the prediction of client motivation and attrition. *Journal of Counselling Psychology, 39*(4): 447–52. https://doi.org/10.1037/0022-0167.39.4.447

Luborsky, L. (1977). Measuring a pervasive psychic structure in psychotherapy: the core conflictual relationship theme. In: N. Freedman & S. Grand (eds), *Communicative structures and psychic structures* (pp. 367–95). Springer.

Luborsky, L. (1994). Therapeutic alliances as predictors of psychotherapy outcomes: factors. In: A.O. Horváth & L. Greenberg (eds), *The working alliance: theory, research, and practice* (pp. 38–48). John Wiley and Sons Inc.

Luborsky, L. & Barrett, M.S. (2007). The core conflictual relationship theme: a basic case formulation method. In: T.D. Eells (ed.), *Handbook of psychotherapy case formulation*, 2nd edn (pp. 105–35). Guilford Press.

Luborsky, L. & Crits-Christoph, P. (1990). *Understanding transference: the CCRT method.* Basic Books.

Luborsky, L. & Crits-Christoph, P. (1998). *Understanding transference: the core conflictual relationship theme method.* American Psychological Association.

Luborsky, L., Barber, J., Schaffer, P. & Cacciola, J. (1990). The narratives told during psychotherapy, and the types of CCRTs within them. In: L. Luborsky & P. Crits-Christoph (eds), *Understanding transference* (pp. 117–32). Basic Books.

Lucariello, J.A. Hudson, R. Fivush & P.J. Bauer (eds) (2004). *The mediated mind: essays in honor of Katherine Nelson*. Erlbaum.

Lyons-Ruth, K. (1999). The two-person unconscious: intersubjective dialogue, enactive relational representation, and the emergence of new forms of relational organization. *Psychoanalytic Inquiry, 19*(4): 576–617. https://doi.org/10.1080/07351699909534267

Lyons-Ruth, K., Bruschweiler-Stern, N., Harrison, A.M., Morgan, A.C., Nahum, J.P., Sander, L., Stern, D.N. & Tronick, E.Z. (1998). Implicit relational knowing: its role in development and psychoanalytic treatment. *Infant Mental Health Journal, 19*(3): 282–89. DOI:10.1002/(SICI)1097-0355(199823)19:3<282::AID-IMHJ3>3.0.CO;2-O.

Lyons-Ruth, K., Dutra, L., Schuder, M.R., Bianchi, I. (2006). From infant attachment disorganization to adult dissociation: relational adaptations or traumatic experiences? *Psychiatric Clinics of North America, 29*(1): 63–86, viii. doi: 10.1016/j.psc.2005.10.011. PMID: 16530587; PMCID: PMC2625289.

MacWhinney, B. (ed.). (2000). The CHILDES database (Version 3.0) [English-North American, Peterson-McCabe dataset]. Carnegie Mellon University.

MacWhinney, B. (2000). *The CHILDES Project: tools for analyzing talk*, 3rd edn. Lawrence Erlbaum Associates.

Mansfield, E.D. & McAdams, D.P. (1996). Generativity and themes of agency and communion in adult autobiography. *Personality and Social Psychology Bulletin, 22*(7): 721–31. https://doi.org/10.1177/0146167296227006

McAdams, D.P. (1988). *Power, intimacy, and the life story: personological inquiries into identity*. Guilford Press.

McAdams, D.P. (1980). A thematic coding system for the intimacy motive. *Journal of Research in Personality, 14*(4): 413–32. https://doi.org/10.1016/0092-6566(80)90001-X

McAdams, D.P. (1982). Experiences of intimacy and power: relationships between social motives and autobiographical memory. *Journal of Personality and Social Psychology, 42*(2): 292–302. https://doi.org/10.1037/0022-3514.42.2.292

McAdams, D.P. (1985). *Power, intimacy, and the life story: personological inquiries into identity*. Dorsey Press.

McAdams, D.P. (1996). Personality, modernity, and the storied self: a contemporary framework for studying persons. *Psychological Inquiry, 7*(4): 295–321. https://doi.org/10.1207/s15327965pli0704_1

McAdams, D.P. (1997). Guided life-story interview (downloaded: 25 March 2021)

McAdams, D.P. (2001). Coding autobiographical episodes for themes of agency and communion (Unpublished Manuscript, Northwestern University).

McAdams, D.P. (2021). Narrative identity and the life story. In: O.P. John & R.W. Robins (eds), *Handbook of personality: theory and research*, 4th edn (pp. 122–41). Guilford Press.

McAdams, D.P., Anyidoho, N.A., Brown, C., Huang, Y.T., Kaplan, B. & Machado, M.A. (2004). Traits and stories: links between dispositional and narrative features of personality. *Journal of Personality, 72*(4): 761–84. https://doi.org/10.1111/j.0022-3506.2004.00279.x

McAdams, D.P. & Cox, K.S. (2010). Self and identity across the life span. In: K.L. Fingerman, C. Berg, J. Smith & T.C. Antonucci (eds), *Handbook of life-span development* (pp. 150–201). Springer Publishing Company.

McAdams, D.P., Hoffman, B.J., Mansfield, E.D. & Day, R. (1996). Themes of agency and communion in significant autobiographical scenes. *Journal of Personality, 64*(2): 339–77. https://doi.org/10.1111/j.1467-6494.1996.tb00514.x

McDonnell, C.G., Valentino, K., Comas, M. & Nuttall, A.K. (2016). Mother–child reminiscing at risk: maternal attachment, elaboration, and child autobiographical memory specificity. *Journal of Experimental Child Psychology, 143*: 65–84. https://doi.org/10.1016/j.jecp.2015.10.012.

McFarquhar, T., Luyten, P. & Fonagy, P. (2018). Changes in interpersonal problems in the psychotherapeutic treatment of depression as measured by the inventory of interpersonal problems: a systematic review and meta-analysis. *Journal of Affective Disorders, 226*: 108–23. doi: 10.1016/j.jad.2017.09.036. Epub 2017 Sep 25. PMID: 28968563.

McLean, K.C., Dunlap, D., Jennings, S.C., Litvitskiy, N.S. & Lilgendahl, J.P. (2022). Stability and change in autobiographical reasoning: a 4-year longitudinal study of narrative identity development. *Journal of Personality, 90*(3): 343–56. https://doi.org/10.1111/jopy.12669

McLean, K.C. & Mansfield, C.D. (2011). To reason or not to reason: is autobiographical reasoning always beneficial? In: T. Habermas (ed.), *The development of autobiographical reasoning in adolescence and beyond: new directions for child and adolescent development, number 131*, vol. 102 (pp. 85–97). John Wiley & Sons.

Meins, E. & Fernyhough, C. (1999). Linguistic acquisitional style and mentalising development: the role of maternal mind-mindedness. *Cognitive Development, 14*(3): 363–80. https://doi.org/10.1016/S0885-2014(99)00010-6

Meins, E., Fernyhough, C., Fradley, E. & Tuckey, M. (2001). Rethinking maternal sensitivity: mothers' comments on infants' mental processes predict security of attachment at 12 months. *Journal of Child Psychology and Psychiatry, 42*(5): 637–48. PMID: 11464968.

Meins, E., Fernyhough, C., Wainwright, R., Clark-Carter, D., Das Gupta, M., Fradley, E. & Tuckey, M. (2003). Pathways to understanding mind: construct validity and predictive validity of maternal mind-mindedness. *Child Development, 74*(4): 1194–211. doi: 10.1111/1467-8624.00601. PMID: 12938713

Meins, E., Fernyhough, C., Wainwright, R., Das Gupta, M., Fradley, E. & Tuckey, M. Maternal mind-mindedness and attachment security as predictors of theory of mind understanding. *Child Development, 73*(6): 1715–26. doi: 10.1111/1467-8624.00501. PMID: 12487489.

Mergenthaler, E. (1996). Emotion–abstraction patterns in verbatim protocols: a new way of describing psychotherapeutic processes. *Journal of Consulting and Clinical Psychology, 64*(6): 1306–15. https://doi.org/10.1037/0022-006X.64.6.1306

Michaelis, L. A. (2020). Tense in English. Aronoff, M., & Rees-Miller, J. (Eds.) *The handbook of linguistics*. 163-181. John Wiley & Sons.

Miskovic, M. (2007). The construction of ethnic identity of Balkan Muslim immigrants: a narrativization of personal experiences. *Qualitative Report, 12*(3): 514–46. DOI: 10.46743/2160-3715/2007.1630.

Mitchell, S.A. (2022). *Relationality: from attachment to intersubjectivity*. Routledge.

Negri, A., Christian, C., Mariani, R., Belotti, L., Andreoli, G. & Danskin, K. (2019). Linguistic features of the therapeutic alliance in the first session: a psychotherapy process study. *Research in Psychotherapy: Psychopathology, Process, and Outcome, 22*(1): 374.

Nelson, K. (1996). *Language in cognitive development*. Erlbaum.

Nelson, K. & Fivush, R. (2004). The emergence of autobiographical memory: a social cultural developmental theory. *Psychological Review, 111*(2): 486–511.

Nelson, K. & Fivush, R. (2020). The development of autobiographical memory, autobiographical narratives, and autobiographical consciousness. *Psychological Reports*, *123*(1): 71–96.

Németh, T.E. (1996). *A szóbeli diskurzusok megnyilatkozás példányokra tagolása* [The segmentation of spoken discourse into utterance units]. Akadémia Kiadó.

Nigro, G. & Neisser, U. (1983). Point of viewing personal memories. *Cognitive Psychology*, *15*: 467–82.

Norcross, J.C. & Lambert, M.J. (2018). Psychotherapy relationships that work III. *Psychotherapy*, *55*(4): 303–15.

Ochs, E. & Capps, L. (2001). *Living narrative: creating lives in everyday storytelling*. Harvard University Press.

Ochs, E., Taylor, C., Rudolph, D. & Smith, R. (1992). Storytelling as a theory-building activity. *Discourse Processes*, *15*(1): 37–72. https://doi.org/10.1080/01638539209544801

Ogden, T.H. (1989). *The primitive edge of experience*. Jason Aronson.

Ogden, T.H. (2018). On potential space. In: M.B. Spelman & F. Thomson-Salo (eds), *The Winnicott tradition: lines of development-evolution of theory and practice over the decades* (pp. 121–33). Routledge.

Onishi, K.H. & Baillargeon, R. (2005). Do 15-month-old infants understand false beliefs? *Science*, *308*(5719): 255–58. doi: 10.1126/science.1107621. PMID: 15821091; PMCID: PMC3357322.

Orange, D.M., Atwood, G.E. & Stolorow, R.D. (2015). *Working intersubjectively: contextualism in psychoanalytic practice*. Routledge.

Palmer, F.R. & Frank Robert, P. (1981). *Semantics*. Cambridge University Press.

Pasupathi, M., Mansour, E. & Brubaker, J.R. (2007). Developing a life story: constructing relations between self and experience in autobiographical narratives. *Human Development*, *50*(2–3): 85–110. https://doi.org/10.1159/000100939

Pawelczyk, J. (2012). 'No stories, no self': co-constructing personal narratives in the psychotherapy session. *Poznań Studies in Contemporary Linguistics*, *48*(1): 1–21. https://doi.org/10.1515/psicl-2012-0002

Perner, J. (2000). Memory and theory of mind. In: E. Tulving & F.I. Craik (eds), *The Oxford handbook of memory* (pp. 297–312). Oxford University Press.

Peterson, C. & McCabe, A. (1983/2013). *Developmental psycholinguistics: three ways of looking at a child's narrative*. Springer.

Peterson, C. & McCabe, A. (1992). Parental styles of narrative elicitation: effect on children's narrative structure and content. *First Language*, *12*(36/3): 299–321. https://doi.org/10.1177/014272379201203606

Phelan, J. (2001). Why narrators can be focalizers—and why it matters. In: W. Van Peer & S.B. Chatman (eds), *New perspectives on narrative perspective* (pp. 51–64). SUNY Press.

Pickering, M.J. & Garrod, S. (2006). Alignment as the basis for successful communication. *Research Language Computation*, *4:* 203–28. https://doi.org/10.1007/s11168-006-9004-0

Pier, J. (2009). Diegesis. In: T.A. Sebeok et al. (eds), *Encyclopedic dictionary of semiotics* (pp. 1, 209–11). Mouton De Gruyter.

Pier, J. (2014). *Narrative levels. The living handbook of narratology*. Hamburg University Press.

Pinsof, W.M. & Chambers, A.L. (2009). Empirically informed systemic psychotherapy: tracking client change and therapist behavior during therapy. In: J.H. Bray & M. Stanton (eds), *The Wiley-Blackwell handbook of family psychology* (pp. 431–46). Wiley Blackwell.

Polya, T.(2005). A narratív perspektíva hatása az elbeszélő személy észlelésére, In: F. Erős (Ed.) Az elbeszélés az élmények kulturális és klinikai elemzésében. Magyar Pszichológiai Szemle Könyvtár. 89-107. Akadémia Kiadó.

Pólya, T., Kis, B., Naszódi, M. & László, J. (2007). Narrative perspective and the emotion regulation of a narrating person. *Empirical Text and Culture Research*, *3*: 50–61.

Prince, G. (1987). *A dictionary of narratology*. University of Nebraska Press.

Prince, G. (2003). *A dictionary of narratology*. University of Nebraska Press.

Quasthoff, U.M. & Becker, T. (eds). (2005). *Narrative interaction*, vol. 5. John Benjamins Publishing.

Quasthoff, U. & Stude, J. (2021). Children's narrative interactions: practices–competences–acquisition. *Narrative Inquiry*, *31*(1): 147–62. https://doi.org/10.1075/ni.20103.qua.

Racsmány, M. & Conway, M.A. (2006). Episodic inhibition. *Journal of Experimental Psychology: Learning, Memory, and Cognition, 32*(1): 44–57. https://doi.org/10.1037/0278-7393.32.1.44

Rapaport, W.J., Segal, E.M., Shapiro, S.C., Zubin, D.A., Bruder, G.A., Duchan, J.F., .. & Yuhan, A.H. (1989). *Deictic centers and the cognitive structure of narrative comprehension*. State University of New York (Buffalo).

Reese, E., Haden, C.A., Baker-Ward, L., Bauer, P.A., Fivush, R. & Ornstein, P. (2011). Coherence of personal narratives across the lifespan: a multidimensional model and coding method. *Journal of Cognition and Development, 12*(4): 424–62. https://doi.org/10.1080/15248372.2011.587854

Reese, E., Meins, E., Fernyhough, C. & Centifanti, L. (2019). Origins of mother–child reminiscing style. *Development and Psychopathology, 31*(2): 631–42. https://doi.org/10.1017/S0954579418000172

Reese, E. & Newcombe, R. (2007). Training mothers in elaborative reminiscing enhances children's autobiographical memory and narrative. *Child Development, 78*(4): 1153–70. https://doi.org/10.1111/j.1467-8624.2007.01058.x

Reese, E., Yan, C., Jack, F. & Hayne, H. (2010). Emerging identities: narrative and self from early childhood to early adolescence. In: K. McLean & M. Pasupathi (eds), *Narrative development in adolescence. advancing responsible adolescent development*. Springer. https://doi.org/10.1007/978-0-387-89825-4_2

Renik, O. & Spillius, E.B. (2004). Intersubjectivity in psychoanalysis. *International Journal of Psychoanalysis.*, *85*(5): 1053–64; discussion 1057–61. doi: 10.1516/0020757042259683. PMID: 15509331.

Rickers-Ovsiankina, M.A., Geller, J.D., Berzins, J.I. & Rogers, G.W. (1971). Patient's role-expectancies in psychotherapy: a theoretical and measurement approach. *Psychotherapy: Theory, Research & Practice, 8*(2): 124–26. https://doi.org/10.1037/h0086637

Rocco, D., Rizzi, L., Dell'Arciprete, G. & Perrella, R. (2022). The functional psychotherapy approach: a process-outcome multiple case study. *Frontiers in Psychology, 12:* 727497. https://doi.org/10.3389/fpsyg.2021.727497

Roth, A. & Fonagy, P. (2006). *What works for whom: a critical review of psychotherapy research*, 2nd edn. Guilford Publications.

Rottenberg, J. & Gross, J.J. (2007). Emotion and emotion regulation: a map for psychotherapy researchers. *Clinical Psychology: Science and Practice*, *14*(4): 323–28. https://doi.org/10.1111/j.1468-2850.2007.00093.x

Rounds, C.H. (2009). *Hungarian: an essential grammar*. Routledge.

Sacks, H. (1986). Some consideration of a story told in ordinary conversations. *Poetics*, *15*(1–2): 127–38.

Safran, J.D. & Muran, J.C. (2001). The therapeutic alliance as a process of intersubjective negotiation. In: J.C. Muran (ed.), *Self-relations in the psychotherapy process* (pp. 165–92). American Psychological Association. https://doi.org/10.1037/10391-007

Sales, J.M. (2009). In: J.A. Quas & R. Fivush (eds), *Creating a context for children's memory: the importance of parental attachment status, coping, and narrative skill for co-constructing meaning following stressful experiences* (pp. 196–217). Oxford University Press.

Sanders, J. & van Krieken, K. (2019). Travelling through narrative time: how tense and temporal deixis guide the representation of time and viewpoint in news narratives. *Cognitive Linguistics, 30*(2): 281–304. https://doi.org/10.1515/cog-2018-0041

Sandler, J. & Sandler, A.M. (1984) The past unconscious and the present unconscious. A contribution to a technical frame of reference. *Psychoanalytic Study of the Child, 49*: 278–92. doi: 10.1080/00797308.1994.11823064. PMID: 7809289.

Scarvaglieri, C. (2020). First encounters in psychotherapy: relationship-building and the pursuit of institutional goals. *Frontiers in Psychology, 11*: 585038. doi: 10.3389/fpsyg.2020.585038.

Schafer, R. (1980). Narration in the psychoanalytic dialogue. *Critical Inquiry*, 7(1): 29–53.

Schafer, R. (1992). *Retelling a life. Narration and dialogue in psychoanalysis*. Basic Books.

Schiffrin, D. (1981). Tense variation in narrative. *Language*, *57*(1): 45–62. https://doi.org/10.2307/414286.

Schiffrin, D. (1994). *Approaches to discourse*. Blackwell.

Schiffrin, D. (1998). Approaches to discourse. *Journal of Pragmatics*, *3*(29): 355–59.

Shipman, K.L. & Zeman, J. (1999). Emotional understanding: a comparison of physically maltreating and nonmaltreating mother–child dyads. *Journal of Clinical Child Psychology, 28*(3): 407–17. doi: 10.1207/S15374424jccp280313. PMID: 10446690.

Shuman, A. (2012). Exploring narrative interaction in multiple contexts. In: J.A. Holstein & J.F. Gubrium (eds), *Varieties of narrative analysis* (pp. 125–50). Sage Publications.

Singer, J.A. & Salovey, P. (1993). *The remembered self: emotion and memory in personality*. Free Press.

Singer, J.A. & Salovey, P. (1996). Motivated memory: self-defining memories, goals, and affect regulation. In: L.L. Martin & A. Tesser (eds), *Striving and feeling: interactions among goals, affect, and self-regulation* (pp. 229–50). Lawrence Erlbaum Associates, Inc.

Sizoo, E. (ed.). (2002). *Women's lifeworlds: women's narratives on shaping their realities*. Routledge.

Smith, B.C. (2016). Proust, the Madeleine and memory. In: S. Groes (ed.), *Memory in the Twenty-First Century*. Palgrave Macmillan. https://doi.org/10.1057/9781137520586_3

Solbakken, O.A. & Abbass, A. (2015). Intensive short-term dynamic residential treatment program for patients with treatment-resistant disorders. *Journal of Affective Disorders, 181*: 67–77. doi: 10.1016/j.jad.2015.04.003. Epub 2015 Apr 13. Erratum in: Journal of Affective Disorders 2015 Sep 15;184:89. PMID: 25917295.

Song, H.J., Onishi, K.H., Baillargeon, R. & Fisher, C. (2008). Can an agent's false belief be corrected by an appropriate communication? Psychological reasoning in 18-month-old infants. *Cognition, 109*(3): 295–315. doi: 10.1016/j.cognition.2008.08.008. Epub 2008 Oct 30. PMID: 18976745; PMCID: PMC2808001.

Sools, A. (2020). Back from the future: a narrative approach to study the imagination of personal futures. *International Journal of Social Research Methodology: Theory & Practice, 23*(4): 451–65. https://doi.org/10.1080/13645579.2020.1719617

Southgate, V., Senju, A. & Csibra, G. (2007). Action anticipation through attribution of false belief by 2-year-olds. *Psychological Science, 18*(7): 587–92. doi: 10.1111/j.1467-9280.2007.01944.x. PMID: 17614866.

Spence, D.P. (1982). Narrative truth and theoretical truth. *Psychoanalytic Quarterly, 51*(1): 43–69. PMID: 7058225.

Spence, D.P. (1984). Perils and pitfalls of free floating attention. *Contemporary Psychoanalysis, 20*(1): 37–59. https://doi.org/10.1080/00107530.1984.10745714

Spence, S.H., O'Shea, G. & Donovan, C.L. (2016). Improvements in interpersonal functioning following interpersonal psychotherapy (IPT) with adolescents and their association with change in depression. *Behavioural and Cognitive Psychotherapy*, *44*(3): 257–72. doi: 10.1017/S1352465815000442. Epub 2015 Aug 21. PMID: 26292976.

Sperber, D. & Wilson, D. (1986). *Relevance: communication and cognition*, vol. 142. Harvard University Press.

Steiner, J. (1984). Some reflections on the analysis of transference: a Kleinian view. *Psychoanalytic Inquiry*, *4*: 443–63. https://doi.org/10.1080/07351698409533556

Stern, D.N. (2018). *The interpersonal world of the infant: a view from psychoanalysis and development psychology*. Routledge.

Stolorow, R., Atwood, G. & Orange, D. (2002). *Worlds of experience: interweaving philosophical and clinical dimensions in psychoanalysis*. Basic Books.

Surian, L., Caldi, S. & Sperber, D. (2007) Attribution of beliefs by 13-month-old infants. *Psychological Science*, *18*(7): 580–86. doi: 10.1111/j.1467-9280.2007.01943.x. PMID: 17614865.

Tannen, D. (2007). *Talking voices: repetition, dialogue, and imagery in conversational discourse*, vol. 26. Cambridge University Press.

Thomä, H. & Kächele, H. (1985). *Lehrbuch der psychoanalytischen Therapie I–II*. Springer-Verlag.

Thomä, H. & Kächele, H. (2007). *Psychoanalytische Therapie: Forschung*, vol. 3. Springer-Verlag.

Thomä, H., Kächele, H., Bilger, A. & Ahrens, S. (2006). *Psychoanalytische Therapie*. Springer Medizin.

Tinsley, H.E., Workman, K.R. & Kass, R.A. (1980). Factor analysis of the domain of client expectancies about counselling. *Journal of Counselling Psychology, 27*(6): 561–70. https://doi.org/10.1037/0022-0167.27.6.561

Todorov, T. (1981). *Introduction to poetics*, vol. 1. University of Minnesota Press.

Tomasello, M. (1999). Having intentions, understanding intentions, and understanding communicative intentions. In: P.D. Zelazo, J.W. Astington & D.R. Olson (eds), *Developing theories of intention: social understanding and self-control* (pp. 63–75). Routledge.

Tompkins, V., Farrar, M.J. & Montgomery, D.E. (2019). Speaking your mind: language and narrative in young children's theory of mind development. In: *Advances in child development and behavior*, vol. 56 (pp. 109–40). JAI.

Trevarthen, C. (1979). Communication and cooperation in early infancy. In: M. Bullowa (ed.), *Before speech: the beginning of interpersonal communication* (pp. 321–47). Cambridge University Press.

Tronick, E.Z. (2003). 'Of course all relationships are unique': how co-creative processes generate unique mother–infant and patient–therapist relationships and change other relationships. *Psychoanalytic Inquiry*, *23*(3): 473–91. https://doi.org/10.1080/07351692309349044

Tulving, E. (1984). Précis of elements of episodic memory. *Behavioral and Brain Sciences*, *7*(2): 223–38. doi:10.1017/S0140525X0004440X

Tulving, E. (2002) Episodic memory: from mind to brain. *Annual Review of Psychology*, *53*: 1–25. doi: 10.1146/annurev.psych.53.100901.135114. PMID: 11752477.

Uehara, I. (2015). Developmental changes in memory-related linguistic skills and their relationship to episodic recall in children. *PLoS One.*, *10*(9): e0137220. doi: 10.1371/journal.pone.0137220. PMID: 26331479; PMCID: PMC4558057.

Ulvenes, P.G., Berggraf, L., Wampold, B.E., Hoffart, A., Stiles, T. & McCullough, L. (2014). Orienting patient to affect, sense of self, and the activation of affect over the course of psychotherapy with cluster C patients. *Journal of Counselling Psychology*, *61*(3): 315–24. https://doi.org/10.1037/cou0000028

Uspenskiĭ, B.A. (1973). *A poetics of composition: the structure of the artistic text and typology of a compositional form*. University of California Press.

van Dijk, T.A. (1975). Action, action description, and narrative. *New Literary History*, *6*(2): 273–94. https://doi.org/10.2307/468420.

van Doeselaar, L., McLean, K.C., Meeus, W., Denissen, J.J.A. & Klimstra, T.A. (2020). Adolescents' identity formation: linking the narrative and the dual-cycle approach. *Journal of Youth and Adolescence*, *49*(4): 818–35. doi: 10.1007/s10964-019-01096-x. Epub 2019 Aug 12. PMID: 31407186; PMCID: PMC7105420.

Van Vreeswijk, M.F. & De Wilde, E.J. (2004). Autobiographical memory specificity, psychopathology, depressed mood and the use of the autobiographical memory test: a meta-analysis. *Behaviour Research and Therapy*, *42*(6): 731–43. doi: 10.1016/S0005-7967(03)00194-3. PMID: 15081887.

Valentino, K. (2011). A developmental psychopathology model of overgeneral autobiographical memory. *Developmental Review*, *31*(1): 32–54. https://doi.org/10.1016/j.dr.2011.05.001

Vermetten, E. & Bremner, J.D. (2003). Olfaction as a traumatic reminder in posttraumatic stress disorder: case reports and review. *Journal of Clinical Psychiatry*, *64*(2): 202–07. doi: 10.4088/jcp.v64n0214.

Vygotsky, L.S. (1930/1993). *Studies on the history of behavior*. Erlbaum.

Walker, S.C. & McGlone, F.P. (2013). The social brain: neurobiological basis of affiliative behaviours and psychological well-being. *Neuropeptides*, *47*(6): 379–93. https://doi.org/10.1016/j.npep.2013.10.008.

Wang, Q. (2001). 'Did you have fun?' American and Chinese mother–child conversations about shared emotional experiences. *Cognitive Development*, *16*(2): 693–715. https://doi.org/10.1016/S0885-2014(01)00055-7

Watson, J.S. (1972). Smiling, cooing, and 'the game'. *Merrill-Palmer Quarterly of Behavior and Development*, *18*(4): 323–39.

Weeks, T.L. & Pasupathi, M. (2010). Autonomy, identity, and narrative construction with parents and friends. In: K.C. McLean & M. Pasupathi (eds), *Narrative development in adolescence: creating the storied self* (pp. 65–91). Springer.

Weiner, I.B. & Exner Jr, J.E. (1991). Rorschach changes in long-term short-term psychotherapy. *Journal of Personality Assessment*, *56*(3): 453–65. doi: 10.1207/s15327752jpa5603_7.

Westen, D., Shedler, J., Durrett, C., Glass, S. & Martens, A. (2003). Personality diagnoses in adolescence: DSM-IV axis II diagnoses and an empirically derived alternative. *American Journal of Psychiatry*, *160*(5): 952–66. DOI: 10.1176/appi.ajp.160.5.952.

Wiebe, J.M. (2012). References in narrative text. In: *Deixis in narrative* (pp. 263–86). Psychology Press.

Williams, D.C. & Levitt, H.M. (2007). Principles for facilitating agency in psychotherapy. *Psychotherapy Research*, *17*(1): 66–82. https://doi.org/10.1080/10503300500469098

Williams, E.N. (2008). A psychotherapy researcher's perspective on therapist self-awareness and self-focused attention after a decade of research. *Psychotherapy Research*, *18*(2): 139–46. doi: 10.1080/10503300701691656. PMID: 18815971.

Williams, J.M.G., Barnhofer, T., Crane, C., Herman, D., Raes, F., Watkins, E. & Dalgleish, T. (2007). Autobiographical memory specificity and emotional disorder. *Psychological Bulletin*, *133*(1): 122–48. https://doi.org/10.1037/0033-2909.133.1.122

Wimmer, H. & Perner, J. (1983). Beliefs about beliefs: representation and constraining function of wrong beliefs in young children's understanding of deception. *Cognition, 13*(1): 103–28. https://doi.org/10.1016/0010-0277(83)90004-5

Winnicott, D.W. (1971). *Playing and reality.* Tavistock Publications.

Wolfson, N. (1976). Speech events and natural speech: some implications for sociolinguistic methodology. *Language in Society*, *5*(2): 189–209. doi:10.1017/S0047404500007028

Wolfson, N. (1979). The conversational historical present alternation. *Language*, *55*(1): 168–82. https://doi.org/10.2307/412521

Yalom, I.D. (1995). *The theory and practice of group psychotherapy.* Basic Books

Yalom, I. & Leszcz, M. (2005). *The theory and practice of group psychotherapy*, 5th edn. Basic Books.

Zilcha-Mano, S. & Fisher, H. (2022). Distinct roles of state-like and trait-like patient–therapist alliance in psychotherapy. *Nature Reviews Psychology*, *1*(4): 194–210. https://doi.org/10.1038/s44159-022-00029-z

Zubin, D.A. & Hewitt, L.E. (1995). The deictic center: a theory of deixis in narrative. In: J.F. Dunchan, G.A. Bruder & L. Hewitt (eds), *Deixis in narrative: a cognitive science perspective* (pp. 129–55). Lawrene Erlbaum Associates.

Index

www.ingramcontent.com/pod-product-compliance
Ingram Content Group UK Ltd.
Pitfield, Milton Keynes, MK11 3LW, UK
UKHW040657080326
468753UK00001B/239

9 781804 130483